The Ultimate Nutrition Guide for Women

How to Stay Healthy with Diet, Vitamins, Minerals and Herbs

Leslie Beck, R.D.

Associate Researcher

Anne von Rosenbach, B.A., M.L.S.

WILEY

John Wiley & Sons, Inc.

For general information about our other products and services, please contact our Customer Care
Department within the United States at (800) 762-2974, outside the United States at (317) 572-3993
or fax (317) 572-4002.

Wiley also publishes its books in a variety of electronic formats. Some content that appears in print may
not be available in electronic books. For more information about Wiley products, visit our web site at
www.wiley.com.

ISBN 0-471-27426-7

Printed in the United States of America

10 9 8 7 6 5 4 3 2 1

This book is dedicated to the memory of

my grandmother, Dorothy Coulter;

ॐ

to the women in my family and

the women I have worked with in

my private practice.

ॐ

I thank you for the incredible learning

you motivate and inspire me

to achieve every single day.

Contents

Introduction   vii

Part 1   Essentials of Nutrition for Women   1
- 1 A Healthy Diet: Standard Advice for All Women   2
- 2 Weight Control and Food Sensitivities   44

Part 2   Low Energy Levels, Fatigue and Pain   61
- 3 Anemia   62
- 4 Chronic Fatigue Syndrome (CFS)   76
- 5 Hypoglycemia   89
- 6 Insomnia   106
- 7 Migraine Headaches   117

Part 3   Breast, Bone and Heart Health   129
- 8 Breast Cancer   130
- 9 Fibrocystic Breast Conditions   151
- 10 Osteoporosis   164
- 11 Heart Disease and High Cholesterol   188

Part 4   Emotional Health   211
- 12 Depression   212
- 13 Eating Disorders   226

Part 5   Conception, Pregnancy and Motherhood   239
- 14 Infertility   240
- 15 Pregnancy   256
- 16 Breastfeeding   286

Part 6   Hormonal Health   301

     17   Premenstrual Syndrome (PMS)   302

     18   Perimenopause   328

     19   Polycystic Ovary Syndrome (PCOS)   346

     20   Thyroid Disease   362

Part 7   Pelvic and Urinary Tract Health   389

     21   Cervical Dysplasia   390

     22   Endometriosis   404

     23   Interstitial Cystitis (IC)   425

     24   Urinary Tract Infections (UTIs)   437

Endnotes   449

Index   459

Introduction

More than 100 million women live in the United States today. And we can expect to live longer than did our grandmothers and great-grandmothers. A woman born in America in 1901 could expect to live, on average, until the age of 50, and a man until the age of 47. A century later, the situation has changed greatly. The average life expectancy for a woman in America today is 79 years, about eight years longer than that of the average man.

The fact that women live longer is partly due to the fact that we practice better health than men. We are more apt to seek medical advice and we are more likely to report that we are making an effort to achieve a healthy weight, to eat better and to exercise more. We are also more interested in nutrition than are men. According to the American Dietetic Association's most recent survey, 89 percent of American women say nutrition is extremely or very important, compared to 79 percent of men.[1]

Over the years, women have always been concerned about nutrition. Every day in my private practice I see women wanting dietary advice for themselves, their children and their partners. As caregivers for their families, women continue to be largely responsible for grocery shopping and meal preparation. At the same time, many women are looking after aging parents, as members of a phenomenon called the "sandwich generation." And as the female baby boomers consider early retirement, there's a strong focus on living an active life, free of aches and pains. As women age, they want to fulfill their life goals with plenty of energy and in good health.

As a professional nutritionist (a Registered Dietitian), I have been giving women and men dietary and supplement advice for the past 13 years. When I see a client, I assess her diet, her medical history and her lifestyle, and then I make recommendations for change. Based on a woman's personal goals, I develop a customized nutrition and eating plan for her. My private practice is located in the heart of downtown Toronto, so many of my clients are baby boomers, women who are taking charge of their health care.

The Nutritional Status of Women

Despite our interest in nutrition and our enthusiasm to live a healthy lifestyle, as women we experience more health problems and visit the doctor more often than men. And some of our nutrition habits receive a failing grade. Studies reveal that North American women are falling short of eating sufficient dairy products, fruit and vegetables. Not surprisingly, many women are not getting the recommended amounts of calcium, folate, iron and zinc, all nutrients essential for maintaining a woman's health. And, although we are eating less fat than we did 25 years ago, we are getting heavier. It's estimated that almost 20 percent of American women are obese, having a Body Mass Index of 30 or greater (see page 45 in chapter 2).

Women Have Unique Needs

It probably comes as no surprise that women have different nutrition needs than do men. The very biology of our bodies increases our need for many nutrients such as calcium and iron. For instance, the hormonal fluctuations that women experience during their reproductive cycle have an impact on what nutrients we need and, often, what foods we eat. You'll also read how the subtle anatomical difference between the male and female urinary tract puts a woman at much greater risk for bladder infections. Pregnancy and breastfeeding are times when a woman needs to consume certain nutrients in greater amounts to nourish her growing baby. If careful attention is not given to diet, these nutrients are taken from a woman's body, leaving her depleted and at risk for health problems.

Women are also at unique risk for major nutrition-related health conditions, including heart disease, osteoporosis, breast cancer and weight-related problems. Some of these diseases are unique to women, whereas others affect women far more often than men. Risk factors for many of these diseases manifest differently for women than for men. For example, for women, having a low level of HDL (good) cholesterol is more predictive of heart disease than having a high level of LDL (bad) cholesterol. In men, high LDLs are more predictive of the disease. Being overweight puts women at risk for many health conditions, especially if excess body fat is stored around the middle.

And of course, women are much more vulnerable to societal pressures to be thin. Day after day we read in magazines and see on television that thin means beautiful, thin means successful. As a result, women are far more likely than men to be dieting, often in a quest to be underweight. The desire to be slim predisposes women to a pattern of losing and gaining weight repeatedly over the years, which can have consequences for long-term health. It also sets the stage for disordered eating, potentially leading to serious eating disorders.

How This Book Can Help You

Ten years ago I was hard-pressed to find good scientific information about how nutrition affected women's health. The fact was, women were less likely to be included in research studies, and the health conditions that afflict women were less likely to be studied. But that has all changed. Over the past decade there has been an explosion in women's health issues. As findings from large trials involving women come to the forefront, scientists are unraveling the link between nutrition and women's health. This growing body of research has made writing this book possible.

American women need nutrition advice that is easy to understand, relevant to their lifestyle and based on scientific evidence. Women don't need a new diet book that offers some far-fetched solution to losing weight. Instead women and girls need to know how food affects their weight, their energy levels and the health of their body. American women need to know how to get more of the key nutrients that their health relies on. In this book, I translate current scientific research into practical food choices with defined serving sizes. When it comes to important nutrients like iron, calcium and folate, I tell you *how much* you need to be getting every day, *what foods* give you the most bang for your buck and, if you don't eat many of these foods, *how to supplement safely*.

This book is written for all women. It's for healthy women who want to stay well and lower their chances of disease. It's also for women who have a certain health condition and want to do whatever they can through diet and supplements to manage, or maybe even treat, their condition. This book is not only for adult women. It also has plenty of important information for younger women—girls and teens—who need to adopt eating habits that will lay the foundation for their future health.

How This Book Is Organized

I have divided this book into seven parts. Parts 2 to 7 are dedicated to certain aspects of women's health—reproductive health, breast and bone health, emotional health and so on. I don't expect you to read this book cover to cover. Instead you should use it as a comprehensive reference guide to all aspects of your nutritional health care. You may be expecting your first baby and find my chapters on pregnancy and breastfeeding particularly relevant. Or you may be a woman in your late 40s experiencing hormonal ups and downs, who's more interested in my chapters on perimenopause, osteoporosis and heart disease. Finally, you may be afflicted with a particular condition, such as endometriosis or migraine headaches, and want to know how nutrition affects your health.

The first part of this book talks about the nutrition concerns of almost all women. Whatever your reason may be for picking up this book, be sure to read chapter 1. In this chapter, I give nutrition advice for *all* healthy women. You'll learn what nutrients are most important for optimal health, how much you need each day and how to get these nutrients in your diet. Chapter 2 deals with topics that concern many women. Here you'll find tools to assess your body weight and determine where you weigh in with respect to future health risks; there is also some information on food sensitivities and allergies.

If you have read my book *The Ultimate Nutrition Guide for Menopause* (John Wiley & Sons, 2002), you are already familiar with my style. Here, too, I've tried to make the information very easy to read and easy to find. I begin each chapter with information you need to know—what causes the particular health condition, its symptoms, risk factors, conventional treatment and prevention strategies. In every chapter, I list my nutrition recommendations in three categories: dietary strategies; vitamins and minerals; herbal remedies. And if you want a quick summary, you can skip ahead to the end of the chapter where I summarize my recommendations in "The Bottom Line."

I hope you and the other women in your family enjoy this book and find it a useful guide to better nutrition and long-lasting health.

Leslie Beck, R.D.
Toronto, Canada

Part 1

Essentials of Nutrition for Women

1

A Healthy Diet: Standard Advice for All Women

If you are like many American women, you may be more concerned about your diet. You may be wondering how your nutritional intake stacks up to that of the average American woman. Like her, are you not meeting your daily targets for calcium, folate, iron and zinc? Is your weight putting your health at risk? To ensure your diet is providing what your body needs to stay healthy and reduce your risk of future health problems, the tables on the following pages will help you make wise food choices.

Every woman should strive to adhere to the following dietary guidelines. These basic eating principles represent a common strategy to help prevent all chronic diseases women face today.

1. *Emphasize plant foods* in your daily diet. Fill your plate with grains, fruits and vegetables. If you eat animal protein foods like meat or poultry, they should take up no more than one-quarter of your plate. Try vegetarian sources of protein, such as beans and soy, more often.

2. *Choose lower-fat foods.* Buy lean cuts of meat and poultry, and lower-fat dairy products. Use added fats and oils—like butter, margarine, salad dressings and spreads—sparingly. Limit your intake of fried foods and high-fat snack foods.

3. *Choose foods and oils that are rich in essential fatty acids,* nutrients our bodies can't make and that must be supplied by our diet. Fish, nuts, seeds, flax and flax oil, canola oil, omega-3 eggs, wheat germ and leafy green vegetables are examples.

4. *Make food choices that are rich in vitamins, minerals, antioxidants and dietary fiber.* Choose whole grains as often as possible. Eat at least three different-colored fruits and three different-colored vegetables every day.

5. As often as possible, *eliminate sources of refined sugar:* cookies, cakes, pastries, frozen desserts, soft drinks, sweetened fruit juices, fruit drinks, candy, etc.

6. *Wash fruits and vegetables* to remove pesticide residues. Or buy organic produce.

7. *Limit foods with chemical additives.*

8. *Limit your intake of caffeine* and *salt.*

9. *Drink at least 9 cups of water* every day.

10. *Avoid alcohol.* If you drink, consume no more than one drink a day, or seven per week.

11. *Take a multivitamin and mineral supplement* each day to ensure you are meeting your needs for most nutrients.

12. *Exercise regularly.* Aim to include aerobic activities (brisk walking, jogging, stair climbing, cycling, swimming, cross-country skiing, aerobic classes) and strength exercises (weights, push-ups, sit-ups) in your weekly routine.

Key Nutrients for Women

Throughout this book, nutrients are presented in roughly alphabetic order—vitamins and then minerals. In the chapters, nutrients are often presented in order of importance or effectiveness.

B VITAMINS

Without B vitamins our bodies would lack energy. These eight nutrients are indispensable for yielding energy compounds from the foods we eat. Many B vitamins serve as helpers to enzymes that release energy from fat, protein and carbohydrate. As you'll read later, an optimal intake of certain B vitamins may help to reduce the risk of heart disease and cancer.

The following lists the B vitamin family, how much you need and where to look for it.

B VITAMIN	RDA FOR WOMEN AGED 19+	BEST FOOD SOURCES
Thiamin (B1)	1.1 milligrams	pork, ham, bacon, liver, whole-grain or enriched breads and cereals, dried peas, beans and lentils, nuts
Riboflavin (B2)	1.1 milligrams	milk, yogurt, cottage cheese, meat, leafy green vegetables, whole-grain or enriched breads and cereals
Niacin (B3)	14 milligrams	milk, eggs, poultry, fish, whole-grain or enriched breads and cereals, nuts, all protein-containing foods
B6	1.3 to 1.5 milligrams	whole grains, bananas, potatoes, legumes, fish, meat, poultry
Folate	400 micrograms	spinach, orange juice, lentils, asparagus, artichokes, avocado, leafy greens, wheat germ, whole grains
B12	2.4 micrograms	meat, poultry, fish, dairy products, eggs, fortified soy and rice milk
Biotin	30 micrograms	widespread in foods
Pantothenic acid	5 milligrams	widespread in foods

Reprinted with permission from Dietary Reference Intakes for Thiamin, Riboflavin, Niacin, Vitamin B6, Folate, Vitamin B12, Pantothenic Acid, Biotin and Choline, *Copyright © 1998 by the National Academy of Sciences. Courtesy of the National Academy Press, Washington, D.C.*

To ensure you are getting your fair share of B vitamins, take a good quality multi-vitamin and mineral supplement each day.

If you're looking for more B vitamins than a regular multi gives you, choose a "high potency" or "super" formula that contains 30 to 75 milligrams of B vitamins (or micrograms in the case of folic acid). You can also take a B complex formula that gives you all eight B vitamins, often combined with vitamin C. One word of caution: the B vitamin niacin could cause flushing of the face and chest when taken in doses greater than 35 milligrams (this can be avoided by taking your supplement just after eating a meal). This symptom is harmless and goes away within 20 minutes, but some people find it uncomfortable. To avoid flushing, look for a formula that contains niacinamide—a non-flushing form of niacin.

Vitamin B6

The body uses B6 to form an important enzyme that's needed to create serotonin, a chemical in the brain that has a calming and relaxing effect. Healthy women need 1.3 to 1.5 milligrams of the vitamin each day. The best sources of B6 are high-protein foods like meat, fish and poultry. Other good sources include whole grains, bananas and potatoes.

B6 in Foods

FOOD	VITAMIN B6 (MILLIGRAMS)
Beef, flank, cooked, 3 oz (90 g)	0.3 mg
Pork center loin, cooked, 3 oz (90 g)	0.3 mg
Chicken breast, cooked, half (140 g)	0.3 mg
Chicken leg, cooked (187 g)	0.2 mg
Salmon, sockeye, cooked, 3 oz (90 g)	0.2 mg
Tuna, canned and drained, 3 oz (90 g)	0.4 mg
100% bran cereal, 1/2 cup (125 ml)	0.5 mg
Cereal, whole-grain flakes, 2/3 cup (160 ml)	0.5 mg
Avocado, Florida, half medium	0.4 mg
Avocado, California, half medium	0.2 mg

| Banana, medium | 0.7 mg |
| Potato, baked, medium with skin | 0.7 mg |

Nutrient Values of Some Common Foods, *Health Canada, Ottawa, 1999.*

B6 SUPPLEMENTS

If you'd like to try a daily supplement, reach for a 50- to 100-milligram pill once a day. Because the eight B vitamins work together, I recommend a B complex supplement. Taking only one B vitamin in high doses could upset the body's balance. Don't take more than 100 milligrams each day, since too much vitamin B6 can cause irreversible nerve damage.

Folate

This B vitamin is critical for all women of childbearing age. Getting adequate amounts of folate before conception and during the first trimester of a woman's pregnancy is an important way to reduce the chances of spinal cord defects in newborns. Folate may also help reduce the risk of heart disease and cervical dysplasia. A deficiency of this important vitamin can increase your risk for these health conditions and can also cause anemia.

Recommended Dietary Allowance (RDA) of Folate for Females

AGE	RDA (MICROGRAMS)
9–13 years	300 mcg
14–18 years	400 mcg
19–30 years	400 mcg
31–50 years	400 mcg
51+ years	400 mcg
Pregnancy	600 mcg
Breastfeeding	500 mcg

Reprinted with permission from Dietary Reference Intakes for Thiamin, Riboflavin, Niacin, Vitamin B6, Folate, Vitamin B12, Pantothenic Acid, Biotin and Choline, *Copyright © 1998 by the National Academy of Sciences. Courtesy of the National Academy Press, Washington, D.C.*

Folate in Foods

FOOD	FOLATE (MICROGRAMS)
Black beans, cooked, 1 cup (250 ml)	270 mcg
Chicken liver, 3.5 oz (100 g)	770 mcg
Chickpeas, cooked, 1 cup (250 ml)	169 mcg
Kidney beans, cooked, 1 cup (250 ml)	242 mcg
Lentils, cooked, 1 cup (250 ml)	378 mcg
Peanuts, 1/2 cup (125 ml)	113 mcg
Sunflower seeds, 2 tbsp (30 ml)	32 mcg
Orange juice, freshly squeezed, 1 cup (250 ml)	79 mcg
Orange juice, frozen, diluted, 1 cup (250 ml)	115 mcg
Orange, 1 medium	40 mcg
Pineapple juice, canned, 1 cup (250 ml)	61 mcg
Asparagus, 5 spears	110 mcg
Artichoke, 1 medium	64 mcg
Avocado, California, half	113 mcg
Avocado, Florida, half	81 mcg
Bean sprouts, 1 cup (250 ml)	91 mcg
Beets, cooked, 1/2 cup (125 ml)	72 mcg
Broccoli, raw, 3 spears	66 mcg
Brussels sprouts, 1/2 cup (125 ml)	83 mcg
Green peas, 1/2 cup (125 ml)	54 mcg
Romaine lettuce, chopped, 1 cup (250 ml)	80 mcg
Spinach, raw, 1 cup (250 ml)	115 mcg
Spinach, cooked, 1 cup (250 ml)	278 mcg

Turnip greens, cooked, 1 cup (250 ml)	180 mcg
Tomato juice, 1 cup (250 ml)	51 mcg
Wheat germ, toasted, 2 tbsp (30 ml)	50 mcg
Whole-wheat bread, 2 slices	28 mcg

Nutrient Values of Some Common Foods, *Health Canada, Ottawa, 1999.*

To help you meet the recommended daily intake of 400 micrograms a day, practice the following:

- Eat spinach, asparagus and artichokes more often. These vegetables have the most folate, with spinach leading the pack.
- Drink a glass of orange juice with your morning meal.
- Use lentils and other legumes in pasta sauces, chilis and tacos.
- Most often, choose whole-grain breads and cereals.

FOLIC ACID SUPPLEMENTS

This B vitamin is called folate when it occurs naturally in foods. It's called folic acid when it's present in vitamin pills and fortified foods. Make sure your multivitamin and mineral supplement offers 0.4 to 1.0 milligrams (400 to 1000 micrograms) of folic acid. If you want to take more folic acid, reach for a B complex formula that gives you all eight B vitamins. B complex supplements offer up to 1000 micrograms of folic acid. The daily upper limit for this B vitamin is 1000 micrograms.

If you decide to take a folic acid supplement, make sure to buy one with vitamin B12 since these two nutrients work closely together (that's why I prefer a high-potency multi or a B complex). The body uses folic acid to activate B12 and vice versa. So a deficiency of one vitamin will eventually lead to a deficiency of the other. If you supplement with folic acid and don't pay attention to meeting your B12 requirements, you can hide an underlying B12 deficiency.

Folic acid is well tolerated. It is generally recommended that you do not exceed the tolerable upper limit of 1000 micrograms per day. However, if you suffer from a malabsorption problem, higher doses can be safely used (be sure to take vitamin B12, too!). Doses above 15,000 micrograms are associated with nerve and intestinal damage.

Vitamin B12

As you read above, vitamin B12 and folate work very closely together in the body. Without enough B12, your body is unable to use folate. Without any help from folate, vitamin B12 maintains the protective covering of nerve fibers. Your bones also rely on this B vitamin for normal metabolism.

Recommended Dietary Allowance (RDA) of Vitamin B12 for Females

AGE	RDA (MICROGRAMS)
9–13 years	1.8 mcg
14–18 years	2.4 mcg
19–30 years	2.4 mcg
31–50 years	2.4 mcg
51+ years	2.4 mcg
Pregnancy	2.6 mcg
Breastfeeding	2.8 mcg

Reprinted with permission from Dietary Reference Intakes for Thiamin, Riboflavin, Niacin, Vitamin B6, Folate, Vitamin B12, Pantothenic Acid, Biotin and Choline, *Copyright © 1998 by the National Academy of Sciences. Courtesy of the National Academy Press, Washington, D.C.*

This vitamin is found exclusively in animal foods. (Some soy and rice beverages are fortified with B12.) If you eat meat, poultry and dairy products on a regular basis, you're probably not at risk for a B12 deficiency.

B12 in Foods

FOOD	VITAMIN B12 (MICROGRAMS)
Beef, cooked, 3 oz (90 g)	2.8 mcg
Pork, center loin, cooked, 3 oz (90 g)	0.5 mcg
Poultry breast, cooked, 5 oz (150 g)	0.3 mcg

Salmon, sockeye, cooked, 3 oz (90 g)	4.9 mcg
Tuna, canned and drained, 3 oz (90 g)	2.5 mcg
Mussels, cooked, 3 oz (90 g)	20 mcg
Milk, 1 cup (250 ml)	0.9 mcg
Yogurt, 3/4 cup (175 ml)	0.9 mcg
Cottage cheese, 1%, 1/2 cup (125 ml)	0.7 mcg
Cheddar cheese, 1.5 oz (45 g)	0.3 mcg
Egg, 1 whole	0.6 mcg
Fortified soy beverage, 1 cup (250 ml)	1.0 mcg
Fortified rice beverage, 1 cup (250 ml)	1.0 mcg

Nutrient Values of Some Common Foods, *Health Canada, Ottawa, 1999.*

B12 SUPPLEMENTS

If you are a strict vegetarian who eats no animal products and you don't drink a fortified soy or rice beverage, I strongly recommend a B12 supplement. In fact, anyone over the age of 50 should be getting their B12 from a supplement or fortified foods. That's because up to one-third of older adults produce inadequate amounts of stomach acid and are inefficient at absorbing B12 from food.

If you take certain medications you should consider taking extra B12 in the form of a supplement. If you suffer from reflux or ulcers and take acid blockers (e.g., Tagamet®, Zantac®, Pepcid®) your body may not absorb enough B12 (as well as iron). Metformin®, used to manage type 2 diabetes and polycystic ovary syndrome, can also deplete B12 levels. If you take these medications, your doctor should monitor your blood periodically for signs of anemia.

To get your B12, I recommend a good multivitamin and mineral supplement or a B complex supplement that contains the whole family of B vitamins. If you take a single B12 supplement, take 500 to 1000 micrograms once daily.

If you are taking a high-dose B12 supplement to correct a deficiency, don't take it with a vitamin C pill. Large amounts of vitamin C can destroy B12. Take your vitamin C supplement one hour after you take your B12.

ANTIOXIDANTS

Over the past decade, scientists have discovered the importance of dietary antioxidants, including vitamin C, vitamin E, selenium and beta-carotene. It's well accepted that oxidative damage caused by free radical molecules contributes to disease. We generate free radicals every day as a result of normal metabolism, and the body has a built-in antioxidant system that mops up free radicals. But pollution, cigarette smoking and heavy exercise can increase free radical production and overwhelm the body's ability to neutralize them. It appears that a daily intake of antioxidants is necessary to protect our health. A growing body of evidence suggests that dietary antioxidants can help ward off heart disease, cancer, cataracts and even Alzheimer's disease.

VITAMIN C

Scientists have learned that the antioxidant powers of vitamin C might reduce the risk of cataracts and heart disease. Vitamin C may also keep you healthy by enhancing your body's immune system. This vitamin also plays an important role in collagen synthesis, an important tissue for breast and bone health.

Recommended Dietary Allowance (RDA) of Vitamin C for Females

AGE	RDA (MILLIGRAMS)
9–13 years	45 mg
14–18 years	65 mg
19+ years	75 mg
Pregnancy	85 mg
Breastfeeding	120 mg
Smokers	Add 35 mg to your RDA

Reprinted with permission from Dietary Reference Intakes for Vitamin C, Vitamin E, Selenium and Carotenoids, *Copyright © 1999 by the National Academy of Sciences. Courtesy of the National Academy Press, Washington, D.C.*

Vitamin C in Foods

FOOD	VITAMIN C (MILLIGRAMS)
Cantaloupe, 1/4 medium	56 mg
Orange, 1 medium	70 mg
Orange juice, fresh, 1 cup (250 ml)	131 mg
Grapefruit, red or pink, half	47 mg
Kiwi, 1 large	68 mg
Mango, 1	49 mg
Strawberries, raw, 1 cup (250 ml)	89 mg
Broccoli, raw, 1 spear	141 mg
Brussels sprouts, cooked, 1/2 cup (125 ml)	50 mg
Cauliflower, raw, 1/2 cup (125 ml)	38 mg
Potato, baked with skin, 1	27 mg
Red pepper, raw, 1/2 cup (125 ml)	95 mg
Tomato juice, 1 cup (250 ml)	47 mg

Nutrient Values of Some Common Foods, *Health Canada, Ottawa, 1999.*

VITAMIN C SUPPLEMENTS

Keep in mind that fruits and vegetables contain many other natural chemicals that may work with vitamin C to keep you healthy. So even if you do take a vitamin C pill, I recommend that you still add foods rich in vitamin C to your daily diet. If you don't eat at least two vitamin-C-rich foods each day, a supplement is a good idea.

- If you're looking for the most C for your money, choose a supplement labeled Ester C. Studies in the lab have found this form of vitamin C is more available to the body.

- If you don't like to swallow pills and prefer a chewable supplement, make sure it contains calcium ascorbate or sodium ascorbate. These forms of vitamin C are less acidic to the enamel of your teeth.

- Take a 500 or 600 milligram supplement, once or twice a day. Taking more than 200 milligrams of vitamin C at once won't increase your blood levels further. I've recommended 500 or 600 milligrams because these are the most common doses you'll find. If you want to take more, you're better off splitting your dose over the course of the day.

- The daily upper limit for vitamin C has been set at 2000 milligrams to avoid diarrhea.

VITAMIN D

Along with calcium, this vitamin plays a key role in preventing osteoporosis. Many women living in the northern states are at risk for developing a deficiency in vitamin D. Our skin is able to make plenty of vitamin D if it's exposed to sunlight. But if you live in an area where you see little sunshine for much of the year, dietary sources of this vitamin become extremely important. Elderly women who don't get outside often need to pay extra attention to their vitamin D intake. As we get older, our skin becomes less efficient at producing the vitamin from sunlight. You'll see below that very few foods contain vitamin D.

Recommended Dietary Allowance (RDA) of Vitamin D for Females

AGE	RDA (INTERNATIONAL UNITS)
0–50 years	200 IU (5 micrograms)
51–70 years	400 IU (10 micrograms)
71+ years	600 IU (15 micrograms)
Pregnancy & Breastfeeding	200 IU (5 micrograms)

Reprinted with permission from Dietary Reference Intakes for Calcium, Phosphorus, Magnesium, Vitamin D and Fluoride, *Copyright © 1999 by the National Academy of Sciences. Courtesy of the National Academy Press, Washington, D.C.*

Vitamin D in Foods

FOOD	VITAMIN D (INTERNATIONAL UNITS)
Herring, 3.5 oz (100 g)	680 IU
Salmon, canned, 3.5 oz (100 g)	500 IU
Sardines, 3.5 oz (100 g)	290 IU
Milk, fluid, 1 cup (250 ml)	100 IU
Soy beverage, fortified, 1 cup (250 ml)	100 IU
Rice beverage, fortified, 1 cup (250 ml)	100 IU
Egg, 1 whole	24 IU
Margarine, 1 tsp (5 ml)	15 IU

USDA Nutrient Database for Standard Reference, Release 14. USDA Nutrient Data Laboratory, Agricultural Research Service.

VITAMIN D SUPPLEMENTS

Most multivitamin and mineral formulas offer 400 IU of the vitamin. If you take calcium supplements, buy one with vitamin D added. The daily upper limit for vitamin D is 2000 IU.

VITAMIN E

This vitamin is a powerful antioxidant. Once consumed, vitamin E makes its way to the liver where it is incorporated into cell membranes and lipoproteins that transport cholesterol. It is here that vitamin E works to protect these compounds from oxygen damage caused by free radicals, possibly reducing the risk of heart disease. This powerhouse nutrient has been touted to ward off certain cancers, cataracts and Alzheimer's disease, and to boost the immune system.

Recommended Dietary Allowance (RDA) of Vitamin E for Females

AGE	RDA* (INTERNATIONAL UNITS)
9–13 years	16 IU (11 mg)
14 years through adulthood	22 IU (15 mg)
Pregnancy	22 IU (15 mg)
Breastfeeding	28 IU (19 mg)

*The RDA is your daily requirement for natural vitamin E found in foods (alpha-tocopherol).

Reprinted with permission from Dietary Reference Intakes for Vitamin C, Vitamin E, Selenium and Carotenoids, Copyright © 1999 by the National Academy of Sciences. Courtesy of the National Academy Press, Washington, D.C.

Wheat germ, nuts, seeds, soybeans, vegetable oils, corn oil, whole grains and kale are all good sources of vitamin E, so be sure to include a few of these in your daily diet. But it can be a challenge to reach the daily recommended intake of 22 IU when you consider that adding 2 tablespoons of wheat germ to your morning smoothie gives you only 4 IU of the vitamin—and wheat germ is one of the best sources. For this reason many women opt for a daily supplement to help them meet their target intakes.

VITAMIN E SUPPLEMENTS

To help you choose the right vitamin E supplement, consider the following suggestions:

- Take 100 to 400 IU per day. There's no evidence to warrant taking more.

- Buy a natural source vitamin E supplement (or look for *d-alpha-tocopherol* on the label; synthetic forms are labeled *dl-alpha tocopherol*). Although the body absorbs both synthetic and natural forms equally well, your liver prefers the natural form. It incorporates more natural vitamin E into transport molecules. Studies have shown that twice as much vitamin E ends up in the blood of people taking natural E as in those taking the same amount of synthetic E.[1]

- If you're taking a blood-thinning medication like Coumadin® (warfarin), don't take vitamin E without your doctor's approval, since it has slight anti-clotting properties.
- The daily upper limit for vitamin E is 1500 IU of natural vitamin E or 2200 IU of the synthetic form.

CALCIUM

No doubt you know how important this mineral is in keeping your bones healthy. Osteoporosis cannot be cured, but you can prevent it by building strong bones early in life by eating a calcium-rich diet. This is especially important for young girls between the ages of 8 and 16, when most bone density is formed. Calcium may also help ease some of the symptoms of premenstrual syndrome. And if you're taking a medication that causes bone loss, you need to get plenty of this important mineral each and every day.

Recommended Dietary Allowance (RDA) of Calcium for Females

AGE	RDA (MILLIGRAMS)
Children, aged 4–8 years	800 mg
Children, aged 9–12	1300 mg
Teenagers, 13–18 years	1300 mg
Adults, aged 19–50 years	1000 mg
Adults over 50 years	1200 mg
Pregnant women	1000 mg
Breastfeeding	1000 mg

Reprinted with permission from Dietary Reference Intakes for Calcium, Phosphorus, Magnesium, Vitamin D and Fluoride, *Copyright © 1999 by the National Academy of Sciences. Courtesy of the National Academy Press, Washington, D.C.*

Calcium in Foods

FOOD	CALCIUM (MILLIGRAMS)
Dairy Foods	
Milk, Lactaid, 1 cup (250 ml)	300 mg
Milk, calcium enriched, 1 cup (250 ml)	420 mg
Carnation Instant Breakfast, with 1 cup milk (250 ml)	540 mg
Chocolate milk, 1 cup (250 ml)	285 mg
Cheese, cheddar, 1.5 oz (45 g)	300 mg
Cheese, Swiss or Gruyere, 1.5 oz (45 g)	480 mg
Cheese, mozzarella, 1.5 oz (45 g)	269 mg
Cheese, cottage, 1/2 cup (125 ml)	75 mg
Cheese, ricotta, 1/2 cup (125 ml)	255mg
Evaporated milk, 1/2 cup (125 ml)	350 mg
Light sour cream, 1/4 cup (60 ml)	120 mg
Pudding, low-fat Healthy Choice, 1/2 cup (125 ml)	110 mg
Skim milk powder, dry, 3 tbsp (45 ml)	155 mg
Yogurt, plain, 3/4 cup (175 ml)	300 mg
Yogurt, fruit, 3/4 cup (175 ml)	250 mg
Non-Dairy Sources of Calcium	
Soybeans, 1 cup cooked (250 ml)	175 mg
Soybeans, roasted, 1/4 cup (60 ml)	60 mg
Soy beverage, 1 cup (250 ml)	100 mg
Soy beverage, fortified (So Good), 1 cup (250 ml)	330 mg
Baked beans, 1 cup (250 ml)	150 mg
Black beans, 1 cup (250 ml)	102 mg
Kidney beans, 1 cup cooked (250 ml)	69 mg
Lentils, 1 cup cooked (250 ml)	37 mg

Tempeh, 1 cup cooked (250 ml)	154 mg
Tofu, raw, firm, with calcium sulphate, 4 oz (120 g)	260 mg
Tofu, raw, regular, with calcium sulphate, 4 oz (120 g)	130 mg
Sardines, 8 small (with bones)	165 mg
Salmon, 1/2 can drained (with bones)	225 mg
Broccoli, 1 cup raw (250 ml)	42 mg
Broccoli, 1 cup cooked (250 ml)	94 mg
Bok choy, 1 cup cooked (250 ml)	158 mg
Collard greens, 1 cup cooked (250 ml)	357 mg
Kale, 1 cup cooked (250 ml)	179 mg
Rutabaga, 1/2 cup cooked (125 ml)	57 mg
Swiss chard, 1 cup raw (250 ml)	21 mg
Swiss chard, 1 cup cooked (250 ml)	102 mg
Okra, 1 cup cooked (250 ml)	176 mg
Currants, 1/2 cup (125 ml)	60 mg
Figs, 5 medium	135 mg
Orange, 1 medium	50 mg
Almonds, 1/4 cup (60 ml)	100 mg
Brazil nuts, 1/4 cup (60 ml)	65 mg
Hazelnuts, 1/4 cup (60 ml)	65 mg
Blackstrap molasses, 2 tbsp (30 ml)	288 mg
Fancy molasses, 2 tbsp (30 ml)	70 mg
Calcium-fortified orange juice, 1 cup (250 ml)	360 mg

Nutrient Values of Some Common Foods, *Health Canada, Ottawa, 1999.*

CALCIUM SUPPLEMENTS

Many women must rely on a supplement to meet their calcium needs. To help you decide if you need a calcium supplement, use my 300 Milligram Rule. One milk serving gives you 300 milligrams of calcium. For every serving you're missing and not replacing with other calcium-rich foods, you need to get 300 milligrams of elemental calcium through a supplement. Here's how to choose a high-quality supplement:

1. Look at the source of calcium. There are many types of calcium supplements on the shelf. Some of the more common types include the following:

   - *Calcium carbonate* is only about 10 to 30 percent absorbed by the body. The amount you absorb depends on the how much stomach acid is present. As people age, their stomachs produce less hydrochloric acid. Because of this calcium carbonate is not the best choice for older adults or for people on medications that block acid production. If you do take this form of calcium, take it with meals to increase its absorption. Do not take calcium carbonate at bedtime, unless you take it with a snack. On the plus side, this is the most inexpensive type of calcium supplement.

   - *Calcium citrate* is about 30 percent absorbed by the body, so it is a better choice for anyone over the age of 50. Calcium citrate malate is one of the most highly absorbable (and expensive) forms of calcium. Calcium citrate supplements are well absorbed either with meals or on an empty stomach.

   - *Calcium chelates* (HVP chelate) are supplements that contain calcium that's bound to an amino acid. In the case of HVP chelate, the amino acid is from vegetable protein. Some manufacturers claim that up to 75 percent of calcium in the chelate form is absorbed by the body.

   - *Effervescent calcium supplements* contain calcium carbonate and often other forms of more absorbable calcium. Because they get a head start on disintegrating they may be absorbed in the intestinal tract more quickly. Dissolve these in water or orange juice.

   - *Bone meal* or *dolomite* or *oyster shell* are not recommended because some products have been found to contain trace amounts of contaminants such as lead and mercury.

2. Know how much "elemental calcium" each pill gives you. Look on the list of ingredients for this information. The amount of elemental calcium is what you use to calculate your daily intake. Calcium carbonate or calcium chelates may not be 100 percent elemental calcium. The front label may state 500 milligrams, but when you look carefully at the ingredient list you may find the product contains only 350 milligrams of elemental calcium. This will determine how many tablets you need to take to get your recommended dose.

3. Choose a formula with vitamin D and magnesium. These nutrients work in tandem with calcium to promote optimal bone health. For instance, vitamin D increases calcium absorption in your intestine by as much as 30 to 80 percent.

4. Spread larger doses throughout the day. Since all calcium sources (including food sources) are not 100 percent absorbed, it makes sense to split a higher dose over two or three meals. If you've been advised to take 600 milligrams of calcium a day, take a 300 milligram tablet with breakfast and another one at dinner.

5. Take your calcium supplements with a large glass of water.

The daily upper limit for calcium intake is 2500 milligrams from food and supplements. In most healthy people, this amount will not cause any side effects. The major risks from getting too much calcium include kidney stones (in people with a history of stones), constipation and gas.

MAGNESIUM

Magnesium is found in abundance in the body (second only to calcium), with about 24 grams of this mineral contained half in the bones and half in your tissues. It is found in all the body's cells, where it maintains fluid balance by pumping sodium and potassium in and out. More than 300 enzymes rely on a steady supply of magnesium for optimal activity. Magnesium is part of adenosine triphosphate (ATP), the active energy compound that's used by every cell in your body.

Research suggests that only 25 percent of the United States population is meeting their daily magnesium needs.[2] I am sure we could all use a magnesium boost in our daily diet. Here's what you should be striving for each day.

Recommended Dietary Allowance (RDA) of Magnesium for Females

AGE	RDA (MILLIGRAMS)
14–18 years	360 mg
19–30 years	310 mg
31+ years	320 mg
Pregnancy	
<18 years	400 mg
19–30 years	350 mg
31–50 years	360 mg
Breastfeeding	
<18 years	360 mg
19–30 years	310 mg
31–50 years	320 mg

Reprinted with permission from Dietary Reference Intakes for Calcium, Phosphorus, Magnesium, Vitamin D and Fluoride, *Copyright © 1999 by the National Academy of Sciences. Courtesy of the National Academy Press, Washington, D.C.*

The best sources of magnesium are whole foods, including unrefined grains, nuts, seeds, legumes, dried fruit and green vegetables.

Magnesium in Foods

FOOD	MAGNESIUM (MILLIGRAMS)
Wheat bran, 2 tbsp (30 ml)	46 mg
Wheat germ, 1/4 cup (60 ml)	91 mg
Almonds, 1 oz (24 nuts)	84 mg
Brazil nuts, 1 oz (8 nuts)	64 mg

Peanuts, 1 oz (35 nuts)	51 mg
Sunflower seeds, 1 oz	100 mg
Black beans, cooked, 1 cup (250 ml)	121 mg
Chickpeas, cooked, 1 cup (250 ml)	78 mg
Lentils, cooked, 1 cup (250 ml)	71 mg
Kidney beans, cooked, 1 cup (250 ml)	80 mg
Navy beans, cooked, 1 cup (250 ml)	107 mg
Soybeans, cooked, 1/2 cup (125 ml)	131 mg
Tofu, raw, firm, 1/2 cup (125 ml)	118 mg
Dates, 10	29 mg
Figs, 10 dried	111 mg
Green peas, 1/2 cup (125 ml)	31 mg
Spinach, cooked, 1/2 cup (125 ml)	81 mg
Swiss chard, cooked, 1/2 cup (125 ml)	76 mg

Nutrient Values of Some Common Foods, *Health Canada, Ottawa, 1999.*

MAGNESIUM SUPPLEMENTS

If you want to take a supplement, buy magnesium citrate. Compared to other forms of the mineral (e.g., magnesium oxide), magnesium citrates are more easily absorbed by your body. You can also get supplemental magnesium from your calcium pills if you buy one that has magnesium added.

The daily upper limit for magnesium has been set at 350 milligrams from a supplement. That's because doses higher than this can cause diarrhea and stomach upset, common side effects of magnesium supplementation. To prevent these side effects, you can split a larger dose over the course of the day.

IRON

Iron is one of the most common nutrient deficiencies among women. Women who diet to lose weight, shy away from red meat and animal food, or engage in heavy exercise are all at risk for missing out on this important mineral. Women need more iron than men because they lose an average of 15 to 20 milligrams each month during their menstrual period. A woman's iron needs increase during her pregnancy. The consequences of iron deficiency are low energy, fatigue, listlessness, poor motivation to exercise and difficulty concentrating.

Recommended Dietary Allowance (RDA) of Iron for Females

AGE	RDA (MILLIGRAMS)
9–13 years	8 mg
14–18 years	15 mg
19–50 years	18 mg
50+ years	8 mg
Pregnancy	27 mg
Breastfeeding	9 mg

Reprinted with permission from Dietary Reference Intakes for Vitamin A, Vitamin K, Arsenic, Boron, Chromium, Copper, Iodine, Iron, Manganese, Molybdenum, Nickel, Silicon, Vanadium, and Zinc, *Copyright © 2001 by the National Academy of Sciences. Courtesy of the National Academy Press, Washington, D.C.*

Iron in Foods

FOOD	IRON (MILLIGRAMS)
Lean beef, cooked, 3 oz (90 g)	3.0 mg
Beans in tomato sauce, 1 cup (250 ml)	5.0 mg
Kidney beans, 1/2 cup (125 ml)	2.5 mg

Apricots, dried, 6	2.8 mg
Prune juice, 1/2 cup (125 ml)	5.0 mg
Spinach, cooked, 1 cup (250 ml)	4.0 mg
All-Bran, Kellogg's, 1/2 cup (125 ml)	4.7 mg
All-Bran Buds, Kellogg's, 1/2 cup (125 ml)	5.9 mg
Bran flakes, 3/4 cup (175 ml)	4.9 mg
Just Right, Kellogg's, 1 cup (250 ml)	6.0 mg
Raisin bran, 3/4 cup (175 ml)	5.5 mg
Special K, Kellogg's, 3/4 cup (175 ml)	3.2 mg
Cream of Wheat, 1/2 cup (125 ml)	8.0 mg
Oatmeal, instant, 1 pouch	3.8 mg
Wheat germ, 1 tbsp (15 ml)	2.5 mg
Blackstrap molasses, 1 tbsp (15 ml)	3.2 mg

Nutrient Values of Some Common Foods, *Health Canada, Ottawa, 1999.*

Read the section on iron in chapter 3, "Anemia." You'll learn that animal foods contain the most absorbable form of the mineral (called heme iron), whereas plant foods contain iron that's less efficiently absorbed.

IRON SUPPLEMENTS

Unless you are diagnosed with anemia, there is no need to take single iron supplements. In fact, this can be dangerous, since large amounts of iron can be toxic. In addition to making iron-rich food choices, a multivitamin and mineral supplement should provide 10 to 15 milligrams of the mineral.

ZINC

This trace mineral has many vital roles in the body. It is a critical component of many enzymes and hormones, and it assists in immune function and growth and development. It's also an important part of male sperm. Among the many consequences of zinc deficiency are retarded growth development, diarrhea, more frequent infections than usual, slow wound healing and impaired thyroid gland activity. Pregnant women, young girls, vegetarian women and elderly women are at greatest risk for short-changing their body of this mineral.

Recommended Dietary Allowance (RDA) of Zinc for Females

AGE	RDA (MILLIGRAMS)
4–8 years	5 mg
9–13 years	7 mg
14–18 years	9 mg
19–50 years	8 mg
51+ years	8 mg
Pregnancy	11 mg
Breastfeeding	12 mg

Reprinted with permission from Dietary Reference Intakes for Vitamin A, Vitamin K, Arsenic, Boron, Chromium, Copper, Iodine, Iron, Manganese, Molybdenum, Nickel, Silicon, Vanadium, and Zinc, *Copyright © 2001 by the National Academy of Sciences. Courtesy of the National Academy Press, Washington, D.C.*

Zinc in Foods

FOOD	ZINC (MILLIGRAMS)
Beef, cooked, 3 oz (90 g)	4.5 mg
Chicken, cooked, 3 oz (90 g)	1.5 mg
Turkey, cooked, 3 oz (90 g)	1.0 mg
Lamb, cooked, 3 oz (90 g)	1.0 mg
Pork, cooked, 3 oz (90 g)	2.3 mg
Crab, king, cooked, 3 oz (90 g)	6.8 mg
Oysters, eastern, 3 oz (90 g)	150 mg
Milk, 1 cup (250 ml)	1.0 mg
Cheddar cheese, 1 oz (30 g)	0.9 mg
Yogurt, 3/4 cup (175 ml)	1.4 mg
Egg, 1 whole	0.5 mg
Bran flakes, 3/4 cup (175 ml)	1.2–3.7 mg
Wheat germ, 2 tbsp (30 ml)	2.3 mg
Baked beans, 1 cup (250 ml)	4.0–7.2 mg
Black beans, cooked, 1 cup (250 ml)	3.6 mg
Garbanzo beans, cooked, 1 cup (250 ml)	5.0 mg
Lima beans, 1/2 cup (125 ml)	1.9 mg
Lentils, cooked, 1 cup (250 ml)	5.0 mg
Soybeans, cooked, 1 cup (250 ml)	2.0 mg
Soy/rice beverages, fortified, 1 cup (250 ml)	1.0 mg
Tofu, 1/2 cup (125 ml)	2.0 mg
Veggie burger, 1	1.1–5.5 mg

Green peas, 1/2 cup (125 ml)	1.0 mg
Cashews, 1/4 cup (60 ml)	1.9 mg
Pumpkin seeds, 1/4 cup (60 ml)	2.6 mg
Sunflower seeds, 1/4 cup (60 ml)	1.8 mg

Nutrient Values of Some Common Foods, *Health Canada, Ottawa, 1999.*

ZINC SUPPLEMENTS

Your diet plus a good multivitamin and mineral supplement will give you all the zinc you need to stay healthy. Most multivitamin and mineral formulas provide 10 to 20 milligrams. Separate zinc supplements are rarely appropriate. Too much zinc has toxic effects: consuming amounts greater than 50 milligrams per day can depress your immune system, making you more susceptible to infection. Do not exceed 40 milligrams per day.

⟋⟍

Other Elements of a Healthy Diet

Of course we don't eat vitamins and minerals in isolation. These nutrients are packaged in whole foods that contain many other protective compounds. Fruits, vegetables, whole grains, legumes and other plant foods provide dietary fiber and plant chemicals known as phytochemicals. These phytochemicals protect our health in many ways. Some act as antioxidants, others trigger enzymes that inactivate cancer-causing substances, and others boost the body's immune system. Most importantly, scientists are learning every day that whole foods offer a package of nutrients and health-enhancing ingredients that likely work together to keep us healthy. More than 200 studies from around the world have shown that a diet plentiful in fruits and vegetables lowers the risk of many cancers, but this association has not been found when nutrients are consumed all by themselves. Here's the bottom line: taking a pill is no substitute for the benefits of a diet containing a variety of nutritious foods.

DIETARY FIBER

Dietary fiber is actually made up of two types of fiber, *soluble* and *insoluble*. Both types are present in varying proportions in different plant foods, but some foods may be rich in one or the other. And the two types of fiber function differently in your body to promote health.

Soluble fibers, as their name suggests, dissolve in water. Dried peas, beans and lentils, oats, barley, psyllium husks, apples and citrus fruits are good sources of soluble fiber. When you consume these foods, the soluble fibers form a gel in your stomach and slow the rate of digestion and absorption.

Foods like wheat bran, whole grains and some vegetables contain mainly insoluble fibers. Although these fibers do not dissolve in water, they do have a significant capacity for retaining water. In this way they act to increase stool bulk and promote regularity.

It's estimated that Americans are getting 11 to 14 grams of fiber each day, only one-half of what is recommended. Experts agree that a daily intake of 25 grams of total dietary fiber is needed to reap its health benefits. To help you sneak more fiber into your diet, try the following:

- Eat a variety of foods every day to get the benefits of both soluble and insoluble fiber.

- Strive for five or more servings of fruits and vegetables each day. Leave the peel on fruits and vegetables whenever possible.

- Eat at least five servings of whole-grain foods each day.

- Buy high-fiber breakfast cereals. Aim for at least 4 grams of fiber per serving. (Check the nutrition information panel.)

- Top your breakfast cereal with banana, berries or raisins.

- Add 2 tablespoons of natural wheat bran, oat bran or ground flaxseed to cereals, yogurt, casseroles and soup.

- Eat legumes more often—add white kidney beans to pasta sauce, black beans to tacos, chickpeas to salads, lentils to soup. Start with small portions to minimize gas.

- Add a few tablespoons of walnuts, soy nuts, sunflower seeds or raisins to salads.

- Reach for high-fiber snacks like popcorn, dried apricots or dates.

Fiber in Foods

FOOD	FIBER (GRAMS)
Cereals	
100% bran cereal, 1/2 cup (125 ml)	10.0 g
Bran flakes, 3/4 cup (175 ml)	6.3 g
Grape-Nuts, 1/2 cup (125 ml)	6.0 g
Kellogg's All-Bran Buds, 1/3 cup (75 ml)	13.0 g
Quaker Corn Bran, 1 cup (250 ml)	6.3 g
Oat bran, 1 cup, cooked (250 ml)	4.5 g
Oatmeal, 1 cup, cooked (250 ml)	3.6 g
Red River Cereal, 1 cup, cooked (250 ml)	4.8 g
Shredded Wheat, 1 biscuit (175 ml)	3.2 g
Bread and Other Grain Foods	
Pita pocket, whole wheat	4.8 g
Whole wheat bread, 100%, 2 slices	4.0 g
Spaghetti, whole wheat, 1 cup, cooked (250 ml)	4.8 g
Rice, brown, 1 cup, cooked (250 ml)	3.1 g
Wheat bran, 2 tbsp (30 ml)	2.4 g
Fruits	
Apple, 1 medium with skin	2.6 g
Apricots, dried, 1/4 cup (60 ml)	2.6 g
Banana, 1 medium	1.9 g
Blueberries, 1/2 cup (125 ml)	2.0 g
Figs, 5 dried	8.5 g
Orange, 1 medium	2.4 g
Pear, 1 medium with skin	5.1 g
Prunes, 3 dried	3.0 g
Raisins, seedless, 1/2 cup (125 ml)	2.8 g
Strawberries, 1 cup (250 ml)	3.8 g

Vegetables

Broccoli, 1/2 cup (125 ml)	2.0 g
Brussels sprouts, 1/2 cup (125 ml)	2.6 g
Carrots, 1/2 cup (125 ml)	2.2 g
Corn niblets, 1/2 cup (125 ml)	2.3 g
Green peas, 1/2 cup (125 ml)	3.7 g
Lima beans, 1/2 cup (125 ml)	3.8 g
Potato, 1 medium baked with skin	5.0 g
Sweet potato, 1/2 cup mashed (125 ml)	3.9 g

Legumes & Nuts

Almonds, 1/2 cup (125 ml)	8.2 g
Beans and tomato sauce, canned, 1 cup (250 ml)	20.7 g
Black beans, 1 cup, cooked (250 ml)	13.0 g
Chickpeas, 1 cup, cooked (250 ml)	6.1 g
Kidney beans, 1 cup, cooked (250 ml)	6.7 g
Lentils, 1 cup, cooked (250 ml)	9.0 g
Peanuts, dry roasted, 1/2 cup (125 ml)	6.9 g

Nutrient Values of Some Common Foods, *Health Canada, Ottawa, 1999.*

Use the list above to gradually add higher-fiber foods to your diet. Too much fiber too soon can cause bloating, gas and diarrhea. Spread fiber-rich foods out over the course of the day. And don't forget that fiber needs fluid to work, so drink at least eight ounces of fluid with each high-fiber meal and snack.

FRUITS AND VEGETABLES

Dark green and orange vegetables and fruits appear to be powerful protectors against illness. Spinach, kale, rapini, collard greens, Swiss chard, romaine lettuce, squash, carrots, sweet potatoes, cantaloupe and peaches are good sources of beta-carotene, an antioxidant nutrient that might protect cells from damage caused by harmful free radical molecules. (Free radicals roam the body and damage the genetic material of cells, which may lead to cancer development.) Many also contain folate and vitamin C.

Scientists are learning that there's more to fruits and vegetables than vitamins, minerals and fiber. They also contain thousands of phytochemicals, naturally occurring compounds that act as antioxidants and natural antibiotics. Experts believe that phytochemicals probably work together with vitamins and minerals in the food.

Make sure you get *at least five to ten servings of fruits and vegetables each day*. Aim for a minimum of three fruits and three vegetables. Here are a few ways to get more "green" into your diet:

Spinach One-half cup (125 ml) of cooked spinach provides your full day's requirement for vitamin A and offers plenty of folate. Spinach is also an excellent source of vitamin C. One-half cup (125 ml) cooked has more nutrition than 1 cup (250 ml) raw because it contains 2 cups (500 ml) of leaves and heating makes the protein in spinach easier to break down. Steam, braise or stir-fry with a little garlic. Add a splash of balsamic vinegar at the end of cooking.

Kale Just 1 cup (250 ml) of this member of the cabbage family provides more than twice the daily requirements for beta-carotene and vitamin C. Kale is also a good source of calcium and vitamin E, another important antioxidant. Steam or stir-fry this green with other vegetables, or throw kale into soup and simmer. Kale shrinks a lot during cooking; 3 cups (750 ml) raw will give you 1 cup (250 ml) cooked.

Collard greens In addition to plenty of vitamins and minerals, this vegetable contains natural sulfur compounds that may prevent certain cancers. Stir-fry collard greens. Once it's cooked, add a dash of roasted sesame oil and a handful of cashews.

Beet greens The next time you buy fresh beets, save the greens and eat them, too. The green tops of root vegetables have more nutrition when it comes to vitamins and minerals than the root. These greens are a good source of vitamins A and C, as well as calcium and iron. Prepare them as you would any green.

Swiss chard Here's another great vegetable that provides calcium, beta-carotene and vitamin C. Use both the leaves and the stalks when cooking, but add the leaves at the end of cooking, as the stalks take longer to soften. Stir-fry Swiss chard with a little olive oil and garlic. Or add lemon juice and Parmesan cheese. It's also great in pasta with a little olive oil and red pepper flakes.

PROTEIN FOODS

It's important to be meeting your daily requirement for protein. Dietary protein is needed by the body to build muscle tissue, enzymes, hormones and immune compounds. A diet that's chronically low in protein can weaken the immune system, making you more susceptible to infection. If you're looking for results in the gym, an optimal protein intake is important for building and repairing muscle tissue.

Protein is made up of building blocks called amino acids. There are 20 amino acids, and nine of these are essential—that means the body cannot synthesize them at all, or it cannot make them in sufficient quantities to meet its needs. As a result, these nine amino acids must be supplied by the diet. Animal protein foods like meat, dairy, eggs, poultry and fish are considered complete proteins, because they contain all nine amino acids essential for health in adequate amounts. Plant proteins such as legumes, vegetables and grains tend to be limited in one or more essential amino acids.

Complementary Proteins

Vegetarians who eat no animal protein foods must be sure to "complement" their protein foods. By combining two or more vegetarian protein foods so that the essential amino acid missing from one is supplied by the other, vegetarians are able to get all the essential amino acids in their diet. Examples of complementary proteins include beans and rice, peanut butter and whole-wheat bread, and tofu with vegetables and rice. It was once thought that vegetarians had to complement protein foods at every single meal. We now know that if vegetarians eat a variety of protein foods over the course of the day (grains, legumes, nuts, seeds and vegetables) they can fill all their body's needs for amino acids.

Women at risk for protein deficiency include:

- Those who live alone and don't often cook meat, chicken or fish;
- Those who frequently grab quick meals during the day—bagels, pasta, low-fat frozen dinners;
- Vegetarians who do not eat animal foods but do not regularly incorporate high quality vegetable protein sources into their diet;
- Those who engage in heavy exercise and fall into any of the above categories.

Recommended Dietary Allowance (RDA) of Protein for Adult Females

No regular exercise	0.36 grams per lb body weight
Regular exercise	0.55 grams per lb body weight
Heavy exercise	0.55–0.8 grams per lb body weight

Recommended Nutrient Intakes for Canadians, *Health and Welfare Canada, Ottawa, 1983.*

To calculate your actual protein requirements for the day, multiply your weight in pounds by your RDA for protein. For example, a 135-pound woman (61 kg) who does not exercise needs 49 grams of protein each day (135 lb × 0.36). If that same woman was exercising three or four times a week, she would need to eat 74 grams of protein (135 lb × 0.55).[3]

Protein in Foods

FOOD	PROTEIN (GRAMS)
Meat, 3 oz (90 g)	21–25 g
Poultry, 3 oz (90 g)	21 g
Salmon, 3 oz (90 g)	25 g
Sole, 3 oz (90 g)	17 g
Tuna, canned and drained, 1/2 cup (125 ml)	30 g
Egg, 1 whole	6 g
Legumes, 1/2 cup (125 ml)	8 g
Milk, 1 cup (250 ml)	8 g
Yogurt, 3/4 cup (175 ml)	8 g
Cheese, cheddar, 1 oz (30 g)	10 g
Vegetables, 1/2 cup (125 ml)	2 g
Bread, 1 slice	2 g
Rice, pasta, cooked, 1/2 cup (125 ml)	2 g

Nutrient Values of Some Common Foods, *Health Canada, Ottawa, 1999.*

SOY FOODS

Soy foods have potential for helping women in a number of ways. Soy may lower blood cholesterol, slow down bone loss, reduce menopausal hot flashes and possibly reduce your risk of breast cancer if you start eating it at a young age. So you can see there are good reasons to start incorporating this food into your diet. Here are a few ideas to help you get started:

- Pour a calcium-fortified soy beverage on breakfast cereal or in a smoothie; use it in cooking and baking (soups, casseroles, muffins, pancake batters).
- Cube firm tofu and add it to soups—canned or homemade.
- Grill firm tofu on the barbecue. Brush tofu and vegetable kebabs with hoisin sauce or marinate them in teriyaki sauce.
- Substitute firm tofu for ricotta cheese in recipes.
- Use soft tofu in creamy salad dressing or dip recipes.
- Throw canned soybeans in a salad, soup or chili.
- Replace up to one-half of all-purpose flour in a recipe with soy flour.
- Buy roasted soy nuts in health food stores. They come in plain, barbecue, garlic or onion flavors. Enjoy 1/4 cup as a mid-day snack.
- Toss roasted soy nuts in a green salad.
- Replace ground meat with TVP (texturized vegetable protein) in chili, pasta sauce and tacos.
- Try veggie burgers (with soy protein) and veggie dogs on the grill.

Isoflavones

Soybeans contain naturally occurring compounds called isoflavones, a type of plant estrogen. Genistein and daidzein are the most active isoflavones in soy and have been the focus of much research. Isoflavones have a chemical structure similar to estrogen, and this is one reason soy foods are good to include in a woman's diet.

Aim for a daily intake of 40 to 80 milligrams of isoflavones. To keep your blood levels of isoflavones up during the day, consume soy foods twice daily. Depending on the food you eat, your blood isoflavone levels will peak four to eight hours later. Twenty-four hours after eating a soy food, your body will have excreted these isoflavones.

Soy foods vary with respect to the amount of isoflavones they contain. Even the same type of food made by different manufacturers can differ in isoflavone content.

Isoflavones in Soy Foods

SOY FOOD	ISOFLAVONES (MILLIGRAMS)
Roasted soy nuts, 1/4 cup (60 ml)	40–60 mg
Green soybeans, uncooked, 1/2 cup (120 ml)	70 mg
Tempeh, uncooked, 3 oz (90 g)	48 mg
Soy flour, 1/4 cup (60 ml)	28 mg
Tofu, uncooked, 4 oz (120 g)	38 mg
TVP, dry, 1/4 cup (60 ml)	15–60 mg
Soy beverage, So Nice, 1 cup (250 ml)	60 mg
Soy beverage, most brands, 1 cup (250 ml)	25 mg
Soy protein powder, isolate, 2 tbsp (30 ml)	30 mg
Soy sauce	none
Soya oil	none

USDA-Iowa State University Database on the Isoflavone Content of Foods.
U.S. Department of Agriculture, Agricultural Research Service, 1999.

ᕞ

A Healthy Diet Plan

Now you know what nutrients to focus on, and what foods are your best bets for these vitamins and minerals. It's time to put that into practice. To make sure you get your daily share of nutrients, antioxidants and the many other protective chemicals in plant foods, follow the food plan below. Adjust your daily number of servings according to your exercise level. If you work out every day, you'll need to eat the numbers suggested in the upper end of the recommended range. If you are trying to lose weight, stick to the lower end of the range.

Before you start down the road to healthy eating, here are a few pointers to keep in mind:

1. *Make one change at a time.* There's no need to do everything at once. You'll be surprised to find that small changes make a big difference. Set one new goal each week.

2. *Plan ahead whenever you can.* Most of my clients report that their biggest roadblock to eating well is a lack of time. Plan your weekly meals in advance. Grocery shop once a week so you have healthy foods in your fridge and cupboards.

3. Remember that *all foods can be part of a healthy diet.* The occasional splurge on ice cream or deep-fried chicken wings won't upset your healthy eating plan. It's the overall picture that counts.

4. *Periodic overeating, or eating junk foods, does not mean that you have failed.* We're all human. Just return to your usual healthy diet at the next meal.

FOOD GROUP	FOOD CHOICES	RECOMMENDED DAILY SERVINGS
Grain Foods		5 to 12
(Carbohydrate, iron, fiber;	Whole-grain bread, 1 slice	
choose whole-grain*	Bagel, large, 1/4	
as often as possible)	Roll, large, 1/2	
	Pita pocket, 1/2	
	Tortilla, 6", 1	
	Cereal, cold, 3/4 cup (175 ml)	
	Cereal, 100% bran, 1/2 cup (125 ml)	
	Cereal, hot, 1/2 cup (125 ml)	
	Crackers, soda, 6	
	Corn, 1/2 cup (125 ml)	
	Popcorn, plain, 3 cups (750 ml)	
	Grains, cooked, 1/2 cup (125 ml)	
	Pasta, cooked, 1/2 cup (125 ml)	
	Rice, cooked, 1/3 cup (75 ml)	

Vegetables and Fruits		5 to 10
(Carbohydrate, fiber,	Vegetables, cooked, 1/2 cup (125 ml)	
vitamins, minerals)	Vegetables, raw, 1/2 cup (125 ml)	
	Vegetables, leafy green, 1 cup (250 ml)	
	Fruit, whole, 1 piece	
	Fruit, small (plums, apricots), 4	
	Fruit, cut up, 1 cup (250 ml)	
	Berries, 1 cup (250 ml)	
	Juice, unsweetened, 1/2 to 3/4 cup (125–175 ml)	

Milk & Alternatives		2 to 3
(Protein, carbohydrate,	Milk, 1 cup (250 ml)	
calcium, vitamin D,	Yogurt, 3/4 cup (175 ml)	
vitamin A, zinc)	Cheese, 1.5 oz (45 g)	
	Rice beverage, fortified, 1 cup (250 ml)	
	Soy beverage, fortified, 1 cup (250 ml)	

Meat & Alternatives		6 to 9
(Protein, iron, zinc)	Fish, lean meat, poultry, 1 oz (30 g)	
	Egg, whole, 1	
	Egg whites, 2	
	Legumes (beans, chickpeas, lentils), 1/3 cup (75 ml)	
	Soy nuts, 2 tbsp (30 ml)	
	Tempeh, 1/4 cup (60 ml)	
	Tofu, firm, 1/3 cup (75 ml)	
	Texturized vegetable protein, 1/3 cup (75 ml)	
	Veggie dog, small, 1	

Fats & Oils**		4 to 6
(Essential fatty acids,	Butter, margarine, 1 tsp (5 ml)	
vitamin E)		

Mayonnaise, 1 tsp (5 ml)	
Nuts/seeds, 1 tbsp (15 ml)	
Peanut and nut butters, 1.5 tsp (7 ml)	
Salad dressing, 2 tsp (10 ml)	
Vegetable oil, 1 tsp (5 ml)	
Fluid	**8 to 12**
Water, 1 cup (250 ml)	

All serving sizes are based on measures after cooking.

*Whole grains provide more fiber, iron, zinc, vitamin E and antioxidants than refined. Whole-grain foods include barley, brown rice, bulgur, flaxseed, kamut, oatmeal, oat bran, quinoa, whole-wheat bread, whole-rye bread and spelt. When buying bread, look for the words "whole-wheat flour" on the list of ingredients. The terms "wheat flour" and "unbleached wheat flour" mean that refined flour has been used.

**To include sources of essential fatty acids choose canola oil, walnut oil, flaxseed oil and nuts and seeds more often as your fat servings. As you read through the chapters in this book, you will find many mentions of these health-enhancing fats.

Substances to Limit

CAFFEINE

I recommend a daily maximum of 400 to 450 milligrams of caffeine for good health. While your goal is to limit as much caffeine as possible, use this amount as a benchmark to see how much you're consuming now.

Caffeine in Common Beverages, Foods and Medications

FOOD OR MEDICATION	CAFFEINE (MILLIGRAMS)
Coffee (6-ounce cup or 175 ml)	
Regular, drip method	105 mg

Percolator method	75 mg
Instant (1 rounded tsp/5 ml, dry)	60 mg
Espresso (1 fluid ounce)	50 mg
Flavored	25–75 mg
Decaffeinated	
Drip or percolator method	2 mg
Instant (1 rounded tsp/5 ml, dry)	2 mg
Espresso (1 fluid ounce)	5 mg
Tea (6-ounce cup or 175 ml)	
Regular, 3-minute brew	35 mg
Green	25 mg
Bottled (12 fluid ounces)/Instant mix (250 ml)	15 mg
Decaffeinated 5-minute brew	trace
Carbonated Beverages (12 fluid ounces or 350 ml)	
Mountain Dew	55 mg
Colas, regular or sugar-free	35–50 mg
Cherry cola, Dr. Pepper	35–50 mg
Caffeine-free	trace
Chocolate and Cocoa	
Chocolate, baking, unsweetened (25 g)	60 mg
Chocolate, sweet, semi-sweet, dark, milk (25 g)	10–20 mg
Cocoa, unsweetened, dry powder (1 tbsp/15 ml)	10 mg
Chocolate milk (250 ml)	10 mg
Cocoa beverage (250 ml)	5 mg
Chocolate-flavored syrup (25 g)	5 mg
Chocolate pudding (125 ml)	5–10 mg
Chocolate ice cream (125 ml)	2 mg
Chocolate cake, 1 slice	20–30 mg

Medications

Pain relievers (1 tablet)	
Excedrin®	65 mg
Anacin®	32 mg
Excedrin PM®	0 mg
Aspirin, any brand	0 mg
Stay-Awake tablets (1 tablet)	
No Doz®, maximum strength	200 mg
No Doz®, regular strength	100 mg

Reprinted from MayoClinic.com (www.mayoclinic.com/home?id=H000031) with permission of Mayo Foundation for Medical Education and Research, Rochester, MN 55905.

If you have assessed your daily caffeine intake and determined that you're overdoing it, gradually cut back over a period of two to three weeks to minimize withdrawal symptoms such as headaches, tiredness or muscle pain. Start by eliminating caffeine from the latter part of your day. Stick to a "no caffeine" rule after noon. Switch to low-caffeine beverages, like tea or hot chocolate, or caffeine-free alternatives such as decaf coffee, herbal tea, cereal coffee, juice, milk or water. If you're still hooked on coffee, order a latte or cappuccino to get extra calcium. And if your gut is sensitive to lactose in milk, try a soy latte (make sure the soy beverage is calcium fortified).

SODIUM

Sodium is an essential nutrient that our body needs to maintain its fluid balance, but we actually need only a very tiny amount. For sedentary Americans, all it takes is a mere 500 mg (or 1/5 of a teaspoon) of sodium to cover the body's requirement. If you sweat during exercise you need a little more salt, but not much. You might have already guessed that we're getting much more sodium than we need—10 times more, to be precise. Each day the average American consumes about 2 teaspoons of salt.

To help cut back on sodium, avoid the salt shaker at the table, minimize the use of salt in cooking and buy commercial food products that are low in added salt. Eating fewer processed foods is one of the key strategies to de-salt your diet. Most of the salt we consume every day comes from processed and prepared foods; only one-fourth comes from the salt shaker!

The list that follows will help you cut down on foods high in sodium. *Aim for no more than 2400 milligrams of sodium each day (1 teaspoon of salt)*. To season your foods without adding salt, use herbs, spices, flavored vinegars and fruit juices.

Sodium Content of Selected Foods

FOOD	SODIUM (MILLIGRAMS)
Meat & Alternatives	
Fresh meat, poultry, fish, cooked, 3 oz (90 g)	Less than 90 mg
Shellfish, 3 oz (90 g)	100–325 mg
Tuna, canned, 3 oz (90 g)	300 mg
Sausage, 2 oz (60 g)	515 mg
Bologna, 2 oz (60 g)	535 mg
Frankfurter, 1.5 oz (45 g)	560 mg
Lean ham, 3 oz (90 g)	1025 mg
Egg white, 1	155 mg
Whole egg, 1	165 mg
Egg substitute, 1/4 cup (60 ml)	80–120 mg
Dairy Products	
Skim or 1% milk, 1 cup (250 ml)	125 mg
Swiss cheese, 1 oz (30 g)	75 mg
Cheddar cheese, 1 oz (30 g)	175 mg
Blue cheese, 1 oz (30 g)	395 mg
Low-fat cheese, 1 oz (30 g)	150 mg
Processed cheese and spreads, 1 oz (30 g)	75 mg
Cottage cheese, low-fat, 1/2 cup (125 ml)	460 mg
Yogurt, flavored, 1 cup (250 ml)	120–150 mg
Yogurt, nonfat or low-fat, plain, 1 cup (250 ml)	160–175 mg
Vegetables	
Fresh or frozen, 1/2 cup (125 ml)	Less than 70 mg
Canned, no salt, 1/2 cup (125 ml)	Less than 70 mg
Canned, no sauce, 1/2 cup (125 ml)	55–470 mg
Canned, 1/2 cup (125 ml)	215–800 mg
Tomato juice, canned, 3/4 cup (175 ml)	660 mg
Tomato sauce, 1/4 cup (60 ml)	50–370 mg

Grain Foods

Breads, 1 slice	110–175 mg
English muffin, half	130 mg
Bagel, half	190 mg
Baking powder biscuit, 1	305 mg
Cereal: shredded wheat, 3/4 cup (175 ml)	Less than 5 mg
Cereal: puffed wheat and rice, about 1-1/2 cup (375 ml)	Less than 5 mg
Cereal: granola-type, 1/2 cup (125 ml)	5–25 mg
Cereal: flaked, 2/3 to 1 cup (160–250 ml)	170–360 mg
Cereal, cooked, unsalted, 1/2 cup (125 ml)	Less than 5 mg
Cereal, cooked, instant, 1 packet	180 mg
Crackers, saltine type, 5	195 mg
Cooked rice or pasta, unsalted, 1/2 cup (125 ml)	Less than 10 mg
Rice and sauce mix, cooked, 1/2 cup (125 ml)	250–390 mg
Peanut butter, 2 tbsp (30 ml)	150 mg
Peanut butter, unsalted, 2 tbsp (30 ml)	Less than 5 mg
Dry beans, plain, canned, 1/2 cup (125 ml)	350–590 mg

Fats & Oils

Butter, salted, 1 tsp (5 ml)	25 mg
Margarine, unsalted, 1 tsp (5 ml)	Less than 5 mg
Margarine, salted, 1 tsp (5 ml)	50 mg
Mayonnaise, 1 tsp (5 ml)	80 mg
Prepared salad dressing, low-calorie, 2 tbsp (30 ml)	50–310 mg
Prepared salad dressing, 2 tbsp (30 ml)	210–440 mg

Snack Foods

Unsalted nuts, 1/4 cup (60 ml)	Less than 10 mg
Salted nuts, 1/4 cup (60 ml)	120–350 mg
Popcorn, microwave, 3 cups (750 ml)	135–500 mg
Popcorn, air popped, unsalted, 3 cups (750 ml)	1 mg
Unsalted potato chips or corn chips, 1 cup (250 ml)	Less than 5 mg

Salted potato chips or corn chips, 1 cup (250 ml)	170–285 mg
Pretzels, 1 oz (30 g)	500–700 mg
Tortilla chips, 1 oz (30 g)	150–300 mg
Frozen Desserts	
Ice cream, 1/2 cup (125 ml)	5–50 mg
Frozen yogurt, low-fat or nonfat, 1/2 cup (125 ml)	40–55 mg
Ice milk, 1/2 cup (125 ml)	55–60 mg
Condiments & Miscellaneous	
Baking powder, 1 tsp (5 ml)	400–550 mg
Bouillon, 1 cube	1200 mg
Garlic salt, 1 tsp (5 ml)	1480 mg
Mustard, chili sauce, hot sauce, 1 tsp (5 ml)	36–65 mg
Ketchup, steak sauce, 1 tbsp (15 ml)	100–230 mg
Salsa, tartar sauce, 1 tbsp (15 ml)	85–205 mg
Salt, 1/2 tsp (2 ml)	1370 mg
Pickles, sweet or dill, 1 large	330–830 mg
Soy sauce, low sodium, 1 tbsp (15 ml)	600 mg
Soy sauce, 1 tbsp (15 ml)	1030 mg
Convenience Foods	
Canned and dehydrated soups, 1 cup (250 ml)	600–1300 mg
Regular pasta sauce, 1/4 cup (60 ml)	125–275 mg
Lower sodium versions	Read the label*
Canned and frozen main dishes	500–1570 mg
Lower sodium versions	Read the label*

*The sodium content of convenience foods labeled "low sodium" or "reduced salt" can vary, so be sure to check the nutrition information panel. And don't forget to rinse canned vegetables to remove excess salt.

From The Nephrogenic Diabetes Insipidus Foundation, 2000, available at www.ndif.org/na9.html

Reprinted by permission of Cristine Trahms, Head of Nutrition, Center on Human Development and Disability, University of Washington.

2

Weight Control and Food Sensitivities

Now that you have read chapter 1, you have a good idea of the basic nutrients women need for a standard healthy diet. The rest of the book will deal with certain conditions and the part nutrition plays in preventing and managing them. But a large and growing number of women have nutrition concerns apart from, or in addition to, specific health conditions. In this chapter, I'll look at two of these more general concerns: weight control and food sensitivities.

❧

Women and Weight Control

For many women (myself included), weight control has always been important. Since I was a teenager I've had to watch what I eat and exercise regularly in order to maintain a healthy weight. Some women find that staying trim comes naturally and they don't have to work very hard at it (oh, how I envy them!). But as women get older, many find that it becomes more difficult to take off a few unwanted pounds. Many of my perimenopausal clients complain about a "softening around the middle" despite their best efforts at weight control. Luckily, despite the age factor and the challenge of female hormones, weight management is possible through a healthy diet and regular exercise. Over the years, I have helped scores of women lose excess body fat with some sensible advice.

BODY MASS INDEX (BMI)

Being overweight can increase your risk of heart disease, breast cancer and diabetes. It also can complicate your pregnancy and it may even make getting pregnant more difficult. Your health risk is only partially determined by the number you see on the bathroom scale. Once you complete this assessment, you'll get a better idea of how your weight is likely to affect your long-term health.

CALCULATE YOUR BMI (BODY MASS INDEX)	
Divide your weight in pounds by 2.2 = weight in kilograms (kg)	_____
Multiply your height in inches by 2.54 = height in centimeters (cm)	_____
Divide your height (cm) by 100 = height in meters	_____
Square your height in meters	_____
Your BMI = weight (in kg) ÷ height (in meters^2)	_____

Long-term studies show that the overall risk of developing chronic disease is generally related to your BMI as follows:

BMI under 20	may be associated with health problems for some women (e.g., anemia, eating disorder, increased susceptibility to infection)
BMI 20–25	risk is very low; healthy weight
BMI 25–26.9	your risk is starting to increase; caution zone (overweight)
BMI 27–29.9	moderate risk (overweight)
BMI 30+	high risk (obese)

You must remember that there are other factors besides weight that can increase your risk of disease. Poor diet, alcohol, a lack of exercise, smoking and high blood pressure are other important risk factors.

WAIST/HIP RATIO

Another way to assess if you are at a healthy weight is to use the waist/hip ratio.

Using a tape measure, find the circumference of your waist at its narrowest point when your stomach is relaxed.

Waist = _____ inches

Next, measure the circumference of your hips at their widest. (Sorry girls! This is where your buttocks stick out the most.)

Hips = _____ inches

Finally, divide your waist measurement by your hip measurement.

Waist/hip = _____

When it comes to your waist/hip ratio, a healthy target is 0.8 or less. That means you're not carrying excess weight around your middle. It's fat around the abdomen that can lead to health problems.

TIPS FOR LOSING WEIGHT

You may have determined it's time to lose those extra pounds once and for all. Use the food plan in chapter 1 to help you begin. Then move on to use the weight-loss strategies here.

I strongly recommend that you consult with a registered dietitian to help you lose weight safely and effectively. To find a private practice dietitian in your community check out the website at **www.eatright.org**. Working one-on-one with an expert means you will get an eating plan that is customized to your schedule and food preferences. Regular follow-up visits allow you to monitor your progress, adjust your plan as needed and discuss ways to overcome challenges and potential obstacles to success. I see many women in my private practice with polycystic ovary syndrome (PCOS) who successfully lose weight. Here are some strategies that will help you get started losing weight.

1. *Set a realistic goal.* Take a look at what your weight has been for the past 10 to 15 years. If you want to weigh 130 pounds, but you haven't been there since you were 20, keep in mind this might be more difficult to achieve; depending on your current lifestyle, it may be unrealistic. And don't think you have to rely on

the scale to set a goal. I have many clients who choose a size of clothing as their target. If you do decide on a number on the scale, make sure you choose a 5-pound weight range that you plan to stay within. It's not realistic to remain a constant weight. You need a little room for holidays, entertaining and vacations!

2. *Go in with the right mind-set.* Think about making a long-term lifestyle change rather than a short-term quick fix. I can tell you right now that people who approach losing weight with a long-term attitude are far more successful. The right mind-set also means being comfortable with slow and steady weight loss. A safe weight-loss plan shouldn't cause you to lose more than 1 to 3 pounds a week. When you lose weight at a faster rate, there's a good chance you're losing muscle and water. And the more muscle you lose, the slower the rate at which your body burns calories.

3. *Get social support.* If you need help from a spouse, family member, co-worker or friend, ask for it. It often helps to have a workout partner, especially when you're beginning an exercise program. If your roommate pulls out a bag of potato chips every night after dinner, ask him or her to be mindful of your attempt to change your eating habits. If you want positive reinforcement from someone, let that person know.

4. *Start an exercise program.* This is an important step if you're not already active. Exercise burns calories while you do it and, by building up muscle, it helps your body burn more calories at rest. To help lose body fat, aim to get four cardiovascular workouts each week (brisk walking, jogging, stair climbing, swimming, cross-country skiing or aerobics classes). Gradually build up to a minimum of 30 minutes each session. When you're ready, add weight training two or three times a week. Studies have found that adding a weight workout to a weight-loss program speeds up weight loss.

5. *Eat at regular intervals throughout the day.* Eating a meal or snack every four to five hours will help to boost your metabolism, improve your energy level and maintain a consistent blood sugar level. Eating regularly prevents hunger and helps to eliminate mindless snacking and overeating at the next meal.

6. *Don't eat dinner late.* Ideally, sit down to dinner before eight o'clock (the earlier the better). As the evening approaches, your body's metabolism naturally slows down. At the dinner hour, your body actually needs the smallest meal (but of

course this is when most of us consume the majority of our daily calories). If you get home late, tell yourself that you've missed dinner. Just because you walk in the door doesn't mean you have to eat a large dinner. Have a light snack instead—yogurt, a piece of fruit or a bowl of soup.

7. *If your meals are more than five hours apart, plan to have a snack.* Between-meal snacks are important to help keep your energy levels up and prevent snacking on unhealthy foods like sweets. Depending on the meal, your blood sugar will drop three to four hours later. Since your blood sugar is the only source of fuel for your brain, a post-meal dip can make you feel sluggish and tired, and often this is when people go in search of a pick-me-up. So plan this energy boost. But here's my rule—*no snacking on refined starchy foods* like bagels, pretzels, low-fat cookies, low-fat crackers or fat-free muffins. Because these foods are quickly converted to blood glucose, they're more likely to lead to further hunger and cravings for sweets. Better snacks include yogurt, milk, homemade smoothies and whole fruit. Choosing these snacks will also help get more fiber and calcium into your diet.

8. *Be sure to get at least six servings of protein-rich foods each day.* Not only will this help you meet your protein needs, but protein will also help to maintain your blood-sugar levels longer. I recommend splitting your protein servings between lunch and dinner; some people prefer to include some protein at breakfast, too.

   1 protein serving = 1 oz (30 g) lean meat, poultry, fish, hard cheese
   1/4 cup (60 ml) cottage cheese
   1 egg or 2 egg whites
   2 oz (60 g) firm tofu (1/4 cup cubed)
   1/3 cup (75 ml) cooked chickpeas or other legume
   2 tbsp (30 ml) roasted soy nuts

9. *Reduce your portions of carbohydrate-containing foods.* Eating smaller portions of carbohydrates not only reduces your calorie intake, it also helps reduce high levels of blood insulin. That's because, once digested into glucose units, carbohydrate foods trigger the release of insulin in the bloodstream. But following a low-carbohydrate diet does not mean giving up all carbohydrate-containing foods. I do not recommend diets like Dr. Atkins' or Protein Power where followers are told to avoid all starch, fruit and milk products. Over the long run this is not healthy, nor is it sustainable.

Simply reducing your portion size of carbohydrate foods will help you lose weight. Even though bread on its own is low in fat, it still has calories and they add up. For example, one large bagel is equivalent to five slices of bread! Here are a few tips that might help prevent you from overeating starchy foods (something that's very easy to do!):

- Say "no" to the bread basket in restaurants;
- When you have pasta or stir-fries with rice, skip the bread;
- At breakfast, have cereal *or* toast, not both;
- When you eat pasta, your portion should be no larger than 1 cup cooked (appetizer size);
- When you eat rice, your portion should be no larger than 2/3 cup cooked;
- If you tend to overeat foods like pasta, rice or potatoes, consider skipping the starchy food at dinner. You don't have to serve rice or potatoes. Instead, enjoy grilled fish, chicken or lean meat with plenty of vegetables. Or maybe an omelet and salad. In my practice, I find this strategy helps women lose weight and eat more vegetables, and it also reduces bloating.

10. *Get rid of excess sugar—natural and refined.* I certainly don't mind a little jam on your toast or a teaspoon of sugar in your coffee. But drinks like regular soda, fruit drinks and fruit juice only add extra calories to your day, not to mention elevating your blood sugar. I'd rather you quench your thirst with water and get your fruit servings as whole fruit. You'll save calories and boost your fiber intake.

11. *Treat yourself to a serving of sweets, dessert or candy once a week.* Enjoy a "real" serving of whatever you really want once a week. If sweets aren't your thing, make it french fries or chicken wings. Make this weekly treat part of your plan and don't feel guilty about eating it. Remember that any changes you make to lose weight have to be sustainable. Can you really see yourself giving up chocolate for good?

12. *Don't eliminate fat from your diet.* Keep your intake of added fats and oils to a moderate level. Aim to get three to four servings of fat each day.

One fat serving = 1 tsp (5 ml) butter or oil (olive, canola and flaxseed are best)
2 tsp (10 ml) regular salad dressing
4 tsp (20 ml) fat-reduced dressing

1 tbsp (15 ml) cream cheese

2 tbsp (30 ml) low-fat cream cheese

1 tbsp (15 ml) nuts or seeds

1.5 tsp (7 ml) peanut butter

2 tbsp (30 ml) dip (hummus, tzatziki)

8 olives

13. *Limit your alcohol intake to no more than seven drinks a week.* The calories in alcohol—from beer, wine or liquor—add up. What's more, alcohol tends to lower one's willpower, making it more difficult to stick to a healthy meal plan. If you do drink alcohol, one drink a day is not considered harmful to your health. If you're out for an evening, try alternating one alcoholic drink with a low-calorie alcohol-free one (mineral water, club soda, Clamato juice, cranberry and soda). One drink is equivalent to 5 ounces of wine, one bottle of light beer or 1.5 ounces of liquor.

14. *Deal with momentary lapses.* We're all human. Whether you've had a busy social calendar or you've just returned from a wonderful three-week vacation, you're bound to have put on a few pounds. The key to long-term weight maintenance is nipping small weight gains in the bud. That's why I advised you earlier to choose a *weight range* to stay within. If you want to stay trim, you've got to catch that 3- or 5-pound gain before it becomes 10. And if you're not watching it, that 10 pounds can quite easily turn into 20. I'm sure many of you know just what I mean. I recommend monitoring your weight on a regular (i.e., weekly) basis. When you see a few pounds creep on, have a plan of action to take them off: keep a food diary for a few weeks, add an extra workout to your week for a month, or give up your weekly treat until the pounds are back down. Choose something that will work for you.

Leslie's Meal Plan
for Healthy Weight Loss

Breakfast Ideas

Choose one of the following breakfasts:

1. 3/4 cup (175 ml) 100% bran cereal or 1 cup (250 ml) whole-grain cereal (choose a cereal with at least 4 grams fiber per serving)
   1 cup (250 ml) 1% or skim milk or fortified soy beverage
   3/4 cup (175 ml) calcium-fortified orange juice or 1 piece citrus fruit
   Water

2. 2 slices whole-wheat toast with 2 tbsp (30 ml) sugar-reduced jam
   3/4 cup (175 ml) low-fat yogurt (fruit-bottom is okay) or 1 medium-sized skim-milk latte
   3/4 cup (175 ml) calcium-fortified orange juice or 1 piece fruit
   Water

3. 1 cup (250 ml) cooked oatmeal, Red River or Brown Rice cereal (add ground flaxseed, wheat germ or 2 tbsp dried fruit)
   Top with 3/4 cup (175 ml) plain or vanilla-flavored low-fat yogurt or 1 cup (250 ml) milk
   3/4 cup (175 ml) calcium-fortified orange juice

4. Breakfast Blender Smoothie
   Blend together these ingredients:
   1 cup (250 ml) milk or calcium-fortified soy beverage
   1/2 medium-sized banana
   1/2 cup whole frozen strawberries or 3/4 cup (175 ml) calcium-fortified orange juice

Mid-Morning Snack

If lunch is more than five hours after breakfast, choose one of the following:

3/4 cup (175 ml) 1% milk-fat yogurt; or
1 piece fruit

Your Basic Lunch

3 Protein Servings
2 Starchy Food Servings
2 Vegetable Servings
2 Fat Servings
500 ml Water

Lunch Ideas

To meet Basic Lunch needs, choose one of the following lunches:

1. Sandwich on rye, pumpernickel or whole-wheat bread, or pita pocket; made
   with 2–3 oz lean protein (turkey, chicken breast or tuna) and low-fat mayo
   2 tsp (10 ml) mayonnaise or 4 tsp (20 ml) salad dressing if desired
   2 vegetable servings (baby carrots, vegetable soup, green salad or vegetable juice)
   Water

2. 3 oz (90 g) grilled chicken breast or salmon or 3/4 cup (175 ml) cottage cheese
   Large green salad
   4 tsp (20 ml) salad dressing or 2 tsp (10 ml) olive or flaxseed oil
   1 whole-grain roll
   Water

3. Veggie Burger made with soy protein (not a "grain" burger)
   One whole-wheat roll or a small whole-wheat pita pocket
   Mustard, relish, sliced vegetables
   Green salad with 4 tsp (20 ml) salad dressing
   Water

4. 1 cup (250 ml) cooked pasta with tomato sauce with 3 oz (90 g) seafood or chicken or 1 cup (250 ml) legumes (e.g., lentils or kidney beans)
Large green salad
4 tsp (20 ml) salad dressing
Water

Mid-Afternoon Snack

If dinner is more than five hours after lunch, choose one of the following:

1 piece of fruit and 3/4 cup (175 ml) low-fat yogurt; or
1 piece fruit and 2 tbsp (30 ml) roasted soy nuts; or
1 Energy Bar: look for a bar with 14 grams of protein and approximately 200 calories. You'll find a wide selection in health food and sporting-goods stores.

Your Basic Dinner

4 to 5 Protein Servings
0 Starchy Food Servings
2 Vegetable Servings
2 Fat Servings
500 ml Water
Or same as Lunch

Dinner Ideas

To meet Basic Dinner needs, choose one of the following dinners:

1. Large green salad with one of the following:
   2 cups (500 ml) of greens plus raw vegetables; or
   1 can tuna or salmon in water, drained; or
   1 grilled chicken breast
   4 tsp (20 ml) salad dressing
   Water

2. Two-egg omelet (use omega-3 eggs*)
   Add chopped vegetables, 2 tbsp grated low-fat cheese, salsa if desired
   Steamed vegetables or large green salad
   4 tsp (20 ml) salad dressing
   * Omega-3 eggs are available in all grocery stores.

3. 5 oz (150 g) baked salmon filet (wrap in foil with lemon juice and fresh chopped
   dill; bake at 450°F for 25–30 minutes)
   Steamed vegetables and/or green salad
   4 tsp (20 ml) salad dressing
   Water

4. 4–5 oz (120–150 g) roasted pork tenderloin (brush with hoisin sauce; bake at 375°F
   for 30 minutes)
   Steamed vegetables and/or salad
   4 tsp (20 ml) salad dressing or 2 tsp (10 ml) oil
   Water

5. 4–5 oz (120–150 g) grilled lean beef
   Large green salad and/or steamed vegetables
   4 tsp (20 ml) salad dressing or 2 tsp (10 ml) oil
   Water

6. 5 oz (150 g) white fish; e.g., halibut, swordfish, sea bass, grouper (marinate with
   your favorite dressing or brush with hoisin sauce; bake at 450°F for 15 minutes)
   Steamed or stir-fried vegetables or salad
   Water

Your Daily Food Servings

All serving sizes are measured *after* cooking.

Protein Foods   6 or 8 servings

1 serving = 1 oz lean meat, poultry, fish
- 1 oz (30 g) hard cheese
- 1 egg or 2 egg whites
- 1/4 cup (60 ml) cottage cheese
- 2 oz (60 g) firm tofu
- 2 tbsp (30 ml) roasted soy nuts

Starchy Foods   4 or 6 servings

1 serving = 1 slice bread
- 1/2 cup (125 ml) pasta or corn
- 1/3 cup (75 ml) rice
- 1/2 cup (125 ml) hot cereal
- 3/4 cup (175 ml) cold cereal
- 1/2 potato or 1/2 cup (125 ml) sweet potato

Fruit   3 servings

1 serving = 6 oz (180 g) unsweetened fruit juice or 1 medium-sized fruit

Vegetables   3+ servings

1 serving = 1/2 cup (125 ml) cooked or raw vegetables
- 1 cup leafy vegetables (e.g., salad)

Milk   2 servings

1 serving = 1 cup (250 ml) milk
- 3/4 cup (175 ml) low-fat yogurt
- 1 cup (250 ml) fortified soy beverage

Fats & Oils   3–4 servings
1 serving = 1 tsp (5 ml) vegetable oil, butter or margarine
            2 tsp (5 ml) salad dressing
            1 tbsp (15 ml) nuts/seeds
            1.5 tsp (7 ml) peanut butter
            2 tbsp (30 ml) dip

∽

Food Sensitivities

Over the past five years, I have seen an increasing number of women who complain of food sensitivities. While traditional allergy testing may turn up nothing, these women often complain of bloating, gas and abdominal distention after eating certain foods. Other women with specific health issues find that they are unable to properly digest foods that once posed no problem.

True *food allergies* involve your body eliciting an immune response to a food. Food allergies are usually due to the protein component of the offending food. For some reason, some of the food protein is absorbed from the intestine intact instead of being digested as most proteins are. Once the intact protein is in the bloodstream, it is recognized as a foreign protein to the body. Your body's immune system produces antibodies to halt the "invasion." As your immune system attempts to fight off the problem food, symptoms appear throughout the body. The most common symptoms can include swelling of the lips; stomach cramps, vomiting, diarrhea; hives, rashes or eczema; and/or wheezing or breathing problems.

True food allergies are uncommon but they can involve any food. Common foods that cause allergic reactions include eggs, shellfish, fish, wheat, nuts, dairy and soybeans. Food allergy symptoms vary from person to person. Symptoms can begin within minutes or a few hours after eating the offending food.

Most allergic reactions to food are relatively mild. However, a small percentage of allergic individuals have severe, life-threatening reactions called *anaphylaxis*. Anaphylaxis occurs when an offending food overwhelms the individual, causing several different parts of the body to experience reactions at the same time—hives, swelling of the throat and difficulty breathing. If not treated immediately (by an injection of adrenaline), this severe form of food allergy can be fatal.

If you suspect that you have a food allergy, speak to your doctor about allergy testing. Several types of tests are available, including skin-prick testing and blood testing. The elimination diet I discuss below can also help you to determine which foods you may be allergic to.

Not all unpleasant reactions to foods are caused by an allergy. A *food intolerance* is much more common than a food allergy. "Food intolerance" is the term used to describe a druglike reaction to a food component. A reaction to a food can be caused by a number of chemicals, which may be present in food as natural or added components. Food chemicals that have been implicated in these types of adverse reactions include naturally occurring salicylates, amines and benzoates. Other chemicals include a number of food additives used in the processing and preservation of foods. Compounds most frequently tied to adverse reactions are yellow dye number 5, monosodium glutamate (MSG), and sulfites.

Another cause of food intolerance is a *lactase deficiency*. Lactase is an enzyme found in the lining of the gut. This enzyme breaks down lactose, the natural sugar found in milk. If a person does not have enough lactase in his or her intestine, the body cannot properly digest lactose. Instead, the lactose remains undigested in the gut, pulling water into the intestine, which can lead to diarrhea. Bacteria then ferment the lactose causing bloating, gas and pain.

Sometimes natural substances that occur in foods can cause a reaction similar to an allergic reaction. For instance, histamine can reach high levels in cheese, some wines and in certain kinds of fish, particularly tuna and mackerel. Eating one of these foods can lead to a reaction called *histamine toxicity* in susceptible individuals.

Some of the symptoms caused by a food intolerance can be very similar to those caused by a food allergy, so it may be difficult to tell if you have an allergy or an intolerance. One way to tell is by your symptoms. Food intolerances often cause more general symptoms like drowsiness, fatigue, irritability, headache and muscle aches and pains.

THE ELIMINATION/CHALLENGE DIET

If you are having difficulty identifying what foods are causing you grief, use the elimination diet to pinpoint your trigger foods. It may pose a short-term hassle but you'll find it's worth the effort. This process should help you decide what foods to avoid and what foods you can continue to enjoy.

The mainstay of this diet is the demonstration of relief of symptoms on removal of a given food item and recurrence of symptoms on its reintroduction (elimination/challenge testing). You might consider enlisting the help of a registered dietitian (**www.eatright.org**) to help you follow this diet.

Because milk, soybeans, eggs, wheat, peanuts, nuts, shellfish and corn are the main culprits for the majority of people who have food sensitivities, these foods are usually not included in the starting diet. Make sure that these foods are not in other foods you eat. For example, egg or milk may be in mayonnaise or salad dressings. Stay on this elimination diet for 10 to 14 days.

During this period, keep a food and symptom diary. Record everything you eat, amounts eaten and what time you ate the food or meal. Document any symptoms, the time of day you started to feel the symptom, and the duration of time you felt the symptom. You might want to grade your symptoms: 1 = mild, 2 = moderate, 3 = severe. If your symptoms do not subside, eliminate additional foods until your symptoms stop.

Once your symptoms disappear, the challenge phase begins: suspect foods are reintroduced to the basic diet until symptoms reappear. Do this gradually, introducing them one at a time. I recommend the following procedure for testing foods:

Day 1: Introduce the food in the morning, at or after breakfast. If you do not experience symptoms, try it again in the afternoon or with dinner.

Day 2: Do not eat any of the test food. Follow your elimination diet. If you do not experience a reaction today, the food is considered safe and can be included in your diet.

Day 3: If no symptoms occur, try the next food on your list, according to the above schedule.

You may find that you can tolerate some foods if you eat them once every few days, but not if they are consumed every day. You may also learn that some troublesome foods are better tolerated if eaten in small portions. The good news is you don't have to completely eliminate all problematic foods from your diet, especially if you enjoy them.

Determining what foods you need to stay away from can take time. If allergy testing or an elimination/challenge diet reveals that you have to avoid certain foods altogether, consult a registered dietitian in your community who can work with you to plan a healthy diet that meets all of your nutritional needs.

Part 2

Low Energy Levels, Fatigue and Pain

3

Anemia

Anemia literally means "too little blood." It is the most common disorder of the blood, and the most prevalent nutritional problem in the world today. Anemia is any condition in which too few red blood cells are present, or in which the red blood cells are too small or contain too little hemoglobin (the pigment that transports oxygen throughout your body).

Anemia lowers the oxygen-carrying capacity of the blood and starves tissues in your body of the energy they need to function properly. Anemia affects the whole body, causing fatigue, shortness of breath, lack of energy and many other complications.

There are several kinds of anemia, but the most common and severe type is iron-deficiency anemia. Women are especially at risk of developing iron-deficiency anemia throughout their reproductive years. In fact, iron deficiency is the most common nutrient deficiency in American women. It's estimated that up to 84 percent of American women do not meet their daily requirement for iron.[1] In some studies, the prevalence of low iron stores has ranged from 25 to 39 percent.

Deficiencies of folate and vitamin B12 can also cause anemia. Short-changing your body of these vitamins affects your red blood cells differently than a lack of iron. You will read how to prevent these types of anemia later in this chapter.

Anemia is not a disease itself, but it can be a symptom of many different conditions including nutrient deficiencies, bleeding, excessive red blood cell destruction and defective red blood cell formation. Anemia is treated by stopping the source of blood loss and/or rebuilding your body's nutrient stores through the use of supplements and diet.

👋

What Causes Anemia?

Blood is essential to human life. It carries nutrients, oxygen, hormones, cellular waste and other substances to and from all parts of your body. Almost 50 percent of your blood is composed of red blood cells, which contain an essential oxygen-carrying protein called hemoglobin. To stay healthy, your body requires a steady supply of oxygen to nourish tissues and keep them functioning efficiently. The red blood cells circulate in your bloodstream, transporting oxygen from your lungs to the working muscle cells and tissues of your body.

Many nutrients are required for red blood cell production. Iron, vitamin B12 and folic acid are the most important nutrients, but small quantities of vitamin C, riboflavin and copper are also necessary, along with a specific balance of hormones. If your body doesn't have adequate amounts of these nutrients and hormones, red blood cell production slows down and eventually causes anemia.

Anemia develops when there is a reduction in the number and the size of red blood cells or when the amount of hemoglobin contained in the red blood cells is too low. Anemia limits the amount of oxygen your blood can deliver to your body. Essentially your cells become starved for energy.

The most common and severe type of anemia is iron-deficiency anemia. The mineral iron is essential for making hemoglobin, the main component of red blood cells. Your body uses its iron supply very efficiently. Iron is recycled from dead red blood cells to produce new ones. Consequently, the recommended dietary intake for iron is relatively low (to learn how much iron you need each day, refer to the RDA table on page 23 of chapter 1). If you eat a healthy, well-balanced diet, chances are you are getting enough iron to ensure healthy red blood cell production.

There are, however, circumstances when normal dietary intake is not sufficient to maintain your iron stores. In adults, the main cause of iron deficiency is blood loss. Conditions that result in chronic or repeated bleeding, such as nosebleeds, hemorrhoids, certain cancers, ulcers or other gastrointestinal problems, will deplete iron stores and may eventually lead to anemia. Anemia can also develop because of a sudden blood loss caused by an injury or surgery.

Women are particularly vulnerable to iron-deficiency anemia, especially during their reproductive years. Because of the regular blood loss that occurs during menstruation, women have higher iron requirements than men. Pregnancy also depletes iron stores at a much faster rate than normal. The growing fetus and placenta require a higher blood volume and a larger supply of iron. Pregnant women need additional iron and are very likely to develop iron deficiency unless they supplement their dietary intake. A traumatic childbirth can also cause a sudden blood loss, which can lead to anemia, low blood pressure and other complications.

While excessive blood loss is the main cause of iron-deficiency anemia, your dietary intake of iron is extremely important for maintaining your body's iron stores. A diet that chronically lacks the proper amount of iron will lead to iron deficiency, and ultimately anemia.

Diet may not be the only culprit behind a case of iron deficiency. You may be consuming enough iron every day, but your body may not be absorbing it properly. Poor iron absorption will have a negative effect on your iron stores and could easily lead to anemia. Certain factors in your diet can impair your body's ability to absorb iron from food, discussed in the section below. Thyroid hormones and certain drugs may also interfere with your ability to utilize iron effectively.

Anemia is often a side effect of chronic disease, especially in the elderly. Health conditions such as infection, inflammation and cancer will suppress red blood cell production and deprive the developing cells of much needed iron. In rarer instances, anemia can develop when the destruction of red blood cells exceeds the rate of production. This type of anemia can result from many conditions, including an enlarged spleen, various auto-immune disorders, red blood cell abnormalities and cancer. Elderly people with a chronic disease may also be taking medication that is known to destroy red blood cells prematurely.

In addition to iron deficiency, there are several other nutritional factors that can cause anemia. Deficiencies in vitamin B12, vitamin C or folate (folic acid) can cause abnormalities in red blood cell production. A lack of vitamin B12 in your diet or impaired absorption can lead to *pernicious anemia*. If your diet lacks folate, another B vitamin, *megaloblastic anemia* can result.

Symptoms

Iron-deficiency anemia is a progressive condition. It usually develops in stages, so it can take months or even years before symptoms appear. The main symptoms of anemia include fatigue, weakness, loss of appetite, loss of energy, shortness of breath and increased susceptibility to infection. Many of my clients complain of difficulty performing exercise that once posed no problem for them. In the presence of iron deficiency, it is not uncommon to lack motivation to work out. It's important to keep in mind that you may feel these symptoms even if you are not classified as anemic. A marginal iron deficiency can affect your energy levels, too, although not as severely.

Tongue irritation, cracks at the side of the mouth and spoonlike deformities in the fingernails also may result from iron deficiency. Some people with anemia develop pica, a craving for non-food substances such as ice, dirt or pure starch. In young children, iron deficiency may cause irreversible abnormalities in brain development, resulting in impaired attention span, cognitive function and learning ability. However, scientists don't know the severity of iron deficiency necessary to produce these developmental changes.

Anemia ranges from mild to severe, and the symptoms also vary accordingly. Mild anemia does not have any significant long-term consequences. It may simply result in dizziness, faintness, thirst, sweating or a rapid pulse. These symptoms usually disappear when iron supplies are restored. More severe cases of anemia may lead to medical problems involving the heart. Because anemia lowers the amount of oxygen in the bloodstream, the heart must beat faster and deliver more blood to the tissues. If the heart is unable to keep up with this increased demand, symptoms of heart failure may develop, including difficulty in breathing, swollen legs and angina.

The speed at which blood is lost will also affect the symptoms of anemia. When blood loss is sudden and occurs over several hours or less, the loss of only one-third of the body's blood volume causes death. If bleeding takes place over a longer period, such as days or weeks, the body can tolerate a loss of up to two-thirds of its blood volume, often without suffering anything more than a feeling of fatigue or weakness.

Who's at Risk?

If you fall into any of the following categories you're at risk for developing iron-deficiency anemia:

- You're female
- You're pregnant
- You engage in regular endurance exercise (e.g., long-distance running, triathlons)
- You follow a low-calorie diet (less than 1300 calories)
- You're a vegetarian

All women of reproductive age are at risk of developing iron deficiency, and at even greater risk if their diet lacks iron-rich foods. Women who are pregnant or breastfeeding are also predisposed to anemia because of the additional demands of the growing baby and placenta. Female runners or triathletes lose iron through sweat and can become iron deficient, especially if their diet lacks iron. Any woman who reduces her calorie intake to lose weight or eats an unbalanced vegetarian diet is also at risk.

Teenage girls are another high-risk group due to the onset of menstruation, increased growth requirements and a diet that often has an inadequate dietary intake of iron.

Infants are born with sufficient stores of iron, but this iron supply becomes depleted during the first few months of life. Exclusively breastfed babies and babies fed on whole cow's milk are especially at risk of developing iron deficiency. For this reason, pediatricians recommend that infants receive additional iron from iron-fortified cereals or formulas from the time that they are six months of age.

Surveys indicate that young children also fall into a high-risk category for iron deficiency. Children from low-income families or from ethnic groups such as Chinese and Native American peoples may not eat sufficient quantities of iron-rich foods to maintain a healthy iron supply.

Diagnosis

Blood tests are used to diagnose anemia. Your doctor will look at the level of hemoglobin in your blood to determine the degree of iron deficiency. A simple blood test can also determine the amount of iron that's stored in your liver. On rare occasions it may be necessary to examine a sample of bone marrow to assess the iron content of your red blood cells.

Blood tests that identify the size, shape, color and number of red blood cells are used to identify anemia that is caused by deficiencies in other vitamins, such as vitamin B12, vitamin C and folate (folic acid). Anemia that is a result of chronic disease or other physical disorders will normally be identified as part of the diagnosis of the underlying medical condition.

Conventional Treatment

Excessive bleeding is often a primary cause of anemia, so the first step in treatment usually involves locating and stopping the source of the bleeding. In most cases, iron supplements are prescribed as a short-term therapy for iron deficiency (read more about this below).

When anemia is severe or the blood loss is rapid, you may need a blood transfusion to immediately replenish your iron supplies. If excessive menstrual bleeding or another uterine problem causes your anemia, your doctor may prescribe oral contraceptives to reduce your monthly blood flow.

The other types of vitamin-deficiency anemia are also treated with a daily regimen of vitamin supplements. People with vitamin B12 and folic acid deficiency must take supplements for their entire life. Anemia caused by medical disorders or chronic disease usually disappears once the underlying cause of the condition is addressed.

Preventing and Treating Iron-Deficiency Anemia

In most chapters in this book, the format involves discussing food/dietary strategies first, then vitamins and minerals, and finally herbal remedies, if applicable. In the case of anemia, I must start off with vitamins and minerals since they are key strategies to both preventing and treating the different types of anemia. Certain foods are important for enhancing the body's absorption of these nutrients, especially in the case of iron. So, let's begin with the mighty "micro" nutrients, the vitamins and minerals.

VITAMINS AND MINERALS

Iron

Most of the body's iron is found in two proteins: hemoglobin in red blood cells and myoglobin in muscle cells. As a component of these two proteins, iron helps carry oxygen throughout the body and release it to tissues where it is used for energy. To help prevent the signs and symptoms of an iron deficiency, it is critical that women consume adequate amounts of iron every day: see the RDA table on page 23 of chapter 1.

The richest sources of iron are beef, fish, poultry, pork and lamb. They supply heme iron, the type that can be absorbed and utilized the most efficiently by your body. Heme sources of iron make up about 10 percent of the iron we consume each day. Even though heme iron accounts for such a small proportion of our intake, it is so well absorbed that it actually contributes a significant amount of iron.

The rest of our iron comes from plant foods such as dried fruits, whole grains, leafy green vegetables, nuts, seeds and legumes. These are nonheme sources of iron, and the body is much less efficient in absorbing and using this type of iron. Vegetarians may have difficulty maintaining healthy iron stores because their diet relies exclusively on nonheme sources. The rate at which your body is able to absorb nonheme iron is strongly influenced by other factors in your diet, as you will read in the sections that follow.

To boost your intake of iron, aim to include in your diet some of the foods from the Iron in Foods table on page 23 in chapter 1.

Over the years, our dietary preferences have changed considerably. Today, we eat more grains, fruits and vegetables and less meat than we did 20 years ago. This trend towards a plant-based diet has affected our overall intake of iron. Women often restrict the amount of meat they eat, in an attempt to lose weight or to watch their blood cholesterol level. This can make it very difficult to achieve the recommended daily requirements for iron. Statistics indicate that adolescent girls also tend to limit their meat intake.

MULTIVITAMIN/MINERAL AND IRON SUPPLEMENTS

To help you meet your daily iron requirements, a multivitamin and mineral supplement is a wise idea. Most formulas provide 10 milligrams of iron, but you can find multivitamins that provide up to 18 milligrams of the mineral.

If you are diagnosed with iron-deficiency anemia, your doctor will prescribe single iron pills. Depending on the extent of your iron deficiency, you may take one to three iron tablets (each containing 50 to 100 milligrams of elemental iron) per day. If you are advised to take an iron pill, take it on an empty stomach to enhance absorption. Many people find that taking their iron supplement before bed instead of during the day reduces stomach upset. Iron can be constipating, so I recommend you make a special effort to boost your fiber and water intake to prevent this side effect.

A supplementation period of 6 to 12 weeks is usually sufficient to treat your anemia. However, you may need to take the supplements for up to six months in order to completely restore your body's iron reserves. As your iron levels improve, your symptoms will gradually disappear.

While taking iron you may notice that your stools turn black. There's no need to worry—this is a normal and harmless side effect of the treatment. Your doctor will perform occasional blood tests to ensure that the bleeding has stopped or that your iron supply has increased to a healthy level.

When it comes to iron supplements, it is important to remember that more is *not* better. Your intestine can absorb only a limited amount of iron, so the benefits do not increase with larger doses. On the contrary, too much iron may cause indigestion and constipation. Excessive doses of iron can actually be quite toxic, causing damage to your liver and intestines. An iron overload can result in death. To avoid these problems, do not take iron supplements without having a blood test to confirm that you are suffering from an iron deficiency.

ENHANCING ABSORPTION OF NONHEME IRON

Animal Foods Meat, poultry and fish contain the most bio-available heme iron, most easily absorbed and utilized by the body. These sources also contain a special component, called MFP factor, that promotes the absorption of nonheme iron from other foods eaten with them. So, if you're wanting to absorb more iron from your brown rice stir-fry, throw in a little lean beef. This trick will work for those of you who don't follow a vegetarian diet.

Vitamin C If you are a vegetarian, here's a strategy worth noting. Including a little vitamin C in your plant-based meal can enhance the body's absorption of nonheme iron four-fold. In fact, vitamin C is the most potent promoter of nonheme iron absorption. The acidity of the vitamin converts iron to the ferrous form that's ready for absorption (your stomach acid enhances iron absorption in the same way). Here are some winning combinations:

- Whole-wheat pasta with tomato sauce
- Brown rice stir-fry with broccoli and red pepper
- Whole-grain breakfast cereal topped with strawberries
- Whole-grain toast with a small glass of orange juice
- Spinach salad tossed with orange or grapefruit segments

Calcium Chances are you've heard that calcium can interfere with iron absorption, especially when iron and calcium are taken simultaneously. It is true that these minerals (as well as magnesium and zinc) are absorbed the same way in the intestinal tract, so they can compete with one another for transport across the intestinal tract. But recent research has shown that taking a calcium supplement with meals for up to six months does not affect iron levels in healthy adults. However, if you are taking calcium supplements *and* iron pills to treat anemia, it is advisable to take them at separate times.

Tea and Coffee Natural compounds called tannins can bind with iron and make it unavailable for absorption. Tannins are found in black tea and, to a lesser extent, in coffee, nuts and some fruits and vegetables. If you are a tea drinker, enjoy your cup of tea between meals. Or add a little milk or lemon to your cup of tea, since both inactivate its iron-binding properties.

Phytate-Rich Foods Another compound in plant foods called phytic acid (phytate) can attach to iron and inhibit its absorption. These compounds are found in dietary fiber, nuts, spinach and other leafy vegetables. The recommended intake for dietary fiber (25 grams per day) is not associated with impaired iron absorption. You would have to be eating a diet that is extremely high in fiber (50 grams or more each day) before you would interfere with the body's absorption of minerals.

Cooking vegetables such as spinach releases some of the iron that's bound to phytates. For this reason, cooked vegetables are always a better source of minerals than their raw counterparts.

ॐ

Preventing and Treating Other Types of Anemia

VITAMINS AND MINERALS

Folate

An ongoing deficiency of this important B vitamin leads to what is known as macrocytic or megaloblastic anemia. Folate is needed to synthesize DNA, the genetic material that's required by all cells. When your body lacks folate as a result of poor diet, impaired absorption or an unusually high need for the vitamin, the DNA metabolism is harmed, especially in rapidly dividing cells like red blood cells.

The anemia of folate deficiency is characterized by large, immature red blood cells. Without folate, DNA production slows and red blood cells lose their ability to divide. These immature cells are enlarged and oval shaped. As such, they cannot carry oxygen or travel through the tiny blood vessels (capillaries) as efficiently as normal red blood cells.

To help prevent anemia associated with a folate deficiency, aim to meet your recommended daily allowance: see the RDA table on page 6 in chapter 1. If you are pregnant, your folate requirement rises considerably to cover the needs of rapidly multiplying cells.

For a look at some of the top dietary folate sources, see the Folate in Foods table on page 7 in chapter 1. You will notice that some of the best sources of folate are leafy green vegetables. In fact, the vitamin's name is derived from the word "foliage." Foods deliver folate in a bound form; because your intestine prefers folate in its free form, special enzymes located on the surface of your intestine must first break down the bound folate. The free folate is then absorbed into your bloodstream and delivered to your body's cells.

Sounds fine so far. The problem is that this complicated system of handling folate from the diet is vulnerable to injuries in the intestinal tract. If your intestinal cells are harmed, then folate is lost from the body. Alcohol abuse and chronic use of aspirin and antacids can disrupt the absorption of folate. If you use the occasional aspirin to relieve a headache you need not be concerned, but if you rely heavily on these medications you are at risk of developing a folate deficiency. The medication Azulfidine® (sulfasalazine), used to treat inflammatory bowel disease such as Crohn's disease or ulcerative colitis, also interferes with folate absorption.

Other medications that can affect folate levels in the body include oral contraceptives, barbiturates, Metformin® (for type 2 diabetes) and certain anticonvulsant drugs. If you take any of these prescription drugs, check with your pharmacist for possible nutrient interactions.

FOLIC ACID SUPPLEMENTS

Folate refers to the B vitamin in its natural form found in foods. Folic acid describes the synthetic vitamin found in vitamin supplements or fortified foods like breakfast cereal. It can be challenging to meet your daily folate requirements through diet alone. You must be sure to include in your diet at least two or three folate-rich foods from the table on page 7. A good start to making sure you are meeting your RDA is a daily multivitamin and mineral. When choosing a brand, select a product that has 0.4 to 1.0 milligrams (400–1000 micrograms) of folate. B complex supplements that provide all eight B vitamins in one pill will also give you this amount of folic acid.

If you decide to take a folic acid supplement, make sure to buy one with vitamin B12, since these two nutrients work closely together (that's why I prefer a high-potency multi or a B complex). The body uses folic acid to activate B12 and vice versa. So a deficiency of one vitamin will eventually lead to a deficiency of the other. Supplementing with folic acid and neglecting to meet your B12 requirements can hide an underlying B12 deficiency. Folic acid supplementation will correct the anemia, and a blood test will find your red blood cells normal, but the nerve symptoms of a B12 deficiency can still progress.

Folic acid is well tolerated. It is generally recommended that you do not exceed the tolerable upper limit of 1000 micrograms per day. However, if you suffer from a malabsorption problem, higher doses can be safely used (be sure to take vitamin B12, too). Doses above 15,000 micrograms are associated with nerve and intestinal damage.

Vitamin B12

Vitamin B12 and folate work very closely together in the body. Without enough B12, your body is unable to use folate, leading eventually to a folate deficiency and megaloblastic anemia (your blood test will show large, immature red blood cells). Alone, vitamin B12 maintains the protective covering of nerve fibers. Your bones also rely on this B vitamin for normal metabolism.

In addition to developing the anemia related to a folate deficiency, a lack of B12 can lead to pernicious anemia. This type of anemia is caused by impaired B12 absorption, not by poor dietary intake. After you consume B12 from your diet, the acid in your stomach helps to release the vitamin from proteins in food. The vitamin then binds to an intrinsic factor that enables B12 to be absorbed into the bloodstream.

A vitamin B12 deficiency can occur for two reasons. Some people produce an insufficient amount of hydrochloric acid in their stomach. This condition, called atrophic gastritis, is common in older adults. Without enough stomach acid, B12 can't be released from food proteins and it won't be absorbed into the blood.

Some people inherit a defective gene for intrinsic factor. They don't produce this necessary factor that attaches to B12 and transports it into the bloodstream. A B12 deficiency caused by a lack of intrinsic factor leads to pernicious anemia. This anemia is characterized by a deficit of red blood cells, muscle weakness and nerve damage. Most doctors prefer to treat pernicious anemia with injections of vitamin B12, although oral supplements may also be effective. A recent study found that taking a B12 supplement dissolved under the tongue, twice daily, was as effective as shots in restoring B12 levels.[2]

For the amount of B12 women need on a daily basis, see the RDA table on page 9 in chapter 1. This vitamin is found exclusively in animal foods. If you eat meat, poultry and dairy products on a regular basis you're probably not at risk for a B12 deficiency. See the B12 in Foods table on page 10 in chapter 1 for some of the best food sources of vitamin B12.

B12 Supplements

If you are a strict vegetarian who eats no animal products and you don't drink a fortified soy or rice beverage, I strongly recommend a B12 supplement. In fact, anyone over the age of 50 should be getting their B12 from a supplement or fortified foods. That's because the bodies of up to one-third of older adults produce inadequate amounts of stomach acid and are therefore inefficient at absorbing B12 from food.

If you take certain medications you should consider taking extra B12 in the form of a supplement. If you suffer from reflux or ulcers and take acid blockers (e.g., Tagamet®, Zantac®, Pepcid®) your body may not absorb enough B12 (as well as iron). Metformin®, used to manage type 2 diabetes and polycystic ovary syndrome, can also deplete B12 levels. If you take these medications, your doctor should monitor your blood periodically for signs of anemia.

To get your B12, I recommend a good multivitamin and mineral supplement or a B complex supplement that contains the whole family of B vitamins. If you take a single B12 supplement, take 500 to 1000 micrograms once daily. If you are taking a high-dose B12 supplement to correct a deficiency, don't take it with a vitamin C pill. Large amounts of vitamin C can destroy B12. Take your vitamin C supplement one hour after you take your B12.

The Bottom Line...
Leslie's recommendations for preventing and managing anemia

1. To prevent iron-deficiency anemia, be sure to include iron-rich foods in your daily diet.

2. To maximize the absorption of nonheme iron (the type of iron predominant in grains, legumes, vegetables and fruit), include a source of vitamin C with each meal.

3. If you are not a vegetarian, include a little meat, poultry or fish with meals rich in nonheme iron.

4. If you're a tea drinker and you rely on nonheme sources of iron to meet your needs, enjoy your tea apart from your meals.

5. To ensure you're meeting your daily iron requirement, consider taking a multivitamin and mineral supplement that contains 10 to 18 milligrams of iron. If you

are no longer menstruating, there's no need to get more than 8 milligrams of iron in your supplement since your daily needs have declined.

6. If you are iron deficient or you have anemia, take 50 to 100 milligrams of elemental iron one to three times a day or as directed by your doctor. Get your blood retested after four to eight weeks of treatment. When your iron stores are replenished, stop taking iron supplements. High doses of iron are toxic when taken for a long period of time.

7. If you are taking supplemental iron pills and you already take calcium pills each day, don't take these supplements at the same time.

8. To prevent megaloblastic anemia, ensure you meet your daily requirement for folate. The best food sources include lentils, kidney beans, black beans, cooked spinach and orange juice.

9. To help you reach your daily target of folate, choose a multivitamin and mineral pill that contains 0.4 to 1.0 milligrams of folic acid. Or, if you prefer, take a B complex supplement.

10. If you take single folic acid supplements, be sure to buy one that has vitamin B12 added. That's because folic acid supplementation can mask a B12 deficiency.

11. To prevent anemia caused by a folate deficiency, make sure you're getting your daily vitamin B12 requirements. B12 is needed to activate folate.

12. If you are a complete vegetarian (vegan) who eats no animal products, be sure to include a B12-fortified soy or rice beverage in your daily diet. Take a 500- or 1000-microgram B12 supplement.

13. If you are diagnosed with pernicious anemia, your doctor will likely prescribe monthly vitamin B12 injections. If shots aren't your thing, consider taking 1000 micrograms of sublingual B12 twice daily.

4

Chronic Fatigue Syndrome (CFS)

Relentless fatigue . . . punishing exhaustion . . . limited energy. This daunting list represents only a few of the symptoms commonly associated with the disabling disease known as Chronic Fatigue Syndrome (CFS). CFS is an enigma—a largely misunderstood illness that saps vitality and steals mental acuity. Very little is known about the causes of CFS and even less about the possible cures. We do know, however, that most cases of CFS occur in white, middle- to upper-class women.

CFS is a disease characterized by profound fatigue that is not improved with bed rest. People with CFS are easily exhausted by the slightest physical or mental activities. Because there is no cure, CFS can persist for years, dramatically altering the lives of women who suffer from it.

What Causes CFS?

Chronic fatigue syndrome is a complicated disorder defined by symptoms of severe, debilitating fatigue. Over the years, doctors have diagnosed chronic tiredness under a variety of different names, including nervous exhaustion, Yuppie flu, Epstein-Barr virus disease or myalgic encephalomyelitis. In 1988, a committee of experts studying the illness selected a new name, Chronic Fatigue Syndrome, to represent the most noticeable and consistent symptom of the disease.[1] Since then, CFS has become an important social and public health issue and is currently the focus of intense research.

There doesn't seem to be one single cause for CFS. Instead, research indicates that there could be a number of different factors, working alone or in combination, which might cause CFS. Initially, CFS was thought to be produced by a virus infection. Scientific attention was focused on the Epstein-Barr virus, herpes-type viruses and infections that cause polio. But extensive studies were unable to establish a direct connection between CFS and these or any other infectious agents. Despite this, scientists still speculate that a virus may help trigger the disease.

There is little argument among experts that a disturbed immune system plays an important role in CFS. Scientists believe that CFS is caused when an infection or virus attacks someone with a weakened immune system. Once the infection has passed, the immune system doesn't return to its normal state. Instead, it remains active, continuously producing excess immune-activating factors. As these factors circulate through the bloodstream, they may cause profound fatigue. Studies find that many people with CFS have chronically overactive immune systems. Many people with CFS are shown to have white blood cells that are less able to fight off viruses.

Often people with CFS have a history of allergies, which, for some unknown reason, seems to predispose them to the disease. But scientists realize that allergy isn't the only source of the problem, because some CFS sufferers have no allergy symptoms at all. There is also the possibility that a severe metabolic dysfunction may be the culprit behind the debilitating symptoms of CFS. Many CFS sufferers show evidence of extreme shifts in metabolism that limit heart and lung functions, making it difficult and even physically damaging to carry out normal activities. Research has also linked brain abnormalities with CFS, especially those associated with sleep-related disorders.

In the hunt for the origins of CFS, research is beginning to assign an important role to the central nervous system. Certain malfunctions of the nervous system can produce racing heartbeats or sudden drops in blood pressure. These conditions seem to be associated with the development of CFS in ways that are not yet fully understood. Periods of physical or emotional stress also have an impact on the nervous system. Stressful events stimulate the brain to produce cortisol and other stress hormones. These hormones affect the immune system by suppressing inflammation. Because stress may be a trigger for the development of CFS, it's possible that there is a connection between the disease and the altered levels of stress hormones.

Most recently, developments in CFS research have led to the exciting discovery of a new human enzyme. This abnormal enzyme may affect the body's ability to control common viruses and maintain energy in body cells. Early studies indicate that the enzyme is present in most people with CFS and may be the cause of the low energy levels.

❧

Symptoms

The most obvious symptom of CFS is extreme fatigue that interferes with your ability to carry out daily activities. This level of fatigue goes far beyond the exhausted, over-tired feelings that we all get from time to time. The fatigue that characterizes CFS is relentless and does not go away for weeks, months or years at a time, despite your best efforts to get adequate rest and relaxation.

CFS sufferers may also have a variety of other symptoms. Muscle weakness, sleep disturbances, lightheadedness, fainting and dizziness are all common problems associated with the disease. CFS may also cause impaired thinking, forgetfulness, confusion, difficulty concentrating, depression and anxiety. Because the disease involves a faulty immune system, it's common for people with CFS to experience food allergies, other fungal infections (e.g., yeast infections) and frequent bouts of the common cold. (If you suffer recurrent vaginal yeast infections, I discuss their management in chapter 15, "Pregnancy.")

CFS symptoms and their duration vary widely from individual to individual. Approximately 50 percent of people with CFS return to a fairly normal lifestyle within five years. The other half will still be dramatically ill even after ten years. Some people recover from the disease in two to three years, only to suffer a relapse at a later time. CFS can be cyclical, producing alternating periods of illness and relatively good health.

❧

Who's at Risk?

In the United States, estimates indicate that there may be as many as half a million people suffering from some form of CFS. Studies from the early 1980s revealed that it was mainly well-educated, affluent Caucasian women, between the ages of 25 and 45 years, who suffered from CFS. However, recent studies have brought an end to that modern stereotype. As a growing number of doctors recognize CFS as a legitimate disorder, newly gathered data shows that the illness can occur in all income, racial and age groups.[2] Women still seem to report the condition two to four times more often than men, possibly because women are more willing to seek medical treatment for fatigue.[3]

✌

Diagnosis

Fatigue is a primary symptom of many health conditions. In 95 percent of cases, fatigue is caused by a medical or psychiatric illness that can be diagnosed and treated. Before you can be diagnosed with CFS, your doctor will attempt to rule out diseases such as fibromyalgia, mononucleosis, hypothyroidism, cancer, depression and hormonal dysfunction, as well as related disorders.

At this time there is no specific diagnostic test for CFS. To determine whether you have the disease, a thorough evaluation of your health will be necessary. This will include an examination of your medical history, a physical examination and a review of your mental status. Because CFS is diagnosed through a process of elimination, your doctor will order a series of laboratory and x-ray screening tests to rule out other possible causes of your chronic fatigue. Once these other medical conditions have been eliminated, your doctor will consider CFS if you meet the following criteria:

1. Unexplained, persistent or relapsing fatigue that lasts for at least six months; fatigue that is not the result of ongoing exertion; fatigue that is not alleviated by rest and is debilitating enough to restrict previous levels of activity.

2. The presence of at least four of the following symptoms:

   - substantial impairment of short-term memory or concentration

   - sore throat

   - tender lymph nodes

   - muscle pain

- multi-joint pain without swelling or redness
- headaches of a new type, pattern or severity
- unrefreshing sleep
- post-exertion fatigue that lasts more than 24 hours

༉

Conventional Treatment

Medications prescribed for CFS are intended to provide relief of symptoms. They are not considered to cure the disease. Today doctors use a combination of therapies and a gradual approach to rehabilitation in treating this disease.

Low-dose *tricyclic antidepressants* seem to have a positive effect on some people with CFS, possibly because they improve the quality of sleep. Another form of antidepressant, known as *SSRIs* (serotonin reuptake inhibitors), has also provided treatment benefits. In some cases, *benzodiazepines,* a type of drug used to treat anxiety and sleep problems, will improve the quality of life for CFS sufferers. *NSAIDs* (nonsteroidal anti-inflammatory drugs) will help fight the aches and pains, and *antihistamines* may relieve the allergy symptoms associated with the condition. You will probably need to try more than one type of drug before you find the right combination for you.

Learning to manage your fatigue will help improve your ability to function, despite your symptoms. Through behavior therapy you might find effective ways to plan your activities, so that you can take advantage of your peak energy levels. Exercise is also important in the management of CFS. Although exercise may seem to aggravate your symptoms, it is essential that you continue to maintain some muscle strength and conditioning. A moderate exercise program that takes into account your personal tolerance levels will help you keep your illness from robbing you of your physical strength and endurance. Throughout the course of this disease, you must learn to pace yourself physically, emotionally and mentally, because extra stress will inevitably make your symptoms much worse.

Managing CFS

If you have CFS, nutrition plays an important role in your recovery to good health. As you'll read below, scientists have found that a number of vitamins and minerals are deficient in many people with CFS. This seems to be mostly due to the illness itself, rather than a poor diet. Even marginal nutrient deficiencies can contribute to your fatigue symptoms, and the lack of important nutrients can also delay your healing process.

DIETARY STRATEGIES

The *quality* of the foods you eat seems to be most important in helping to restore your energy levels. In a nutshell, follow a wholesome, healthy diet:

1. *Emphasize plant foods* in your daily diet. Fill your plate with grains, fruits and vegetables. If you eat animal-protein foods like meat or poultry, they should take up no more than one-quarter of your plate. Try vegetarian sources of protein like beans and soy more often.

2. *Choose foods and oils that are rich in essential fatty acids.* Fish, nuts, seeds, flax and flax oil, canola oil, Omega-3 eggs, wheat germ and leafy green vegetables are examples.

3. *Make food choices that are rich in vitamins, minerals and protective plant compounds.* Choose whole grains as often as possible. Eat at least three different-colored fruits and three different-colored vegetables every day.

4. *Eliminate sources of refined sugar* as often as possible: cookies, cakes, pastries, frozen desserts, soft drinks, sweetened fruit juices, fruit drinks, candy, etc.

5. *Buy organic produce* or *wash fruits and vegetables* to remove pesticide residues.

6. *Limit foods with chemical additives.*

7. *Avoid caffeine,* which can worsen fatigue by interrupting sleep patterns.

8. *Drink at least 9 cups of water every day.*

9. *Avoid alcohol.* If you drink, consume no more than one drink a day, or seven per week.

10. *Take a multivitamin and mineral supplement each day* to ensure you are meeting your needs for most nutrients. Buy a product that contains no artificial preservatives, colors and flavors, or added sugar, starch, lactose or yeast. This should be declared in small print below the ingredient list. If you experience gastrointestinal upset when taking a multivitamin, try a "professional brand" supplement available at certain health food stores. These products contain no binding materials and they are suitable for people with food sensitivities; however, they're expensive and you have to take three to six capsules a day to meet your recommended intake levels. Brand names include Genestra® and Thorne Research®.

To help you follow these principles, follow my dietary guidelines in chapter 1. You'll learn what foods you should be eating more often. You'll also learn how many servings of these foods you should be striving for each day.

If you experience bloating, cramps, gas, diarrhea or skin rashes after eating, it's a good idea to be tested for food allergies. Ask your family doctor for referral to an allergy specialist.

Because no single cause has been identified for CFS, there is no single diet or supplement program that can be said to cure the condition. However, there is research to suggest that the vitamins, minerals and herbs I discuss below can improve CFS symptoms. Since these supplements are all considered safe in the amounts indicated, it makes sense to try one or more of these for a trial period. You should always make an effort to boost your intake of these nutrients through your food choices, too.

VITAMINS AND MINERALS

B Vitamins

Without B vitamins our bodies would lack energy. These eight nutrients are indispensable for yielding energy compounds from the foods we eat. Many B vitamins serve as helpers to enzymes that release energy from fat, protein and carbohydrates. Compared to healthy people, patients with CFS often have lower levels of B vitamins in their blood. One study also found that enzymes dependent on B vitamins were less active in people with CFS. I could not find any published studies that tried to determine if taking vitamin B supplements could improve fatigue symptoms. For information on the family of B vitamins—how much you need and where to look for it—see the table on page 4 in chapter 1.

To ensure you are getting your fair share of B vitamins, take a good quality multi-vitamin and mineral supplement each day. If you're over 50, you should be getting your B12 from a supplement anyway. That's because as we age we become less efficient at producing stomach acid, a necessary aid for B12 absorption from food.

If you're looking for more B vitamins than a regular multi gives you, choose a "high potency" or "super" formula that contains 30 to 75 milligrams of B vitamins (or micrograms in the case of folic acid). You can also take a B complex formula that gives you all eight B vitamins, often combined with vitamin C. If you supplement with these products, you should know that niacin might cause flushing of the face and chest when it's taken in doses greater than 35 milligrams (this is easily avoided if you take your supplement just after eating a meal). This symptom is harmless and goes away within 20 minutes, but some people find it uncomfortable. To avoid flushing, look for a formula that contains *niacinamide* instead of niacin. Niacinamide is a non-flushing form of niacin.

Magnesium

More than 300 enzymes rely on a steady supply of magnesium for optimal activity. Magnesium is part of adenosine triphosphate (ATP), the active energy compound that's used by every cell in your body. It's believed that a deficiency in magnesium can lead to the decreased energy and weakness seen in CFS. Some investigations have found low levels of magnesium in the red blood cells of patients with CFS. When these patients are regularly given magnesium by injection, they report more energy, less pain and more balanced emotions. Other studies have found evidence of a magnesium deficiency in people afflicted with CFS.

Although there is no concrete evidence to support the use of extra magnesium in CFS, there is no harm done by increasing your intake of this mineral. In fact, research suggests that only 25 percent of the population is meeting their daily magnesium needs. I am sure we could all use a magnesium boost in our daily diet. To see what you should be striving for each day, see the RDA table on page 21 in chapter 1. Also see the Magnesium in Foods chart on page 21 for the foods that will help you meet these daily targets.

MAGNESIUM SUPPLEMENTS

There is no definite dose of magnesium for the treatment of CFS. Doses of 200 to 300 milligrams have been used to reduce the muscle pain and joint tenderness associated with fibromyalgia. If you want to take a supplement, buy magnesium citrate.

Compared to other forms of the mineral (e.g., magnesium oxide), magnesium citrates are more easily absorbed by your body. You can also get supplemental magnesium from your calcium pills if you buy one that has magnesium added.

The daily upper limit for magnesium has been set at 350 milligrams from a supplement. That's because doses higher than this can cause diarrhea and stomach upset, common side effects of magnesium supplementation.

HERBAL REMEDIES

The following herbs have been shown to boost the body's production of infection-fighting immune compounds. Of the three I discuss, Echinacea and Panax ginseng have been shown to enhance the activity of immune cells in people with CFS. Echinacea can be beneficial to help treat bothersome colds, while ginseng and aged garlic extract can be used longer term for immune stimulation.

Echinacea

If you suffer from frequent colds, studies have found that this herb can reduce the duration of your symptoms by as much as 50 percent. Echinacea's active ingredients enhance the body's immune system by increasing production of certain white blood cells that fight off viruses and bacteria.

Three species of Echinacea are found in products—Echinacea pupurea, Echinacea angustifolia and Echinacea pallida—and all have medicinal benefits. Buy a product that's standardized to contain 4 percent echinacosides (Echinacea angustifolia) and 0.7 percent flavonoids (Echinacea pupurea), two of the herb's active ingredients. Unless you're allergic to plants in the Asteracease/Compositae family (ragweed, daisy, marigold and chrysanthemum), take Echinacea at the first sign of cold or flu symptoms. Take 900 milligrams of Echinacea, three to four times daily. Limit daily use to eight consecutive weeks due to concern that long-term use of Echinacea might depress the immune system.

Panax Ginseng

This ginseng goes by many names, including Asian, Korean and Chinese. Studies have shown the herb to have strong immune-enhancing properties. A large Italian study found that individuals taking 100 milligrams of a standardized ginseng product (G115 extract) had significantly higher levels of antibodies in response to a flu shot compared to those who did not take the herb.[4] Killer white blood cells were nearly twice as high in the ginseng group after eight weeks of supplementation. These and other white blood cells are an important part of the body's defense against viruses and foreign molecules.

The benefits of Panax ginseng on the immune system can be attributed to active compounds in the root called ginsenosides. Many ginsenosides have been identified, but ginsenosides Rg1 and Rb1 have received the most attention. Scientific research has focused on ginseng extracts standardized to contain 4 to 7 percent ginsenosides.

If you're going to add ginseng to your remedy list, buy a product with a statement of standardization or with G115 on the label. Ginsana® from Pharmaton® Natural Health Products contains the G115 extract that's been used in clinical studies. The typical dosage of a standardized extract is 100 or 200 milligrams once daily. Take ginseng for three weeks to three months, and then follow with a one- to two-week rest period before you resume taking the herb.

Ginseng is relatively safe at the 100 or 200 milligram dosage. In some people, it may cause mild stomach upset, irritability and insomnia. To avoid overstimulation, start with 100 milligrams a day, and avoid taking the herb with caffeine. Ginseng should not be used during pregnancy or breastfeeding, or in individuals with uncontrolled high blood pressure.

Siberian Ginseng

Unlike Panax ginseng, this herb has a much milder effect and fewer reported side effects. Pregnant and nursing women can safely take Siberian ginseng, and it is much less likely to cause overstimulation in sensitive individuals. To ensure quality, choose a product standardized for eleutherosides B and E. The usual dosage is 300 to 400 milligrams once daily for six to eight weeks, followed by a one- to two-week break.

Garlic

You may want to add fresh garlic to your meals more often. A daily intake of garlic and its accompanying sulfur compounds has been used to enhance the body's immune system and kill many types of bacteria and fungi (including the Candida organism that causes yeast infections). One-half to one clove a day is recommended.

When it comes to garlic pills, buy *aged* garlic extract. The aging process used to make this supplement increases the concentration of the special sulfur compounds that stimulate the immune system. In fact, animal studies have found that the amount of garlic equivalent to three aged garlic extract capsules dramatically increases activity of white blood cells (killer cells, macrophages and leukocytes). Generally, two to six capsules a day (one or two with meals) are recommended. You can also take aged garlic in a liquid form (Kyolic® brand) that you add to foods.

OTHER NATURAL HEALTH PRODUCTS

Essential Fatty Acids

The fat in foods or in body fat is made up of individual building blocks called fatty acids. The body can make all but two fatty acids: *linoleic acid* and *alpha-linolenic acid (ALA)*. Because these two fatty acids are essential to our health and well-being, they must be supplied by the diet. Linoleic acid is considered an omega-6 fatty acid, and is found in leafy vegetables, seeds, nuts, grains and vegetable oils made from corn, safflower, sunflower, soybean and sesame. Alpha-linolenic acid belongs to the omega-3 family of fats; good food sources include canola oil, flaxseed and flaxseed oil, walnuts and walnut oil, wheat germ and soybeans.

When we consume these fatty acids, the body uses them to make other fatty acids—GLA, DHA and EPA are a few important ones. These fatty acids are needed to maintain the structure of cell membranes and make hormonelike compounds called prostaglandins. Prostaglandins, in turn, help regulate blood pressure, blood clot formation and our immune response to infection.

It's thought that people with CFS don't metabolize essential fatty acids properly, and this leads to a faulty immune system. One of the body's natural anti-virus agents, called interferon, requires essential fatty acids in order to exert its virus-fighting effect. Some studies have determined that many CFS sufferers have lowered levels of essential fats in their body.

Based on this evidence, it certainly makes sense to include sources of these very important nutrients in your diet. Perhaps you have cut all types of fat from your diet, thinking this is healthy, only to deprive your body of essential fats. Your daily diet should include at least 4 teaspoons of fats or oils rich in essential fatty acids. I recommend that you emphasize sources of alpha-linolenic acid, since this particular fatty acid is emerging as a very healthy part of the diet.

Should you take a supplement of essential fatty acids? There certainly are plenty available in the health food store. Capsules of evening primrose oil (containing GLA), fish oil (containing DHA and EPA) and flaxseed oil (containing ALA) are all examples. Well, it turns out there is some evidence to support their use. In one study from

Scotland, 63 adults with CFS were given either fish oil (eight 500-milligram capsules per day) or placebo capsules for three months. When the study was over, 85 percent of those given fish oil had a significant improvement in their symptoms.[5] As would be expected, there was also an increase in cellular levels of essential fatty acids. I should point out that researchers from the United Kingdom tried to replicate these results and could not. Their study, conducted among 50 patients with CFS, found no difference in symptoms between the fish-oil group and the placebo group.

Despite these mixed findings, you may still want to give these supplements a try. If so, buy a product that offers a combination of EPA and DHA. A good quality fish-oil supplement should also contain vitamin E. This nutrient is added to help stabilize the oils. Avoid fish *liver* oil capsules. Supplements made from fish livers are a concentrated source of vitamins A and D. Too much vitamin A and D can be toxic when taken in large amounts for long periods of time.

Fish oil has a blood-thinning effect; if you take other medication that thins the blood, be sure to check with your physician first. Follow your healthcare practitioner's advice for dosage.

L-Carnitine

This compound is not considered an essential nutrient because the body makes it in sufficient quantities. Carnitine helps all cells in the body generate energy, especially muscle cells. It's possible that a deficiency of this compound can cause the fatigue associated with CFS. Studies have shown that CFS patients tend to have lower levels of carnitine in their blood, and higher levels are linked with less severe symptoms.

Researchers from Chicago took the carnitine-and-CFS hypothesis one step further. They gave 30 people with CFS either carnitine or a drug treatment for two months. After a two-week rest period, the treatments were switched; those who originally got the drug were given carnitine, and vice versa. The researchers found a significant improvement in those taking the carnitine supplements after eight weeks.[6] The greatest improvement took place between one and two months.

L-carnitine is found in meat and dairy products. As a general dietary supplement, the recommended dose is 1 to 3 grams per day. The supplement is considered safe. Occasional side effects of gastrointestinal upset have been reported. Avoid products that contain D-carnitine or DL-carnitine—these forms compete with L-carnitine in the body and could lead to a deficiency.

THE BOTTOM LINE...

Leslie's recommendations for managing CFS

1. First and foremost, implement the healthiest diet possible.

2. If your intestinal tract or skin reacts to certain foods, make an appointment with a specialist to have food-allergy tests performed. Often food sensitivities are the result of a weakened immune system.

3. To ensure you are meeting your daily targets for essential nutrients, especially the B vitamins, take a multivitamin and mineral supplement each day. If you are sensitive to many foods, buy a "professional brand" that contains no binding ingredients.

4. In addition to eating wholesome, nutrient-dense foods, some evidence suggests that taking certain natural health products might ease the symptoms of CFS. Consider adding the following to your daily regime:
   - B complex vitamin formula
   - Magnesium citrate, 200 to 300 milligrams
   - Essential fatty acids (fish or flax oil), 5 to 8 capsules
   - L-carnitine, 1 to 3 grams

5. To stimulate your body's immune system, consider adding the following herbal remedies to your daily plan:
   - Panax ginseng (G115 extract), 100 to 200 milligrams
   - Aged garlic extract, 2 to 6 capsules

6. If you suffer from frequent bouts of the common cold, try a standardized extract of Echinacea at first sign of infection. Take 900 milligrams of Echinacea three to four times daily until your cold disappears. Avoid using this herb if you are allergic to members of the Asteracease/Compositae plant family (ragweed, daisy, marigold and chrysanthemum).

5

Hypoglycemia

Hypoglycemia develops when the glucose (sugar) levels in your blood fall below normal. Low glucose or blood sugar can cause many body organs to malfunction. The brain is the most susceptible because glucose is its main energy source.

People with diabetes often develop hypoglycemia because of an imbalance between their medication and their diet or exercise levels. But hypoglycemia can also occur in people who don't have diabetes. A low blood-sugar level can be caused by a variety of other factors, including stress, poor diet, alcohol consumption and certain medical conditions.

Consuming sugar in any form, be it fruit juice or hard candy, can quickly relieve the hypoglycemic symptoms of headache, dizziness, weakness, confusion and shakiness. In most cases, following the right diet can prevent hypoglycemia altogether.

❦

What Causes Hypoglycemia?

Your body relies on a form of sugar known as glucose as its main source of fuel for daily activities. During the process of digestion, the carbohydrates (sugars and starches) that you eat are converted into glucose. Glucose is often referred to as blood sugar because it is absorbed by your bloodstream and carried to every cell in your body. Unused glucose is stored in your muscles and liver as glycogen. Your body draws on these sugar stores for energy when your blood sugar drops.

Whenever you eat food, the breakdown of carbohydrates into glucose causes your blood-sugar level to rise. This triggers your pancreas, an organ located in your upper abdomen, to release a hormone called insulin. Insulin helps glucose enter body cells, where it supplies the energy to fuel most bodily functions. As glucose is absorbed into the cells, your blood-sugar level gradually drops back to a normal range.

A few hours later, when most of the available glucose supply is consumed, your blood-sugar levels start to fall below normal, indicating that your body needs more fuel. Your pancreas responds to the falling glucose levels by releasing a different hormone, called glucagon. Glucagon stimulates your liver to release its stored supply of glucose into the bloodstream, where it is circulated to the cells. Once again, your blood-sugar levels rise back to normal.

Every day your body performs this delicate balancing act over and over. By relying on insulin, glucagon and several other hormones, your body is able to keep your blood-glucose levels under constant control and regulate your daily energy supply.

Hypoglycemia occurs when your blood-glucose levels drop too low, and you no longer have enough energy to fuel your daily activities. Hypoglycemia develops most often as a complication of diabetes. Diabetes occurs when your body can't use glucose as fuel because your pancreas produces insufficient amounts of insulin, or because your cells are resistant to the action of insulin. Many people with diabetes have to take insulin or other drugs to keep their blood-sugar level in the normal range. When people with diabetes eat too little food, exercise too strenuously, drink too much alcohol or take too much medication, they are at risk of developing hypoglycemia. Because so many people with diabetes depend on medication to lower their blood sugar, they may experience episodes of hypoglycemia throughout their lifetime.

You can still have hypoglycemia if you don't have diabetes. If you develop low blood-sugar symptoms after eating a meal, you may have what's called *reactive* hypoglycemia. This type of low blood-sugar reaction occurs when your pancreas releases too much insulin at once, causing your blood-sugar level to fall below normal. Symptoms usually develop within two to five hours after eating a meal. If you are prone to reactive hypoglycemia, eating too many starchy or sweet foods can aggravate the condition. That's because large portions of carbohydrate-rich foods cause your blood sugar to rise very rapidly, triggering excessive insulin production and a dramatic drop in your glucose levels. This roller coaster sequence of events will upset your natural hormonal balance and leave you feeling sweaty, anxious, hungry and shaky.

Other possible causes of hypoglycemia include

- stress and anxiety
- an unbalanced diet that is high in refined grains and/or sugars
- drinking alcohol
- early pregnancy
- prolonged fasting
- long periods of strenuous exercise
- exercising while you are on beta blocker medication (e.g., propranolol)
- certain medications, especially pentamidine (used to treat AIDS-related pneumonia)
- liver disease
- gastric surgery that disrupts the balance between digestion and insulin release
- hereditary intolerance of foods that contain the natural sugars fructose and galactose (rare childhood conditions)

While there are many conditions that may cause hypoglycemia, it is important to remember that only 1 percent of hypoglycemia cases occur in people who do not have diabetes. Studies indicate that it is actually quite a rare disorder.

Symptoms

When your blood-sugar level falls, your body responds by releasing a hormone called epinephrine (adrenaline) from your adrenal glands. This hormone stimulates your liver to release its stored glucose into your bloodstream. But this adrenaline rush also produces the unpleasant symptoms that are characteristic of hypoglycemia, which include sweating, nervousness, rapid heartbeat, anxiety, hunger, faintness and trembling.

If your blood-sugar level continues to fall, the reduced glucose supply will begin to affect your brain. When hypoglycemia interferes with brain activities, you may experience headache, dizziness, rapid heartbeat, sweating, confusion, blurred vision, difficulty concentrating, anxiety, agitation, weakness or fainting and abnormal behavior that could be mistaken for drunkenness. If your condition continues to worsen, convulsions, loss of consciousness and coma may result. Keep in mind that such life-threatening symptoms are usually caused by too much medication in people with diabetes.

Symptoms of hypoglycemia vary in severity among individuals and may progress from mild to severe in a short period of time.

❧

Who's at Risk?

Hypoglycemia is most common among people who have diabetes and take blood-sugar lowering medication. Other factors that can predispose you to hypoglycemia include fasting, following a low-calorie diet, being pregnant, having certain medical disorders and taking certain medications.

For some people, hypoglycemia develops when they drink alcohol after a long period without eating food. As their blood-glucose levels fall, they develop a hypoglycemia-induced stupor, which makes them appear drunk and confused. This type of stupor can develop even when blood-alcohol levels are well below the legal driving limit.

❧

Diagnosis

If you have symptoms of hypoglycemia and you do not have diabetes, your doctor may conduct some simple blood tests to measure your blood-sugar and insulin levels. Ideally, this test will be done while you are experiencing an episode of hypoglycemic symptoms. The diagnosis of hypoglycemia will be confirmed if the blood test indicates that your blood-sugar levels are below normal and your symptoms improve when you consume sugar.

Your doctor will also take your medical history and conduct a physical examination, and may test you for diabetes. Depending on the cause of your hypoglycemia, additional laboratory tests may be required.

For years doctors used the oral glucose tolerance test to diagnose hypoglycemia. However, its use has fallen out of favor because it can produce misleading results. It is now recognized that the signs and symptoms of hypoglycemia can occur in individuals who have blood-glucose levels within the normal range. And 10 percent of people who don't have any symptoms of hypoglycemia show low blood-sugar levels when they take the oral glucose tolerance test. So relying on blood-sugar levels alone is often not enough to diagnose hypoglycemia.

One of the most useful ways to determine if you suffer from hypoglycemia is to assess your symptoms. In general, when symptoms appear three to four hours after eating and disappear after you've consumed food, hypoglycemia is a likely cause. The following questionnaire is a useful tool to help you determine if you are suffering from hypoglycemia.

Hypoglycemia Questionnaire

SYMPTOM	NO	MILD	MODERATE	SEVERE
Crave sweets	0	1	2	3
Irritable if meal is missed	0	1	2	3
Feel tired or weak if meal is missed	0	1	2	3
Dizziness if you stand suddenly	0	1	2	3
Frequent headaches	0	1	2	3
Poor memory or concentration	0	1	2	3
Feel tired an hour or so after eating	0	1	2	3
Heart palpitations	0	1	2	3
Feel shaky at times	0	1	2	3
Afternoon fatigue	0	1	2	3
Vision blurs on occasion	0	1	2	3
Depression or mood swings	0	1	2	3
Overweight	0	1	2	3

Often anxious or nervous	0	1	2	3
Total Score				

SCORING

<5	hypoglycemia is not a likely factor
6–15	hypoglycemia is a likely factor
>15	hypoglycemia is extremely likely

Murray, M. and J.E. Pizzano, Hypoglycemia. Textbook of Natural Medicine Volume 2, *Edinburgh: Churchill Livingstone, 1999.*

Conventional Treatment

In most cases, the symptoms of hypoglycemia will quickly improve when you consume sugar in any form. Eating candy, sugar cubes, glucose or dextrose tablets or drinking a glass of fruit juice, milk or sugar water will immediately raise your blood-sugar levels, making you feel much better. If you do experience a low blood-sugar reaction, treat it immediately by consuming 10 to 15 grams of carbohydrates such as 5 Life Savers, a half banana, or 1/2 to 3/4 cup (125 – 175 ml) fruit juice.

If you have diabetes or you are prone to recurring episodes of hypoglycemia, you should always carry some candy or other type of sugar. Glucose tablets are widely available in drugstores in the diet section. They are handy to have in the event of a low blood-sugar reaction when you are away from home and don't have access to food; three tablets give you 10–15 grams of carbohydrates. In severe cases of hypoglycemia, an injection of glucagon or intravenous glucose may be necessary to restore blood-sugar levels.

Hypoglycemia that develops after gastrointestinal surgery can often be managed by eating small, frequent meals and following a high-protein, low-carbohydrate diet. A hereditary intolerance of fructose (fruit sugar) or galactose (milk sugar) is treated by eliminating the foods that cause hypoglycemic symptoms.

~

Managing Hypoglycemia

This section focuses on nutritional strategies that will help you maintain a consistent blood-sugar level, and so be less vulnerable to hypoglycemia. While some of my recommendations are helpful for women with diabetes, for the most part they are intended for women who have hypoglycemia that is not related to medication that lowers blood sugar.

Over the years, I have had many clients seek my help for managing their hypoglycemia. They have learned that following the proper diet is key to preventing hypoglycemia. Instead of relying on fast-acting carbohydrates to treat a low blood-sugar reaction, use the strategies below to prevent a sugar low from occurring in the first place.

DIETARY STRATEGIES

Meal Timing

One of the first and most important ways to prevent a low blood-sugar reaction is to eat regularly throughout the day. After eating a meal, your blood sugar will peak in 45 to 90 minutes. After this point, your sugar level starts its decline. If you suffer from hypoglycemia, you should *eat every three hours*. That means eating *three meals and three snacks*. Here's what a meal and snack schedule might look like if you work during the day from nine o'clock to five o'clock (note that time spans are to show approximate time of meal or snack, not duration):

Breakfast:	7:30–8:00 a.m.
Snack:	10:00–10:30 a.m.
Lunch:	12:00–1:00 p.m.
Snack:	3:00–4:00 p.m.
Dinner:	6:00–7:00 p.m.
Snack:	8:00–9:00 p.m.

Eating at regular intervals sounds simple, yet many people don't make this a priority—they're too busy running from meeting to meeting, working through their lunch hour or racing out the door to pick up children. I can't tell you how often I hear people complain that they don't even have time to eat breakfast before they rush off to work.

Once you get into a consistent pattern of eating, you will feel much better. And if you choose the right foods at your meals and snacks, chances are you'll forget you're vulnerable to hypoglycemic reactions. So now that you have your eating schedule down pat, the next step is choosing foods with longer-lasting energy. Keep reading!

The Glycemic Index

You are already familiar with the fact that carbohydrate-containing foods (e.g., starches, fruits, milk, sugars) eventually wind up as glucose in your bloodstream. So it makes sense that you can prevent hypoglycemia by eating carbohydrates. But not all carbohydrates behave the same way when it comes to raising your blood sugar. Some carbohydrate-rich foods are digested and absorbed into your bloodstream quickly while others are broken down and converted to blood glucose slowly.

Why does this make a difference if you have hypoglycemia? Let's say you eat two slices of white toast for breakfast. White bread (and whole-wheat bread) is digested relatively quickly, causing your blood sugar to rise quickly. This rapid rise in blood glucose triggers your pancreas to release an excessive amount of insulin, causing your blood-glucose level to drop to a very low level. On the other hand, a bowl of high-fiber breakfast cereal with low-fat milk is digested and absorbed more slowly, causing a gradual rise in blood sugar. Because this meal does not result in a fast blood-sugar response, you don't get a surge of insulin. As a result, your blood-sugar level won't plummet. Instead you will experience a smooth, steady blood-sugar level leading to more consistent energy levels.

The rate at which a food causes your blood sugar to rise can be measured and assigned a value. This measure is referred to as the food's glycemic index value. The glycemic index (GI) is a ranking from 0 to 100. The number tells you whether a food raises your blood glucose rapidly, moderately or slowly. Foods that are digested quickly and cause your blood sugar to rise rapidly have high glycemic index values. Foods that are digested slowly, leading to a gradual rise in blood sugar, are assigned low glycemic index values. All foods are compared to pure glucose, which is given a value of 100 (fast acting).

Now let's use the glycemic index to manage your hypoglycemia. The key is to choose carbohydrate foods that do *not* cause large increases in blood sugar.

- Choose low GI foods at your meals and snacks.
- Avoid eating high GI foods as snacks, as they can trigger low blood sugar.
- Combining a high GI food with a low GI food will result in a meal with a medium GI value.

Here's a list of foods ranked by their GI value. To use this table to plan your meals, use the following scale: <55 = low GI; 55 −70 = medium GI; >70 = high GI.

FOOD	GI VALUE
Bread and Crackers	
Baguette, French	95
Kaiser roll	73
Melba toast	70
Pita bread, whole-wheat	57
Pumpernickel, whole-grain	51
Rice cakes	82
Rye bread	65
Soda crackers	74
Sourdough bread	52
Stoned Wheat Thins	67
White bread	70
Whole-wheat bread	69
Breakfast Cereals	
All-Bran, Kellogg's	51
All-Bran Buds with Psyllium, Kellogg's	45
Bran flakes	74
Corn Bran, Quaker	75

Corn flakes	84
Oat bran	50
Oatmeal	49
Raisin bran	73
Shredded Wheat, spoon size	58
Special K	54

Cookies, Cakes and Muffins

Angel food cake	67
Arrowroot	69
Banana bread	47
Blueberry muffin	59
Oat bran muffin	60
Graham crackers	74
Oatmeal cookies	55
Social Tea biscuits	55
Sponge cake	46

Pasta, Grains and Potato

Barley	25
Bulgur	48
Corn, sweet	55
Couscous	65
Fettuccine, egg	32
Potato, french fries	75
Potato, new, unpeeled, boiled	62
Potato, instant, mashed	86
Potato, red-skinned, mashed	91
Potato, red-skinned, boiled	88
Potato, white-skinned, baked	85
Rice, basmati	58

Rice, brown	55
Rice, converted, Uncle Ben's	44
Rice, instant	87
Rice, long grain, white	56
Rice, short grain	72
Spaghetti, whole-wheat	37
Spaghetti, white	41
Sweet potato, mashed	54
Legumes	
Baked beans	48
Black beans	31
Black bean soup	64
Chickpeas, canned	42
Kidney beans	27
Lentils	30
Lentil soup, canned	34
Split pea soup	66
Soy beans	18
Fruit	
Apple	38
Apricot, dried	31
Banana	55
Cantaloupe	65
Cherries	22
Dates, dried	103
Grapefruit	25
Grapes	46
Mango	55
Orange	44

Peach, canned	30
Pear	38
Raisins	64
Watermelon	72
Dairy Products and Alternatives	
Milk, skim	32
Milk, whole	27
Milk, chocolate	34
Ice cream, low-fat	50
Soy beverage	31
Yogurt, flavored, low-fat	33
Snack Foods	
Corn chips	72
Peanuts	14
Popcorn	55
Potato chips	54
Pretzels	83
Sports bar, PowerBar®, chocolate	58
Sugars	
Fructose (fruit sugar)	23
Glucose	100
Honey	58
Lactose (milk sugar)	46
Sucrose (table sugar)	65

Foster-Powell, K. and J. Brand Miller, "International tables of glycemic index," American Journal of Clinical Nutrition *1995;62:871S-93S.*

Soluble Fiber

Many of the foods with a low glycemic index value tend to be higher in a special kind of fiber, called soluble fiber. Dried peas, beans and lentils, oats, barley, psyllium husks, apples and citrus fruits are all good sources of soluble fiber and, as you can see from the GI table, these foods also have a low GI. When you eat these foods, the soluble fiber forms a gel in your stomach and slows the rate of digestion and absorption. That means your blood sugar will rise at a slower rate and your pancreas won't produce excessive amounts of insulin.

If you don't feel like using the GI table to choose foods, you might just plan your meals around foods rich in soluble fiber:

Cereals	Kellogg's All-Bran Buds, oatmeal, oat bran
Grains	barley
Legumes	all (baked beans, bean soups, black beans, chickpeas, kidney beans, lentils, soybeans, etc.)
Fruit	apples, cantaloupe, grapefruit, oranges, pears, strawberries
Vegetables	carrots, green peas, sweet potato

Protein Foods

Choosing foods based on their soluble-fiber content is a great way to lower the glycemic index value of your meal. But there are a couple of other tricks that slow down digestion and influence the rate at which your blood sugar rises. Adding a little protein to your meals slows the rate at which your stomach empties its contents into the small intestine. As a result, the carbohydrate in your meal will enter your bloodstream at a slower rate.

Choose lean protein foods such as lean beef, chicken breast, turkey, pork tenderloin, center-cut pork chops, fish, seafood and eggs. If you are a vegetarian, be sure to include vegetarian protein foods at your meals—tofu, beans, veggie ground round, tempeh, etc.

You don't need to add a lot of protein-rich foods to your meals. For a look at how much protein your body needs each day, see the RDA table on page 33 in chapter 1. Then see the Protein in Foods table on page 33 to see what foods to eat to meet your protein requirements.

To help manage your blood sugar, distribute your protein throughout your day. If you need to eat 60 grams of protein each day, aim for 20 grams at each meal. As for snacks, make sure you choose low GI foods. And don't forget that milk and yogurt have protein as well—they are great low GI snack choices!

One more interesting tidbit—if you enjoy a green salad with your meal, continue doing so. Just make sure you toss it with a vinaigrette dressing. Studies have found that vinegars, especially red wine vinegar, also slow the rate at which food leaves your stomach.

Caffeine and Alcohol

Caffeine is known to cause a low blood-sugar reaction, especially if it has been a few hours since you ate. Researchers from the Yale University School of Medicine found that consuming 400 milligrams of caffeine triggered hypoglycemia when blood-sugar levels were in the low-normal range, as might occur two to three hours after a meal.[1] If you are hypoglycemic, chances are you already know if you are sensitive to caffeine. If you are, make the switch to low-caffeine or caffeine-free beverages. One 6-ounce cup of coffee provides 110 to 175 milligrams of caffeine. Compare that to the same amount of black or green tea at 25 to 35 milligrams. It makes a difference!

Replace coffee with decaf coffee, cereal-based beverages (e.g., Ovaltine), herbal tea, weakly brewed black tea or green teas. If you don't want to part with your daily brew, make sure to drink it with a meal. That way the caffeine will be less likely to bring on low blood sugar. Between meals, stick to vegetable juice, water, milk, herbal tea or decaf lattes.

Drinking alcoholic beverages can also impair blood-sugar control and trigger a hypoglycemic reaction in susceptible individuals. It can induce reactive hypoglycemia by interfering with glucose uptake and promoting the release of insulin from your pancreas. The drop in blood sugar that follows leads to a craving for foods, especially sweets. If you reach for sugary foods in response to this low blood sugar, you'll only aggravate your symptoms.

If you have hypoglycemia, avoid drinking alcohol on an empty stomach. Instead, enjoy your drink with a meal. The presence of food in your stomach will delay the absorption of alcohol. If you do drink, limit yourself to seven alcoholic drinks per week for health protection.

VITAMINS AND MINERALS

Chromium

Supplements of this trace mineral have been promoted to manage hypoglycemia; unfortunately, research studies are few and far between. One small study was conducted in the late 1980s with eight women who had hypoglycemia.[2] Those who took 200 micrograms of chromium for three months experienced a significantly reduced rate of low blood-sugar symptoms and had higher blood-glucose levels two to four hours after eating. Another small study conducted among 20 patients with hypoglycemia found similar results using 125 micrograms of the mineral.[3]

But this is all we have to go on. A greater number of studies have investigated the use of chromium in individuals with type 2 diabetes—and you'll read about this mineral's potential role in insulin resistance and high blood sugar in chapter 19, "Polycystic Ovary Syndrome" (PCOS). Despite the lack of scientific support for the use of chromium in hypoglycemia, it is a wise idea to make sure you get enough of this mineral in your daily diet.

It appears that chromium does play an important role when it comes to regulating blood glucose. Chromium is needed by the body to make glucose tolerance factor (GTF), a compound that interacts with insulin and helps maintain normal blood-sugar levels. With adequate amounts of chromium present, your body uses less insulin to do its job.

The recommended dietary intake for chromium is 25 micrograms (men need 35 micrograms per day). Chromium-rich foods include apples with the skin, green peas, chicken breast, refried beans, mushrooms, oysters, wheat germ and Brewer's yeast. Processed foods and refined (white) starchy foods like white bread, instant rice, white pasta, sugar and sweets all contain very little chromium.

If you're concerned you're not getting enough chromium through food, check your multivitamin and mineral supplement to see how much it contains. If it's less than 25 micrograms, consider taking a separate 200-microgram supplement each day. Studies show that chromium picinolate is absorbed more easily than other forms such as chromium chloride and chromium nicotinate. Chromium supplements are extremely safe.

Keep in mind, though, the most important thing you can do to prevent hypoglycemia is to eat at regular intervals and choose carbohydrate foods high in soluble fiber. If you are not doing this, don't expect chromium to help manage your condition.

OTHER LIFESTYLE FACTORS

Regular Exercise

When it comes to preventing hypoglycemia, I can't neglect to mention the importance of a program of regular, moderate exercise. Exercise improves many aspects of blood-sugar control. Working out enhances your body's sensitivity to insulin, improves glucose uptake by your cells and, interestingly, also increases the concentration of chromium in your tissues.

You don't need to exercise vigorously to reap the benefits. In fact, working out too intensely may bring on hypoglycemia. If you exercise with someone, you should be able to carry on a conversation and be just a little breathless. If you work out at a gym, consult with a certified personal trainer to help you find your target heart-rate zone. Staying within this range while you exercise will prevent you from overdoing it. Good activities include brisk walking, jogging, stair climbing, swimming, rowing and cycling. I usually tell my clients to aim for four workouts a week, each at least 30 minutes long. If you are not doing this much exercise right now, gradually work up to it.

Make sure you plan your snacks around your exercise session. If you eat lunch at noon and exercise at three o'clock (like me), you'll want a snack about 30 minutes before you begin. At two-thirty, try a banana, yogurt or a small sports bar. Depending on what time you eat dinner, you'll likely need to eat another small snack around four o'clock or four-thirty.

THE BOTTOM LINE...

Leslie's recommendations for managing hypoglycemia

1. Eat every three hours to prevent your blood-sugar level from plummeting. If you get so involved in what you are doing that you forget to eat, set a timer on your computer or watch.

2. For the most part, choose carbohydrate foods with a low glycemic index value.

3. Include a source of soluble fiber at meals—oats, dried beans, lentils, citrus fruit or sweet potato. These foods are digested slowly and lead to more sustained energy levels.

4. Include protein foods at your meals, since this nutrient helps to slow down digestion.

5. Enjoy a tossed salad with a vinaigrette dressing at lunch and dinner. Studies have shown that vinegar slows the rate at which food leaves your stomach.

6. As much as possible, avoid caffeinated beverages and alcohol, especially on an empty stomach.

7. Boost your intake of chromium-rich foods such as unpeeled apples, green peas, chicken breast, refried beans, mushrooms, oysters, wheat germ and brewer's yeast. Intakes of 125 to 200 micrograms per day might help reduce symptoms of hypoglycemia. If your multivitamin and mineral supplement contains less than 25 micrograms of chromium, consider adding a 200-microgram supplement to your daily nutrition regime.

8. Exercise at a moderate pace four times a week for at least 30 minutes in duration.

6

Insomnia

Do you wake up after a full night's sleep feeling tired and listless? Do you have difficulty falling asleep despite how tired you feel? Or perhaps you can't seem to stay asleep, tossing and turning throughout the night. If any of these symptoms ring true for you, the chances are good that you're suffering from insomnia.

Insomnia affects up to one-third of all adults and is one of the most common sleep complaints. Women tend to experience insomnia more frequently than men because of our biological factors such as menstruation, pregnancy and menopause.

Most of the time insomnia is a symptom of some other health condition. Insomnia has been linked to a variety of medical and emotional disorders. Studies have shown that insomnia can have a devastating effect on everyday life. It can result in decreased productivity, increased motor vehicle and job-related accidents and higher rates of mental and physical illness. There are a variety of ways to treat insomnia, but the best results come from lifestyle management techniques that improve your ability to relax and manage stress.

What Causes Insomnia?

Sleep is a basic human need. When we sleep, our minds and bodies rest and restore energy, preparing us for another day. Most people need between seven and eight hours of restful sleep each night to maintain good health and to feel mentally alert during the day.

Insomnia, the inability to sleep, is a term that refers to a number of different sleep disruptions and disturbances including

- difficulty falling asleep
- waking up early in the morning and being unable to return to sleep
- waking up frequently during the night or having difficulty staying asleep
- waking up after a full night's sleep and not feeling rested

Every once in a while, we all toss and turn through a sleepless night. This is known as short-term or *transient insomnia*, and is rarely a cause for concern. Only when your sleep habits are disturbed regularly for more than three weeks are you considered to be suffering from *chronic insomnia*. Insomnia usually results from a combination of factors and is often a symptom of some other physical or mental condition that is affecting you.

Insomnia is often associated with psychiatric disturbances and is especially common in people with depression and anxiety disorders. Alzheimer's disease and other forms of dementia can also disturb sleep and cause repeated nighttime awakening. People suffering from arthritis, kidney or thyroid disease, asthma, restless leg syndrome, sleep apnea and gastrointestinal disorders will frequently experience pain and discomfort severe enough to interfere with normal sleep patterns. As well, medications used to treat these and other health conditions may trigger insomnia as an unwanted side effect.

Our sleep patterns change as we age. Research indicates that sleep efficiency decreases from a high of 95 percent in adolescence to less than 80 percent in old age. Consequently, older people have more difficulty falling asleep or staying asleep, and often find that sleep is not as refreshing as it used to be. But there are also many lifestyle and environmental factors that can lead to chronic insomnia. You may suffer from insomnia if you:

- drink excessive amounts of alcohol or take recreational drugs
- drink coffee or caffeinated beverages before bedtime
- smoke cigarettes before bedtime
- take long naps in the daytime or evening
- disrupt your day/night (or sleep/wake) cycle with shift work or travel that results in jet lag
- experience chronic tension or stress, or worry excessively
- sleep in a noisy environment
- sleep in a room that is too warm or too cold

These factors are often responsible for the development of sleep problems and they may also prolong the symptoms of existing insomnia. Simple adjustments in sleep habits and lifestyle can go a long way towards helping you get a good night's sleep.

Insomnia is much more common in women than it is in men. In general, women tend to sleep fewer hours and to experience a poorer quality of sleep, especially as they get older. Fluctuating hormone levels are the primary culprits. As the levels of estrogen and progesterone hormones change in response to menstrual cycles, pregnancy and menopause, women are more likely to suffer ongoing sleep disturbances that rob them of energy, health and mental agility.

1. *Menstruation* Poor quality sleep is often associated with the beginning of the menstrual cycle, when bleeding starts. Some women feel particularly sleepy and fatigued when progesterone levels rise right after ovulation. As the menstrual cycle continues, progesterone levels begin to fall rapidly, signaling the start of menstruation. This is a time when many women are quite wakeful and find it difficult to fall asleep at night.

2. *Premenstrual Syndrome (PMS)* During the latter part of the menstrual cycle, some women struggle with the debilitating symptoms of PMS. In addition to bloating, moodiness, abdominal cramps and irritability, women with PMS may find it hard to get to sleep or to stay asleep or they may sleep excessively. Insomnia and the associated daytime tiredness are common symptoms of PMS.

3. *Pregnancy* The physical and emotional demands of pregnancy often lead women to report more disturbed sleep. Rising levels of progesterone in the first trimester are known to increase sleepiness. In the early stages of pregnancy, sleep patterns may also be disrupted by the need to urinate frequently. In the second trimester sleep quality tends to improve but is still worse than before pregnancy. Most pregnancy-related sleep problems develop during the third trimester, when the fetus puts pressure on the bladder, increasing the need to go to the bathroom during the night. Heartburn, sinus congestion and leg cramps are also common in the later stages of pregnancy and will cause enough physical discomfort to disturb sleep. Once the baby is born, a mother's sleep is interrupted often, and the resulting sleep deprivation may trigger emotional problems such as a mild depression known as *post-partum blues.*

4. *Menopause* As a woman ages, her levels of estrogen and progesterone begin to drop, and eventually she stops menstruating. This transition to actual menopause (cessation of menstruation) is the time when women report the highest levels of sleep disruptions. In many cases, insomnia is brought on by night sweats, which are hot flashes that occur during sleep. Women in menopause often experience daytime tiredness and chronic fatigue.

⤳

Who's at Risk?

According to the National Sleep Foundation, nearly two-thirds of Americans experience sleep problems. Although people of all ages can experience insomnia, it seems that women experience it more frequently than men and are more willing to seek treatment. Insomnia is also common among the elderly. Studies have indicated that people coping with stressful situations, such as divorce or unemployment, or who have medical or emotional conditions, are much more prone to insomnia. Those who have sleep disturbances that persist for more than 12 months are also more likely to develop depression, anxiety disorders and alcohol dependency.

Diagnosis

Insomnia can be difficult to diagnose. The need for sleep varies from individual to individual. Some people require much less sleep to function effectively than others. This makes it challenging to develop sleep standards and norms for effective diagnosis. Generally, you will be diagnosed with insomnia if your sleep disturbances are severe enough to noticeably affect your daytime mood and activities. Determining the frequency, intensity and duration of your sleep disruptions is also helpful in making an accurate diagnosis.

Because insomnia is so often a symptom of another disorder, the American Medical Association recommends that the real emotional, physical or environmental causes of insomnia be diagnosed and treated, before any other steps are taken to treat insomnia complaints. To do this, your doctor will evaluate your sleep patterns, your drug use (including alcohol, nicotine and caffeine), your psychological and physical condition and your level of physical activity. In some cases, you may be sent to a sleep laboratory for further testing.

Conventional Treatment

Naturally, the treatment of insomnia depends on the underlying cause of the condition. Making simple lifestyle changes is often the best way to treat insomnia. Some recommendations for improving your sleep habits include the following:

1. *Exercise* Regular, moderate-intensity exercise is known to improve sleep quality. Take a brisk walk, do some gardening or join an exercise class. You'll find it much easier to fall asleep naturally if you add some activity to your day. Just avoid exercise in the late evening before bedtime because it may overstimulate your body.

2. *Change your diet* Avoid big meals late at night and limit your use of alcohol and tobacco. Foods that are high in sugar or caffeine, such as coffee, tea and caffeinated beverages, should also be restricted. Some people find that their sleep improves

if they avoid eating spicy or high-fat foods in the evening. Limiting fluid intake may also reduce your need to go to the bathroom during the night, allowing you a more restful sleep. You'll read much more about these and other nutritional approaches below.

3. *Control your sleep environment* Keep your bedroom dark and quiet, and make sure it is not too warm or cold. Use your bedroom mainly as a place to sleep and don't use it for watching television, eating, exercising, working or other activities associated with wakefulness.

4. *Establish a regular bedtime routine* Go to bed at the same time each night. Even more important, you should try to get up at the same time in the morning, both during the week and on the weekends. Following a regular routine of brushing your teeth, washing your face, setting your alarm—even when you are away from home—will help you to set the mood for sleep in the evening. Avoid daytime naps that might interfere with your nighttime sleep schedule.

5. *Relax* Stress and worry play an important role in triggering symptoms of insomnia. Relax at bedtime by taking a warm bath, enjoying a cup of herbal tea or reading until you feel sleepy. And try to avoid worrying about daytime problems.

Some people find that alternative therapies, such as biofeedback, muscle relaxation, behavioral therapy or psychotherapy, may help them to achieve a more restful sleep.

If your insomnia can't be managed using these basic techniques, your doctor may recommend medications to help you sleep. These drugs are called hypnotics, but you may hear them referred to as sedatives, barbiturates or tranquilizers. All hypnotics present a risk of overdose, addiction, tolerance and withdrawal symptoms. For this reason, your doctor will prescribe the lowest dose possible. You should use hypnotic drugs only a few times a week and only for a short time (two to four weeks) to avoid future problems.

If you are using hypnotic drugs and suddenly stop taking them you may experience a condition known as *rebound insomnia*. This insomnia is temporary but it can create a vicious cycle of drug use and insomnia symptoms if not properly managed. Hypnotic drugs should be discontinued gradually to avoid this problem.

❧

Managing Insomnia

DIETARY STRATEGIES

Caffeine

This may sound simple—eat and drink less caffeine-containing foods and you'll sleep better. Caffeine does stimulate the central nervous system. While one or two cups of coffee in the morning can give you that gentle lift you were hoping for, the fourth or fifth cup can overstimulate your body and cause insomnia. My first recommendation is to avoid caffeine in the afternoon. Replace caffeinated beverages with caffeine-free or decaffeinated beverages, like herbal tea, mineral water, fruit and vegetable juice or decaf coffee.

The daily upper limit for caffeine is 400 to 450 milligrams per day. This recommendation is based on studies that have investigated the effect of caffeine on blood pressure and other health conditions, not your ability to sleep soundly. It turns out that even less caffeine may keep you up at night. Studies have shown that one or two small cups of coffee in the morning can affect the quality of sleep that night.[1] Caffeine blocks the action of adenosine, a natural sleep-inducing brain chemical. If you're suffering from insomnia, aim for no more than 200 milligrams of caffeine a day, and preferably none. To see where you're getting your caffeine, see the table on page 38 in chapter 1.

Alcohol

The effects of alcohol are detrimental to sleep. Alcohol worsens insomnia and can rob you of a good night's sleep even if you don't have a sleep disorder. Once absorbed into the bloodstream, alcohol is metabolized at a set rate by your liver. If you drink more alcohol than your liver can keep up with (i.e., more than one drink an hour), alcohol arrives in your brain, where it interferes with brain chemicals called neurotransmitters. Alcohol has been shown to impair the REM portion of sleep, the time when your body is in its restorative phase.

Alcohol also dehydrates you, which can make you feel fatigued the next day. It does so by depressing the brain's ability to produce a hormone called antidiuretic hormone. This causes your body to lose water through your kidneys. Water makes it possible for your body to generate energy. You need water to digest, absorb and transport nutrients in your body and to regulate your body temperature. So when you're dehydrated after an evening of drinking alcohol (even a few drinks), your cells and tissues receive nutrients less efficiently and your body can't properly regulate its temperature. Both lead to fatigue.

When it comes to reducing your risk for cancer, women should consume no more than seven drinks per week. But if you're suffering from insomnia, I recommend that you eliminate it from your diet altogether. Instead of having a glass of wine, pour yourself a glass of sparkling mineral water with a slice of lime. Or try some of the non-alcoholic wines or beers available in the supermarket. If you're looking for a cocktail, order a virgin Caesar, a tomato juice or a glass of cranberry and soda.

To lessen alcohol's effect on your ability to sleep, drink alcohol with a meal or snack. If you drink alcohol on an empty stomach, about 20 percent is absorbed directly across the walls of your stomach and reaches the brain within a minute. But when the stomach is full of food, alcohol has a lesser chance of touching the walls and passing through, so the effect on your brain is delayed.

If you're out socially or you are entertaining at home, don't drink more than one alcoholic beverage per hour. Since the liver can't metabolize alcohol any faster than this, drinking slowly will ensure your blood alcohol concentration doesn't rise. To slow your pace, alternate one alcoholic drink with a non-alcoholic drink or a glass of water. One drink is equivalent to 5 ounces of wine, 12 ounces of beer, 10 ounces of wine cooler or 1.5 ounces of liquor.

Carbohydrate before Bed

If you've ever heard that a glass of warm milk can help you sleep, you might give this a try—there is some science to back this claim. A carbohydrate-rich snack like milk, a small bowl of cereal or a slice of toast provides the brain with an amino acid called tryptophan. The brain uses tryptophan as a building block to manufacture a neurotransmitter called *serotonin*. Serotonin has been shown to facilitate sleep, improve mood, diminish pain and even reduce appetite.

If you want to see if eating a little bit of carbohydrate helps you fall asleep, eat something *small* or drink a glass of low-fat milk or soy beverage. Try it for a week. If your insomnia has not improved, look at other factors that may be disrupting sleep.

VITAMINS AND MINERALS

Vitamin B12

Many studies have found that vitamin B12 promotes sleep in people who suffer from sleep disorders. In a randomized double-blind study, Japanese researchers determined that a daily dose of 1.5 to 3 milligrams of the vitamin restored normal sleep patterns in such patients.[2] German researchers have also found that sleep quality, concentration and "feeling refreshed" were significantly correlated with the blood level of vitamin B12 in healthy men and women.[3]

Some researchers believe that B12 helps you sleep by working with melatonin, a natural hormone in the body. Melatonin is involved in maintaining the body's internal clock, which regulates the secretion of various hormones. In so doing, melatonin helps control sleep and wakefulness. Secretion of this hormone is stimulated by darkness and suppressed by light. Vitamin B12 appears to directly influence the action of melatonin and the vitamin may prevent disturbances in melatonin release.

For the daily recommended allowance for vitamin B12 for healthy women, see the RDA table on page 9 in chapter 1. Vitamin B12 is found exclusively in animal foods—meat, poultry, eggs, fish and dairy products are all good sources. Fortified soy and rice beverages also contain vitamin B12. If you want to know exactly how much B12 you're consuming each day, you'll find a list of foods and their B12 content on page 9 in chapter 1.

If you fall into one of the following categories, I recommend you supplement your diet with vitamin B12:

- If you're over 50 years of age. Up to one-third of older adults don't produce enough stomach acid to properly absorb vitamin B12 from their diet. For this reason, it's recommended that you get a daily supplement, or consume foods fortified with the vitamin.

- If you're taking antacid medication for reflux or a stomach ulcer. Any medicine that blocks your body's ability to produce stomach acid will impair your ability to absorb B12 from food (this does not include foods fortified with B12).

- If you're a strict vegetarian who eats no animal foods and you don't drink at least two servings of a fortified soy or rice beverage each day. If this is the case, you're missing out on vitamin B12!

You can get additional B12 from a multivitamin and mineral, a B complex formula or single supplements of the vitamin (these come in 500- or 1000-microgram doses). For sleep disorders due to a deficiency of vitamin B12 (have your doctor measure your B12 stores), a dose of 500 to 1000 micrograms three times daily can be used. If you take vitamin C pills, don't take them with your vitamin B12 supplement—large amounts of vitamin C can destroy B12.

Vitamin B12 is considered safe and nontoxic, even in large amounts. However, there have been some reports of B12 supplements causing diarrhea, itching, swelling, hives and, rarely, anaphylactic reactions. If you are taking high doses of vitamin B12, or any supplement, be sure to inform your healthcare practitioner.

HERBAL REMEDIES

Valerian (*Valeriana officinalis*)

This native North American plant acts like a mild sedative on the central nervous system. Studies show that valerian root makes getting to sleep easier and increases deep sleep. Unlike conventional sleeping pills, the herb does not lead to dependence or addiction. Valerian promotes sleep by interacting with certain brain receptors called GABA receptors and benzodiazepine receptors. Compared to drugs like Valium® and Xanax®, valerian binds very weakly to these receptors.

In one double-blind study from Germany, 44 percent of those taking valerian root reported perfect sleep and 89 percent reported improved sleep compared to those taking the placebo pill.[4] Another small study found that individuals with mild insomnia who took 450 milligrams of valerian experienced a significant decrease in sleep problems.[5] The same researchers studied 128 individuals and found that compared to the placebo, 400 milligrams of valerian produced a significant improvement in sleep quality in people who considered themselves poor sleepers.[6]

Scientists attribute the herb's effectiveness to essential oils in the root. To make sure you are getting a sufficient amount of the active ingredient, buy a product that's been standardized to contain at least 0.5 percent essential oils or 0.8 percent *valerenic acid*. Take 400 to 900 milligrams in capsule or tablet form, 30 minutes to one hour before bedtime. If you wake up feeling groggy, reduce the dose. Don't expect results overnight. The herb works better when it's used over a period of time; it may take two to four weeks to notice an improvement in sleep.

Valerian is not recommended for use during pregnancy or breastfeeding, since it has not been studied in these conditions. Long-term use may result in withdrawal symptoms when the herb is discontinued, similar to those that occur when sleeping pills are discontinued.

THE BOTTOM LINE...
Leslie's recommendations for managing insomnia

1. Cut back your caffeine intake to a daily maximum of no more than 200 milligrams per day. If you've done this and you're still having trouble sleeping, eliminate caffeine completely for two weeks, and see if your sleep and/or your energy level during the day improve.

2. If you drink alcohol and you don't want to give it up (which I do recommend if you're experiencing sleep problems), aim for no more than seven drinks a week or one drink a day. To lessen alcohol's effect on your brain, have your drink with food or a snack.

3. Try a light carbohydrate-rich snack 30 minutes before bed to increase the level of sleep-promoting serotonin in your brain.

4. Make sure you get enough vitamin B12 in your diet. If you can't get enough B12 through food, or if you don't produce enough stomach acid for its absorption, take a daily B12 supplement of 500 micrograms.

5. Consider taking 400 to 900 milligrams of valerian root extract. Buy a product that is standardized to contain at least 0.5 percent essential oils or 0.8 percent valerenic acid. Take the herb 30 to 60 minutes before going to bed.

6. Don't forget to investigate other possible causes of sleep disturbances: a lack of exercise, too much stress or a possible medical problem. If you've tried everything you can and you still have fitful sleep, consult your family physician.

7

Migraine Headaches

Migraine is one of the most common and misunderstood of all diseases. It has disabling effects on millions of people, yet it is very often misdiagnosed and has no definitive cure. Women are three times more likely to suffer from migraines than men—a factor that may be related to the hormonal changes that occur during the menstrual cycle.

A migraine is a type of headache that results from inflammation of the blood vessels and nerves surrounding the brain. The exact causes of migraine headaches are not known, but they seem to be set off by changes in brain activity. Very often, specific substances, actions or stimuli in your body or environment may trigger migraines.

Although the symptoms, frequency and intensity of migraines vary widely, they are often acutely painful and incapacitating. Over 80 percent of migraine sufferers cope with some degree of headache-related disability. Treatment of migraines usually involves a two-pronged approach. Therapies focus on providing relief of symptoms and preventing or reducing future headache attacks.

∗

What Causes a Migraine?

People have been suffering from migraines for hundreds of years, but we still don't clearly understand the underlying causes of this relentless disease. Research indicates that a migraine involves both the nerves around the brain and the blood vessels that feed the brain. Scientists have recorded a spreading pattern of electrical activity within the brains of people with migraines, which may be responsible for some of the classic migraine symptoms. Many people also experience a decrease in blood flow to various parts of the brain, again connected with the onset of migraine. More recently, there has been some evidence that serotonin, a powerful chemical that has the ability to constrict blood vessels, may help stimulate the migraine mechanism.

∗

Symptoms

There are two common types of migraine and they each have slightly different symptoms:

1. *Migraine with aura.* This is referred to as a classic migraine. The aura is a set of neurological symptoms that occur approximately 10 to 30 minutes before the headache starts. During the aura phase, you may experience visual disturbances, such as flashing lights or geometric patterns in front of your eyes, or you may even suffer brief vision loss. It is not uncommon to feel dizzy and confused or to have some facial tingling and muscle weakness as the aura progresses. Migraines with auras affect only 10 to 20 percent of migraine sufferers.

2. *Migraine without aura.* This is known as a common migraine, and it affects many more people than the classic migraine. Although you will not have an aura, you may have mood swings, feel depressed and fatigued or lose your appetite just before the migraine strikes.

A pulsing, throbbing pain characterizes both types of migraine. The pain is often felt only on one side of your head or behind one eye, but it may spread to involve your entire head at a later stage. Migraines are usually aggravated by physical activity and are often accompanied by severe nausea and vomiting. They may also be associated with a wide variety of other symptoms, including heightened sensitivity to light, noise and odor, diarrhea, facial swelling, nasal congestion and scalp tenderness. Once the headache has subsided, it will usually leave you feeling extremely fatigued, listless and irritable.

Although there are some characteristic symptoms of a migraine, most migraines don't conform to a typical pattern. You may be lucky and only suffer a migraine once in a while, or you may be incapacitated by attacks that occur as often as three times a week. The intensity of pain that you feel can vary from reasonably mild to completely debilitating. Migraines also vary in length from a brief, 15-minute episode to an attack that can last a week. On average, the duration of a migraine ranges between 2 and 72 hours.

૪

Who's at Risk?

Migraine is a universal condition that affects approximately 6 percent of men and 15 to 18 percent of women. Although migraines can strike children and adolescents, they most often affect women between 25 and 55 years of age. As many as 50 to 70 percent of all migraine sufferers have a family history of the disease, indicating that these headaches may be hereditary. However, a specific migraine gene has not yet been found.

૪

Diagnosis

Because of the wide variation in symptoms, migraines are quite difficult to diagnose. They can often be confused with other types of headaches, such as tension or sinus headaches. To help doctors make an earlier diagnosis, the American Headache Society has recommended a detailed set of criteria for assessing migraine symptoms. It is reasonable to assume you suffer from migraines if your headaches have some of the following characteristics:

- a sequence of at least five attacks that last between 2 and 72 hours
- pain that is located on one side of your head, sometimes spreading to both sides
- pain that is pulsating or throbbing
- pain that prohibits or limits daily activity
- pain that is aggravated by physical activity
- nausea or vomiting during headache attacks
- sensitivity to light, noise or smell during headache attacks

౨

Migraine Triggers

In some cases, certain stimuli or triggers that you experience as part of your normal life provoke migraines. By avoiding these triggers, you may be able to reduce the frequency or severity of your attacks. Although triggers don't actually cause a migraine, they do seem to influence the activities in your brain that stimulate the disease. Often, you will be sensitive to the combined effect of more than one trigger.

There are many common migraine triggers and you must determine which ones affect you. Keeping a migraine headache diary is a good way to identify the circumstances that set off your migraines.

1. *Diet* Certain foods and food additives are well-known migraine triggers. Alcoholic beverages (especially red wine), foods treated with MSG (monosodium glutamate), foods that contain tyramine (e.g., aged cheeses, soy sauce) or aspartame (NutraSweet™) and foods preserved with nitrates and nitrites all may provoke migraines. Chocolate, caffeine and dairy products are other known culprits.

2. *Lifestyle* Changes in your behavior or your surroundings can encourage migraines. If you alter your eating or sleeping habits, experience high levels of stress or smoke cigarettes, you may find yourself struggling with more frequent migraines.

3. *Environment* Some people find that bright lights or loud noises will bring on a migraine. Weather or temperature changes and physical exertion are common

triggers, and even changing time zones may affect your headache frequency. Strong odors, perfume, high altitudes and computer screens are other recognized triggers.

4. *Female hormones* Women may be more susceptible to migraines because of the estrogen cycles associated with menstruation. Migraines become more prevalent in females after puberty, reaching a peak at age 40, and then declining in frequency as women age. But almost two-thirds of women who suffer from migraines will experience a worsening of their headaches during their period. Up to 15 percent of women will get migraines only during their period, as what is called true menstrual migraine. *Menstrual migraines* are typically without aura and last longer than other migraines. They are also more difficult to treat. To prevent these debilitating headaches, it is extremely important for women to avoid migraine triggers during the premenstrual week (you'll find a list of dietary triggers later in the chapter).

5. *Oral contraceptives and estrogen therapy* also seem to make migraines worse. If you take these medications and suffer from migraines, you may want to speak to your doctor about being on a low-dose estrogen regimen.

6. *Pregnancy* Migraines are more common in early pregnancy but usually improve by the second trimester. In a small group of women, *pregnancy migraines* will worsen throughout their pregnancies. During pregnancy, women should pay special attention to avoiding dietary and environmental triggers, sticking to regular sleeping and eating schedules, getting regular exercise and managing stress (as should all women with migraines).

↝

Conventional Treatment

When a migraine strikes, the light, noise and pain may be overwhelming when you are around other people. Most migraine sufferers retreat to a quiet, dark room and try to sleep through it. The disabling effects of migraines often result in work loss and may seriously curtail social and family activities.

When migraines begin to have a negative impact on your life, your doctor may prescribe drug therapy. People respond to a variety of different medications and you may have to experiment to find the one that works best for you.

MIGRAINE RELIEF MEDICATIONS

These medications target the pain of an attack and should be taken as soon as you sense that a headache is beginning. General analgesics (painkillers) and NSAIDs (non-steroidal anti-inflammatory drugs) are frequently used to relieve the discomfort of mild and moderate migraine attacks. One of the most effective drugs is Imitrex®, a drug that specifically targets the receptors for serotonin and causes blood vessels to constrict. It acts quickly to reduce pain and is effective for over 70 percent of migraine sufferers. Some combination medications may also be useful in cases where other drug therapies are not effective. Because migraines are usually accompanied by extreme nausea, your treatment plan will probably include an anti-nausea drug to relieve these symptoms.

Among other side effects, both analgesics and NSAIDs are known to cause stomach problems that may eventually lead to internal bleeding and ulcers. Overuse of these drugs may also cause you to experience rebound headaches. Rebound headaches are not migraines, but are medication induced and may quickly become chronic.

Severe migraine attacks that result in incapacitating pain may be treated with opiates, which are very powerful painkillers. However, they are also highly addictive and are usually prescribed only in extreme cases.

MIGRAINE PREVENTION THERAPIES

As with migraine relief medications, these drugs will work with varying success. A "good" response to preventive medications is defined as a 50 percent reduction in the severity and frequency of migraine attacks. The main types of prevention medications are

1. *Beta-blockers*—These have a 60 percent success rate. They work to stabilize serotonin levels and reduce the dilation of blood vessels.

2. *Ergot drugs*—These are usually as effective as beta-blockers and also affect serotonin levels and blood vessel dilation.

3. *Calcium channel-blockers*—These are thought to modulate neurotransmitters. The effects are gradual and the success rate is less than with beta-blockers.

4. *Antidepressants*—These have a positive effect on serotonin levels. They are effective but may have serious interactions with other medications.

All of the migraine prevention medications produce side effects that may have serious consequences for your overall health. Most of these drugs are contraindicated during pregnancy. When you are experimenting with preventive therapies, you should try only one drug at a time, so that you and your physician can carefully monitor the positive and negative effects. Dosage should begin at a low level and move upwards only as needed.

ALTERNATIVE TREATMENTS

There is a growing body of evidence to indicate that alternative therapies have a positive effect on the symptoms and frequency of migraine attacks. Resting in a quiet, dark room and applying ice or pressure often helps to relieve pain. Avoiding triggers through diet and lifestyle changes is also very beneficial in preventing the onset of migraines. Other therapies that have shown some success in alleviating migraines are

- relaxation therapy
- biofeedback
- acupuncture
- stress-management training
- psychotherapy
- hypnosis
- physiotherapy, osteopathy and chiropractic therapy

Managing Migraines

DIETARY STRATEGIES

Food Triggers

A number of foods have been reported to trigger a migraine attack. Studies show that when people who suffer migraines eliminate these foods from their diet, about one-third experience fewer headaches, and up to 10 percent become headache free. Here's a list of the most common foods that can trigger a migraine, or make one worse:

- milk
- wine
- chocolate

- coffee, tea
- hot dogs
- garlic

- cheese, especially aged cheese

- eggs
- fish

As well, the following foods and food additives have been reported to bring on a headache:

- alcoholic beverages
- artificial sweeteners
- citrus fruits
- corn
- foods with MSG
- foods with nitrites/nitrates (e.g., processed meats, smoked fish, some imported cheeses, beets, celery, collards, eggplant, lettuce, radishes, spinach, turnip greens)

- lima beans
- lentils
- nuts
- overripe bananas
- peanuts, peanut butter
- red wine
- shellfish
- soybeans
- tomato

Some migraine sufferers have actual food allergies. It's believed that certain immune compounds formed in response to an offending food can trigger a migraine headache. If you find that certain foods are triggering migraines, it might be worthwhile to have your doctor refer you to an allergy specialist for food testing.

Whether it's a food allergy or some other food response that's responsible for your migraines, consult a registered dietitian who specializes in food sensitivities (**www .eatright.org**). He or she can plan an elimination and challenge diet for you, a very useful tool used to identify food triggers. You can also do this on your own. Begin by keeping a food and headache diary. List all foods, beverages, medications and dietary supplements taken. Note the date of your menstrual period, since hormones may precipitate a migraine, too. You should keep this diary for at least two weeks, or long enough to cover at least three migraine attacks. Once you've completed this exercise, look for patterns. Did you eat the same food before each migraine? Did your migraines hit you after a night of drinking wine? You get the idea.

Once you have identified possible culprits, eliminate them from your diet for a period of four weeks, or longer if you experience migraines less frequently. If you are migraine free during this period, it's very likely that you've found your triggers! The next step is to make sure these foods are the actual culprits. One by one, test each food by adding it to your diet. Wait three days before testing the next food on your list. Keep in mind that this exercise may not give you clear-cut results. A combination of events may be required to bring on a migraine. For instance, you may get a migraine only when you eat the food at a specific time in your menstrual cycle. Or, the combination of stress and a food trigger may be required to cause a migraine.

VITAMINS AND MINERALS

Vitamin B2 (Riboflavin)

If you want to prevent a migraine headache from coming on, you might reach for more riboflavin. Riboflavin is needed to facilitate the release of energy from all body cells. In fact, studies reveal that migraine sufferers have less efficient energy metabolism in their brain cells. It's thought that by increasing your riboflavin intake and therefore the potential of your brain cells to generate energy, you might keep migraines at bay. Looks like this strategy might work. In a well-controlled study conducted among 55 patients with migraine, a daily 400-milligram supplement of this B vitamin reduced the frequency of headache attacks in a manner similar to certain drugs used for this condition.[1]

You don't need much riboflavin to prevent a deficiency. The recommended daily intake for women is 1.1 milligrams per day. During pregnancy and breastfeeding you need 1.4 and 1.6 milligrams respectively. Riboflavin is found in many foods including milk, meat, eggs, nuts, enriched flour and green vegetables. If you take a multivitamin or B complex supplement you're getting even more riboflavin, as much as 100 milligrams.

If you're striving to get 400 milligrams each day in the hopes of preventing a migraine, you'll need to buy a separate supplement of this B vitamin. B2 supplements are available in 25-, 50-, 100-, 500- and 1200-milligram doses. Chances are, you won't find this supplement at a drugstore. You'll have to visit your local health food or supplement store. It may make take up to three months to notice an improvement in your headache frequency. Riboflavin supplements are nontoxic and very well tolerated.

Magnesium

Researchers have established an important link between magnesium levels in the body and migraine attacks. Evidence shows that during a migraine headache up to 50 percent of people have low magnesium levels in their brain and red blood cells. It's thought that a deficiency of magnesium in the brain can cause nerve cells to be overly excited, triggering a migraine attack. (A few medications can deplete magnesium stores, including estrogen, estrogen-containing birth control pills and certain diuretics.)

If you increase the amount of magnesium in your tissues and red blood cells, can you prevent a migraine? According to researchers from Germany, the answer is yes. They gave 81 migraine sufferers either 600 milligrams of magnesium or a placebo pill once daily for three months. In the second month of the study, the frequency of migraine attacks was reduced to 42 percent in the magnesium group, compared to only 16 percent in the placebo group. What's more, the duration of a migraine and drug use significantly decreased among those people who took magnesium supplements.[2]

Magnesium is the second most abundant mineral in the body (second only to calcium). It plays a crucial role in over 300 cellular reactions. Among its many roles, magnesium helps cells generate energy, moves important compounds in and out of cells, and transmits impulses from nerve to nerve. To help prevent a low magnesium level and resulting migraines, first make sure you are getting enough from your daily diet by checking the RDA table on page 21 in chapter 1; then consider taking a supplement.

The best sources of magnesium are whole foods including unrefined grains, nuts, seeds, legumes, dried fruit and green vegetables.

Magnesium Supplements

If you're going to try to ward off your migraines by boosting your intake of magnesium, you'll need to take a supplement. The randomized controlled trial I discussed above used 600 milligrams per day. Buy a magnesium citrate supplement; compared to other forms of the mineral (e.g., magnesium oxide), magnesium citrates are more easily absorbed by your body. Split your dose over the course of the day. Take a 300 milligram supplement twice daily, or 200 milligrams three times a day. It will depend on what dose you can find in your health food or supplement store. You may be able to get your extra magnesium from calcium supplements if you buy a 1:1 formula—that means each tablet gives you an equal amount of calcium and magnesium.

The daily upper limit for magnesium has been set at 350 milligrams from a supplement. That's because doses higher than this can cause diarrhea and stomach upset, common side effects of magnesium supplementation. Taking 600 milligrams in divided doses may help ease intestinal upset.

HERBAL REMEDIES

Feverfew (*Tanacetum parthenium*)

Scientific evidence tells us that the leaves of this herb can significantly reduce the frequency and severity of migraine headaches when used properly. The link between feverfew and migraine became popular in England back in the 1970s, when a doctor's wife noticed that her migraines were much improved once she started chewing fresh feverfew leaves. As the story goes, after one year of faithfully taking the leaves, she almost forgot she ever suffered from migraines.

Since then, this herbal remedy has been the focus of a number of studies in people with migraines. Of these trials, one hailing from Nottingham, England, was a randomized controlled trial (the gold standard among researchers). In this study, 76 people who experienced migraines were given either whole feverfew leaf or a placebo for four months, and then the treatments were reversed for another four-month period. The results were impressive. Without knowing what treatment they received, 59 percent of the people taking feverfew identified the treatment during the feverfew period as more effective, compared to 24 percent who chose the placebo period. The herbal remedy reduced the number of classic migraines (with aura) by 32 percent and common migraines (without aura) by 21 percent.[3]

Researchers believe that feverfew reduces the frequency and intensity of migraines by preventing the release of substances called prostaglandins, which dilate blood vessels and cause inflammation. It was once thought that an active ingredient called parthenolide in the herb was responsible for feverfew's beneficial effect. But when researchers made a special alcohol extract that contained the same amount of parthenolide as an effective dose of feverfew leaf, there was no effect on migraine headaches. It seems that other compounds in the leaf of the plant are responsible for feverfew's effect on migraines.

To prevent a migraine, the recommended dose of feverfew is *80 to 100 milligrams daily of powdered feverfew leaf.* We know that whole feverfew leaf is effective, so don't buy an alcohol extract made up of parthenolide. Instead, buy capsules of powdered feverfew leaf. You can also try taking the herb at the onset of a migraine to ease the symptoms.

Feverfew is deemed to be very safe as it rarely causes side effects other than mild gastrointestinal upset. The herb may cause an allergic reaction in people sensitive to members of the Asteracease/Compositae plant family: ragweed, daisy, marigold and chrysanthemum. Like many other herbs, the safety of feverfew has not been studied in pregnant or nursing women, or in those with liver or kidney disease.

THE BOTTOM LINE...
Leslie's recommendations for managing migraines

1. Identify your food triggers. If you are not sure what component of your diet might be a culprit, try an elimination and challenge diet. You might also consider getting tested for food allergies.

2. To prevent a migraine, boost your intake of riboflavin (vitamin B2). Take a 400-milligram supplement each day.

3. Consider supplementing with magnesium to avoid a migraine attack. Research indicates that 600 milligrams of the mineral in supplement form may prevent headaches. Buy magnesium citrate supplements and take 600 milligrams per day in divided doses.

4. If you're looking for an herbal remedy to prevent and lessen the severity of your migraines, reach for feverfew. Take 80 to 100 milligrams of dry powdered leaf once daily. Feverfew may cause allergic reactions in people sensitive to ragweed, daisies, marigolds and chrysanthemums.

Part 3

Breast, Bone and Heart Health

8

Breast Cancer

Breast cancer is the most common type of cancer among American women. The American Cancer Society estimated that 203,500 new cases of breast cancer would develop in 2002, representing 31 percent of all cancers among women. Over her lifetime, a woman has a 10.6 percent chance of getting breast cancer. This lifetime risk does not apply to you as an individual; it represents the average risk for the population of American women. If you have certain risk factors for breast cancer, like a family history or a poor diet, this number underestimates your risk. If you have no risk factors at all for the disease, this lifetime risk overestimates your chances of getting breast cancer.

Sadly, more than 100 American women die every day from breast cancer. But the good news is that the death rate from breast cancer has decreased over the past 15 years. This is largely due to the fact that more and more women are having mammograms, allowing for earlier detection.

ॐ

What Causes Breast Cancer?

Simply put, cancer is a disease in which abnormal cells grow out of control. When enough of these cells accumulate, a tumor forms. Finally, if the cancer cells are able to break away from the tumor, they can circulate through the body and take up residence in another organ, a process called metastasis.

Every cell has a genetic blueprint, called DNA (deoxyribonucleic acid). The DNA of cells contains genes that program cell reproduction, growth and repair, affecting all body processes. Sometimes genes can become damaged and this damage can result in cancer. There are three ways in which your genes can become faulty:

1. A mutation can occur during normal cell division, such that the newly formed cell contains an abnormal gene. This can happen randomly or if the cell is exposed to some other agent.

2. Cells can be exposed to an environmental agent, a carcinogen that harms the DNA. For instance, cigarette smoke is a carcinogen that causes lung cancer.

3. Flawed genes can be inherited from your parents. In fact, very few cancers are actually the result of inherited genes.

Cancer is not explained by genetics alone. Experts agree that cancer is the result of an interaction between genes and environmental factors. For instance, you might have a mutated gene that predisposes you to breast cancer but, because you eat a low-fat diet with plenty of fruits and vegetables, the cancer may never express itself.

The breast is composed of fatty tissue and glands. Within this tissue are milk glands. Lobules are groups of individual milk-forming glands, and each lobule empties into ducts, small passageways that carry milk to the nipple. Breast cancer begins with a single cell that runs amok, usually in the lobule or duct. These are two areas where cells are rapidly dividing during the normal menstrual cycle. Estrogen and progesterone stimulate the breast cells to begin dividing each month, preparing the body for pregnancy. If conception does not occur, breast cell receptors receive a message to stop cell division. The process begins again the following month, and each month until menopause. With cell division regularly occurring for such a span of years, there is a greater chance for a genetic mutation to occur. While most breast cancers are not detected until after menopause, it is believed that they actually begin to develop in the premenopausal years.

Some cases of breast cancer are caused by inherited mutations in the genes BRCA1 and BRCA2. The gene BRCA1 is believed to account for 5 percent of breast cancers, specifically inherited early-onset breast cancer. Families that carry a faulty BRCA1 gene have a high incidence of both breast and ovarian cancer at a young age. Researchers are currently studying BRCA2 and BRCA3 genes.

Who's at Risk?

The clearest risk factors for breast cancer are associated with hormonal and reproductive factors. It is thought that estrogen promotes the growth and development of mutated breast cells. It seems that the longer your breast tissue is exposed to your body's circulating estrogen, the greater the risk for breast cancer.

1. *Age* Breast cancer is more common in women over 50 years of age. More than 75 percent of breast cancers occur in postmenopausal women. Increasing age also makes other risk factors discussed below more likely to occur. When two or more risk factors are combined, your risk is greater than with the one risk factor alone.

2. *Previous breast cancer* A history of breast cancer increases the odds that a woman will get breast cancer again, in the same and in the opposite breast.

3. *Family history of breast cancer* If you have a first-degree relative with breast cancer (a mother, sister or daughter), your risk is approximately doubled. There is an even greater risk if more than one close relative is affected, or if the cancer has occurred at a young age in a family member.

4. *Age of first pregnancy* Women who have children before 30 years of age have a lower risk of breast cancer. Women who have their first child after 30 have a higher risk, and women who never have children are at an even greater risk. Many experts believe that the important factor here is the amount of time between menarche (the age when you began menstruating) and first pregnancy. The theory is that the developing breast tissue is most sensitive to carcinogens during this time. Pregnancy hormones mature the breast cells and make them more resistant to carcinogens. It may be that these same pregnancy hormones stimulate mutated breast cells in a woman who has her first baby after 30 years of age.

5. *Age of first period (menarche)* Onset of your period at a young age—before 12 years of age—is associated with a slightly higher risk of breast cancer. It is believed that the longer breast tissue is exposed to endogenous estrogen (estrogen that's made in your body), the greater the chance for cells to become cancerous.

6. *Late menopause* Women who menstruate for longer than 40 years have a slightly higher risk of breast cancer. Like early menarche, late menopause influences the amount of time breast cells are exposed to estrogen.

The list below describes factors that may play a role in the development of breast cancer, but they are less well understood:

1. *Exposure to radiation* Ionizing radiation from x-rays taken at a younger age may increase the risk for breast cancer later in life. However, experts feel exposure to radiation is probably a minor contributor to your overall risk.

2. *Use of hormones* Studies have failed to show an increased breast cancer risk in young women who take birth control pills. However, the same cannot be said for older women taking hormone replacement therapy (HRT). In July 2002 the Women's Health Initiative (WHI), one of the largest-ever studies of HRT, was abruptly halted because of health risks. The researchers reported that the risk for breast cancer was 26 percent higher in the group of women taking combined HRT (estrogen plus progestin). On average there were about 38 cases of invasive breast cancer per 10,000 women, compared to 30 cases among women taking the placebo. For an individual woman, this translates into an increased risk of less than one tenth of one percent a year. Despite this small increase in risk, the study revealed that the longer a woman stayed on HRT, the more her risk increased. Clearly, the pros and cons of combined HRT need to be discussed with your physician.

3. *Diet* A growing body of research is finding a link between certain diet factors and the risk of breast cancer. Diet affects breast cancer development either by initiating cancer growth and causing a genetic mutation, or by promoting the growth of cancerous cells.

❧

Diagnosis

All American women aged 40 and older should have a screening mammogram every year, in combination with a physical exam of the breasts by a trained health professional. A mammogram is a special x-ray of the breast that shows the location of a lump, its size and certain characteristics that may be suggestive of cancer. If a lump looks suspicious to your physician, further tests will be done to determine if it's malignant and cancerous. Mammograms use very low doses of radiation and do not cause breast cancer, nor do they make an existing cancer worse. A mammogram is a very important screening tool that can catch breast cancer early and lead to a significant improvement in survival.

It is generally accepted that mammograms in women over 50 years of age save lives, but this is less certain in women aged 40 to 49 years. Currently some health professionals do not recommend routine mammograms for this age group, based on results from the Canadian National Breast Screening Study. In this ten-year study of 25,000 women aged 40 to 49 years, there was no difference in breast cancer death rates between women screened and women who were not screened.[1]

The breast self-exam is an important way for you to detect physical changes in your breasts. By the age of 20, all women should routinely perform monthly breast self-exams. Use the pads of your fingers to examine the tissue in your breasts and in your armpits. (Go to **www.cancer.org** for a step-by-step guide to breast self-examination.) Breast self-exams should be practiced at the same time each month. Be sure to also look carefully at your breast for any noticeable physical changes, such as a lump in the breast or underarm area, unusual breast swelling, change in color or texture of skin on the breast, blood leakage from the nipple or inversion of the nipple. Any of these changes should prompt a visit to your family doctor.

Preventing Breast Cancer

When it comes to breast cancer, dietary factors such as fat, alcohol, fiber, fruits and vegetables have all been well studied. Below, I list nutrition recommendations based on our current body of scientific evidence. Some of these strategies have strong research to support their adoption; others have evidence to suggest that they *may* be helpful. While scientists are still learning the role of nutrition in the risk of breast cancer, making these dietary changes will improve your overall well-being, not to mention possibly lowering your chances of getting breast cancer.

DIETARY STRATEGIES

Dietary Fat

Nutrition researchers used to think that a high-fat diet increased the risk of breast cancer. However, it now seems the high-fat diet/breast cancer link is not as clear-cut as we had once thought.

Scientists became interested in the link between fat intake and breast cancer when they noticed that women in countries where diets were low in fat had much lower rates of breast cancer than women in countries with higher-fat diets. It has been hypothesized that dietary fat may increase breast cancer risk by affecting estrogen metabolism. Studies have found that vegetarian women who follow a low-fat, high-fiber diet have lower levels of estrogen and less breast cancer. A high-fat diet may also lead to breast cancer by promoting weight gain and body fat accumulation, which in turn increases the risk of breast cancer.

Most large studies have failed to show a strong relationship between total fat intake and breast cancer risk. A recent 14-year study of 89,000 women found no evidence that a high-fat diet promoted breast cancer, or that a low-fat diet protected against it. It is possible that women in these studies didn't reduce their fat intake enough to see a benefit. The current recommendation of "no more than 30 percent of your daily calories from fat" might be too high to offer protection from breast cancer.

A large Canadian study is underway to determine if a very low-fat diet can prevent breast cancer. So far, one report from this trial found that women who ate a 21 percent fat diet for two years had significantly reduced dense breast areas seen by mammogram (dense breast areas are a risk factor for cancer), compared to women on a 30 percent fat diet.[2] Another report from this research group revealed that women who followed a 15 percent fat diet for two years had lower levels of circulating estrogen, which could offer protection over the long term. Based on these initial reports, I do believe that following a low-fat diet is a wise precautionary measure.

SATURATED FAT

Several studies have looked at the relationship between foods high in saturated fat, such as meat and dairy products, and breast cancer. When it comes to meat, the findings are mixed. Some studies show that higher meat intakes are linked to a greater risk, whereas others don't show any effect. The harmful effect of meat may be due to its saturated fat content, or it may be due to the way it's prepared. Cooking meat at high temperatures forms compounds called heterocyclic amines, which have been shown to cause breast tumors in animals; this may hold true for women, too. A University of Minnesota study found that women who ate hamburger, steak and bacon well-done were more than four times as likely to have breast cancer than women who enjoyed their meat cooked rare or medium.[3] Until we know more about the effect of cooked meat, breast cancer experts advise that we consume no more than 3 ounces (80 grams) of meat each day.

It may be that whole milk offers protection from breast cancer. Finnish researchers studied 4697 women for 25 years, and discovered that the women who had the highest intake of milk had a 48 percent lower risk of developing breast cancer than women who drank the least.[4] Scientists speculate that a special fatty acid called conjugated linoleic acid (CLA) might be responsible for milk's protective effect. CLA occurs naturally in dairy products and meat, and has been shown in a number of animal studies to inhibit breast cancer growth.

Omega-3 Fats

You may want to start eating more fish. In population studies, eating plenty of fish for many years is associated with a lower risk of breast cancer. While no trials have been done in women, one animal study did find that omega-3 fats from fish oil actually suppressed growth of human breast cancer cells and metastases in female mice (scientists inject human breast cancer cells into mice to study the effects of different carcinogens).[5] Despite the lack of strong evidence of fish's protective effect, the existing studies do suggest that you should get more omega-3 fats in your diet. My recommendation is to eat fatty fish three times a week.

Soy Foods

Populations that consume the largest amount of soy in their diet have the lowest rates of breast cancer. Researchers attribute soy's possible protective effect to naturally occurring compounds called isoflavones. When we consume soy foods, bacteria in our intestinal tract convert isoflavones to compounds that have an estrogenlike effect in the body. Acting as weak estrogen compounds, isoflavones are able to attach to estrogen receptors in the body. Genistein and daidzein are the most active soy isoflavones, and have been the focus of much research. Researchers believe that if genistein can bind to estrogen receptors in the breast, they can block the ability of a woman's own estrogen from taking that spot. That means that breast cells have less contact with estrogen.

Studies in the laboratory suggest that isoflavones protect from breast cancer. Studies in animals show that supplementing the diet with soy inhibits the growth of breast tumors; studies on human breast cancer cells have found similar effects. But the question remains: does eating soy on a regular basis lower a woman's risk of breast cancer? No study has been conducted to show what years of eating a high-soy diet does to breast cancer risk. A handful of studies have shown that a regular intake of soy isoflavones may lower circulating levels of estrogen and this might reduce a woman's future risk of breast cancer. Other studies show that consuming a soy-rich diet can lengthen a woman's menstrual cycle, thereby influencing how much estrogen your breast cells are exposed to. Based on what we know today, most experts believe women must consume soy foods over their lifetime to realize the potential benefits of soy isoflavones on breast health.

What if you're at high risk for breast cancer? Or perhaps you're a survivor of the disease, and you're leery about eating foods with so-called plant estrogens. The estrogenlike properties of isoflavones have led some experts to be concerned about the use of soy in women with breast cancer because estrogen may increase this risk. Some preliminary studies show that soy has protective effects for breast cancer, while others suggest soy might increase breast cell growth. Because we lack sufficient reliable information about the effect of soy foods on women with breast cancer, a history of breast cancer or a family history of breast cancer, soy should be treated with caution. Until more is known, I advise women in these situations to avoid consuming large amounts of soy each day. I certainly recommend that these women avoid using soy protein powders and isoflavone supplements. But that doesn't mean you have to give up soy foods. Consuming soy foods three times a week as part of a plant-based diet is considered safe.

If you want to start eating soy foods because they might help reduce your risk of breast cancer, and because they have other health benefits (such as protecting from heart disease), try the following tips to enjoy more soy:

- *Try a calcium-fortified soy beverage.* Pour it on cereal, add it to soups, use it in baking or enjoy it on its own. Find a product that you like—depending on how they are made, brands can taste very different.

- *Snack on roasted soy nuts.* These are crunchy, are full of phytoestrogens and have less fat and more fiber than other nuts. Enjoy them as a snack or sprinkle them over your salad. They also come in flavored varieties.

- *Cook with canned soybeans.* Check out the canned bean aisle of your grocery store for these no-fuss beans. If you can't find them there, look in the ethnic food section. Add them to chilies, pasta sauces, soups and salads. If you have the time, buy them dried, soak them overnight, then simmer for one hour until they're cooked.

- *Use soy deli meats* in place of pepperoni or salami on pizzas and in sandwiches.

- *Try soy ground round* in your next pasta or burrito recipe.

- *Bake with soy flour.* You'll find defatted soy flour at your local health food store. Replace one-quarter to one-half of the all-purpose flour in recipes with soy flour.

- *Try cooking with tofu or tempeh.* For recipes, information and free brochures on soy foods, visit **www.unitedsoybean.org** or write to United Soybean Board, 16640 Chesterfield Grove Road, Suite 130, Chesterfield, MO 63005-1429 (Tel: 1-800-989-8721).

- *Make a morning power shake* with 1 tablespoon (15 ml) of protein powder made from isolated soy protein.

Flaxseed

These tiny whole-grain brown and golden seeds contain a natural compound called lignans. When we eat flaxseed, bacteria in our gut convert these plant lignans to human lignans, which look very much like estrogen in the body. Once in the body, phytoestrogens from flaxseed have a weak estrogen action and they are able to bind to estrogen receptors (just like soy isoflavones). In so doing, they appear to block the action of our body's own estrogen on breast cells.

Animal studies conducted at the University of Toronto have shown that flaxseed has anti-cancer properties.[6] And a recent Canadian study found that flaxseed can slow breast cancer growth in women. Researchers at Princess Margaret Hospital in Toronto and Toronto General Hospital studied 50 women who had been recently diagnosed with breast cancer.[7] While waiting for their surgery, the women were divided into two groups. One group received a daily muffin containing 50 grams of ground flaxseed (about 2 tablespoons) and the remaining women were given an ordinary muffin. When the tumors were removed, the researchers found that the women who had received the flaxseed muffins had slower-growing tumors than the others. These exciting findings suggest that a daily intake of flaxseed might offer protection from breast cancer.

Besides lignans, flaxseed is a source of fiber and of an essential fatty acid our body needs, called alpha linolenic acid. Aim to get 1 to 2 tablespoons of ground flaxseed each day. Grind your flaxseed in a clean coffee grinder or use a mortar and pestle. If you want to spend the extra money, you can also buy flaxseed pre-ground at health food stores. Here are a few ways to add crunch and a great nutty flavor to your meals:

- Add ground flaxseed to hot cereals, muffin batters and cookie mixes. I have clients who even add it to cold breakfast cereal!
- Mix ground flaxseed into a single serving of yogurt.
- Sprinkle flaxseed on salads and soups.
- Add flaxseed to casseroles.
- Try a loaf of flaxseed bread. Check your local bakery or supermarket.
- Try Red River cereal, another good source of flaxseed.

Once you grind flaxseed, store it in an airtight container in the fridge or freezer. The natural fats in flaxseed go rancid quickly if exposed to air and heat.

Fruits and Vegetables

More than 200 studies from around the world have shown that a diet high in fruit and vegetables lowers the risk of many cancers, including breast cancer. Researchers from Harvard University studied more than 89,000 women and found that those who ate more than 2.2 servings of vegetables a day had a 20 percent lower risk of breast cancer than those who ate less than one serving.[8] Another study in premenopausal women found that high total vegetable intake lowered the risk of breast cancer by 54 percent.[9]

It appears that dark green vegetables are most protective. Spinach, kale, rapini, collard greens, Swiss chard and romaine lettuce are good sources of beta-carotene, an antioxidant nutrient that might protect breast cells from damage caused by harmful free radical molecules—free radicals roam the body and damage the genetic material of cells, which may lead to cancer development.

Popping beta-carotene pills does not have the same protective powers. Scientists are learning that there's more to fruits and vegetables than vitamins, minerals and fiber. They also contain thousands of phytochemicals, naturally occurring compounds that act as antioxidants and natural antibiotics, and so may inhibit cancer development. Experts believe that phytochemicals probably work together with vitamins and minerals in the food. In a nutshell, it's the whole food that seems to be most important in cancer prevention.

Make sure you get at least five to ten servings of fruits and vegetables each day. Aim for a minimum of three fruits and three vegetables. Here are a few ways to get more "green" into your diet:

- *Spinach* One-half cup (125 ml) of cooked spinach provides your full day's requirement of vitamin A and offers plenty of folate (read more about the possible role of folate in breast cancer prevention in the section on Vitamins and Minerals on page 145). Spinach is also an excellent source of vitamin C. One-half cup (125 ml) cooked has more nutrition than 1 cup (250 ml) raw because it contains 2 cups (500 ml) of leaves, and heating makes the protein in spinach easier to break down. Steam, braise or stir-fry with a little garlic; add a splash of balsamic vinegar at the end of cooking.

- *Kale* Just 1 cup (250 ml) of this member of the cabbage family provides more than twice the daily requirements of beta-carotene and vitamin C. Kale is also a good source of calcium and vitamin E, another important antioxidant. Steam or stir-fry this green with other vegetables, or throw kale into soup and simmer. Kale shrinks a lot during cooking; 3 cups (750 ml) raw will give you 1 cup (250 ml) cooked.

- *Collard greens* In addition to plenty of vitamins and minerals, this vegetable contains natural sulfur compounds that may prevent certain cancers. Stir-fry collards then add a dash of roasted sesame oil and a handful of cashews.

- *Beet greens* The next time you buy fresh beets, save the greens and eat them, too. The green tops of root vegetables have more nutrition than the root when it comes to vitamins and minerals. These greens are a good source of vitamins A and C, as well as calcium and iron. Prepare them as you would any green.

- *Swiss chard* Here's another great vegetable that provides calcium, beta-carotene and vitamin C. Use both the leaves and the stalks when cooking, but add the leaves at the end of cooking, as the stalks take longer to soften. Stir-fry Swiss chard with a little olive oil and garlic, or add lemon juice and Parmesan cheese; it's also great in pasta with a little olive oil and red pepper flakes.

Fiber and Wheat Bran

Although research is preliminary, there is evidence to suggest that a high fiber intake may offer protection from breast cancer. Toronto researchers found that 20 grams of fiber per day was associated with a modest effect that was statistically significant.[10]

Fiber may help lower your risk of breast cancer by binding to estrogen in the intestine and causing it to be excreted in the stool. Every day, your intestine reabsorbs estrogen from bile, the compound that's released into your intestine from your gallbladder to help digest fat. If dietary fiber can attach to estrogen and facilitate its removal from the body, your body has to take estrogen out of your bloodstream to make more bile. The net result is a lower level of circulating estrogen. It's possible that following a high-fiber diet for many years could lower your risk for breast cancer.

High-fiber diets also tend to be higher in antioxidant vitamins and lower in fat, both of which might protect from breast cancer. People who eat plenty of fiber also tend to maintain a healthy weight. There are many possible explanations for fiber's protective effect. The studies do suggest, however, that dietary fiber works best if you follow a low-fat diet. So adding a little wheat bran to a diet that's high in fat and low in fruits and vegetables probably won't do you much good. More and more we are learning that health protection comes from a combination of healthy foods in the diet.

Dietary fiber is actually made up of two types of fiber, soluble and insoluble. Both types are present in varying proportions in different plant foods, but some foods may be rich in one or the other. And both types of fiber function differently in your body to promote health.

Foods like wheat bran, whole grains and some vegetables contain mainly insoluble fibers. Like their name suggests, these fibers do not dissolve in water, but they do have a significant capacity for retaining water. In this way they act to increase stool bulk and promote regularity. And it's wheat bran (insoluble fiber) that's been studied the most in relation to breast cancer risk.

Soluble fibers do dissolve in water. Dried peas, beans and lentils, oats, barley, psyllium husks, apples and citrus fruits are good sources of soluble fiber. When you consume these foods, the soluble fibers form a gel in your stomach and slow the rate of digestion and absorption.

It's estimated that North Americans are getting 11 to 14 grams of fiber each day, only half of what is recommended. Health authorities agree that a daily intake of 25 grams of total dietary fiber is needed to reap its health benefits. To learn what foods are higher in fiber, see the table on page 29 in chapter 1. To boost your intake of insoluble fiber and wheat bran, try the following:

- Strive for at least five servings of fruits and vegetables every day.
- Leave the peel on fruits and vegetables whenever possible.
- Eat at least five servings of whole-grain foods each day.
- Buy high-fiber breakfast cereals. Aim for at least 4 to 5 grams of fiber per serving (check the nutrition information panel).
- Add 2 tablespoons (30 ml) of natural wheat bran or oat bran to cereals, yogurt, casseroles and soup.
- Add nuts and seeds to salads.
- Reach for high-fiber snacks like popcorn, nuts, dried apricots or dates.

Don't increase your fiber intake overnight; instead, gradually build up to the daily 25 grams of fiber. Too much fiber too soon can cause bloating, gas and diarrhea. And don't forget that fiber needs water to work. Drink 8 ounces of fluid with every high-fiber meal and snack.

Yogurt and Fermented Milk

There is some evidence to suggest that a regular intake of yogurt might protect you from breast cancer. One study, in which researchers compared the diets of women with breast cancer to the diets of women free of the disease, showed that women who ate a low-fat diet with plenty of fiber and fermented milk products had a lower risk for breast cancer.[11] And studies conducted in the lab have shown that fermented milk can slow the growth of breast cancer cells.[12] These foods contain what are called lactic acid bacteria. Once in your intestinal tract, these bacteria form active compounds that suppress the growth of organisms that produce cancer-causing substances.

In America, all commercial yogurts are made using two lactic acid bacteria: L. bulgaricus and S. thermophilus. Some manufacturers add other strains, such as bifidobacteria, L. acidophilus and L. casei. To begin reaping the health benefits of these friendly bacteria, include one serving of yogurt in your daily diet. You might also try kefir or sweet acidophilus milk, fermented milk beverages available in most supermarkets.

PROBIOTIC SUPPLEMENTS

The term probiotic means "to promote life." It refers to living organisms that, upon ingestion in certain numbers, improve the microbial balance in the intestine and exert health benefits. Yogurt and kefir are considered probiotic foods. If you don't eat dairy products, probiotic capsules or tablets are an alternative. In fact, many natural health experts believe that taking a high-quality supplement is the only way to ensure you're getting a sufficient number of friendly bacteria into your intestinal tract. Here are a few considerations when choosing a product:

- *Buy a product that offers 1 to 10 billion live cells per dose.* Taking more than this may result in gastrointestinal discomfort.

- For greater convenience, *choose a product that is stable at room temperature* and does not require refrigeration. This allows you to continue taking your supplement while traveling or at the office. Good manufacturers will test their products to ensure that they maintain their viability over a long period of time.

- *Know the type and source of bacteria in the supplement.* Many experts believe that supplements made from human strains of bacteria are better adapted for growth in the human intestinal tract. When choosing a product, you might ask the pharmacist or retailer if the formula contains human or non-human strains.

- *Always take your supplement with food.* Upon eating a meal, the stomach contents become less acidic due to the presence of food. This allows live bacteria to withstand stomach acid and reach their final destination in the intestinal tract.

Tea (*Camellia sinensis*)

There is a growing body of evidence to suggest that tea protects from certain cancers, including breast cancer. The famous Nurses' Health Study from Harvard found that drinking four or more cups of tea per day (versus one or fewer) was associated with 30 percent lower risk of breast cancer.[13] Animal studies have also revealed that clear tea, tea with milk and extracts of tea can block breast cancer development.

Like fruits and vegetables, tea is a plant food, and as such it contains natural chemicals that act as antioxidants. The antioxidants in tea leaves belong to a special class of compounds called catechins. By mopping up harmful free radical molecules in the body, catechins in tea may prevent damage to the genetic material of breast cells.

There are three main types of tea: green tea, black tea and oolong. All three come from the same tea plant, but they are processed differently. Herbal teas are not made from tea leaves and, as a result, they don't have the antioxidant properties of green and black tea. Here are a few tips to help you get a little tea into your diet.

- If you drink coffee in the afternoon, replace it with tea.
- The next time you're at the grocery store, pick up a box of green tea bags.
- If you're preparing an Asian meal at home, serve it with a pot of green tea. Use the bags or buy it loose.
- Replace all regular and diet soft drinks with tea.
- Enjoy a cup of tea with your mid-day snack. Try different flavors like Earl Grey, apricot or black currant.

The next time you're at your local coffee bar, try chai tea, a spicy hot drink made from tea and spices. To cut down on the sugar content, ask for half the amount of syrup.

Alcoholic Beverages

There is enough evidence to conclude that alcohol probably does increase your risk of breast cancer. In a review of 38 studies conducted up until 1992, researchers concluded that having one, two or three drinks a day all increased the risk of breast cancer.[14] And the more alcohol a woman consumed, the higher her risk. Based on these findings, nutrition and cancer experts recommend that women do not drink alcohol. If consumed at all, alcoholic drinks should be limited to one a day or seven per week.

Alcohol may make breast cells more vulnerable to the effects of carcinogens, or it may enhance the liver's processing of these substances. Alcohol may inhibit the ability of cells to repair faulty genes. Alcohol may also increase estrogen levels in the body.

If you need to lower your daily intake of alcohol, replace alcoholic beverages with sparkling mineral water, Clamato or tomato juice or soda with a splash of cranberry juice. Eliminate alcoholic beverages on evenings that you are not entertaining. Save your glass of wine or cocktail for social occasions.

Weight Control

A number of studies have determined that gaining weight after menopause is linked with a higher risk of breast cancer.[15] Obesity may influence breast cancer risk by increasing circulating estrogen levels, since estrogen is produced in body fat cells. If you are overweight, or if you have gained weight since menopause, I strongly advise that you take steps to lose weight. Start by determining your body mass index (BMI) to get a sense of how your current weight is affecting your health—see chapter 2 to calculate your BMI and to find strategies and a meal plan to help get you started.

VITAMINS AND MINERALS

Carotenoids

In my discussion of fruits and vegetables, I told you that green vegetables high in beta-carotene are thought to be more protective than other vegetables. Toronto scientists estimated that women who get the most beta-carotene in their diet reduce their risk of breast cancer by 15 percent.[16] Researchers have also learned that a diet rich in beta-carotene fruits and vegetables may improve breast cancer survival.

Beta-carotene has two roles in the body. It has an antioxidant effect, which can help protect our genes from oxidative damage caused by free radicals. But beta-carotene is also converted to vitamin A inside the body. Vitamin A is essential for proper cell growth and development, and it also enhances our body's immune system. Both roles may help keep breast cancer at bay.

More than 600 different carotenoid compounds exist in plants. While beta-carotene is the most plentiful, other important carotenoids include lutein and lycopene. Researchers are investigating the link between these carotenoids and breast cancer risk. The Harvard Nurses' Health Study from Harvard University found that premenopausal women who ate five or more servings of high-carotenoid fruits and vegetables had a lower risk of breast cancer than women who ate less than two servings a day.[17]

Dietary carotenoids aren't that well absorbed. But you'll absorb more of them if you eat these foods with a little fat. Try a yogurt dip with carrot sticks, a little olive oil in lycopene-rich pasta sauce or a splash of salad dressing on your roasted red pepper.

Use my list below to increase your intake of carotenoid-rich fruits and vegetables. Every day, aim for five servings of 1/2 cup (125 ml) each.

BETA-CAROTENE	LYCOPENE	LUTEIN
Carrots	Tomatoes	Beet greens
Squash	Tomato sauce	Collards
Sweet potato	Tomato juice	Corn
Red pepper	Guava	Kale
Cantaloupe	Grapefruit, red and pink	Okra
Peach	Watermelon	Red pepper
Nectarine	Romaine lettuce	
Mango	Spinach	
Papaya		

Vitamin C

Although the research findings on vitamin C are less consistent than for beta-carotene, there is evidence to suggest you should be getting more in your diet. The vitamin may keep women healthy by acting as an antioxidant or it may work by enhancing the body's immune system. Vitamin C also plays an important role in the synthesis of collagen, an important tissue in the breast.

For women, the daily recommended intake for vitamin C is 75 milligrams (if you smoke you need 110 milligrams). This amount is easy to get from your diet. For a look at your best bets for vitamin C, see the Vitamin C in Foods table on page 12 in chapter 1.

VITAMIN C SUPPLEMENTS

At this time, there is no evidence to warrant vitamin C supplements for breast cancer prevention; it won't do harm if you're already taking one. But before you pop a pill every day, make sure you add one or two vitamin-C-rich foods to your daily diet. Don't forget that fruits and vegetables have plenty of other protective compounds that may work in tandem with vitamin C to keep you healthy. If you find your diet lacks these foods, or you want to increase your vitamin C intake further, use the following guide when taking vitamin C supplements.

- Take 500 or 600 milligrams of vitamin C, once or twice daily. Taking more than 200 milligrams of vitamin C at once won't increase your blood levels further. I've recommended 500 or 600 milligrams because these are the most common doses you'll find. If you want to take more, you're better off splitting your dose over the course of the day.

- Look for a brand that states "Ester C" on the label. This is a patented form of vitamin C that laboratory studies have found to be up to four times more available to the body than regular vitamin C (ascorbic acid or ascorbate).

- If you prefer a chewable supplement, make sure it's made from calcium ascorbate or sodium ascorbate. These forms of the vitamin are less acidic, so they're easier on the enamel of your teeth.

Vitamin B12

Although preliminary, one recent study suggests that a deficiency of vitamin B12 may increase the risk of breast cancer.[18] It's thought that depleted levels of vitamin B12 can cause damage to DNA molecules. In the body, vitamin B12 works very closely with folate, an important B vitamin that's needed to synthesize DNA in cells. Folate is needed to activate B12 and vice versa.

Most B12 deficiencies are caused by impaired absorption, not a poor diet. After we consume B12 in our diet, the acid in our stomachs helps to release the B12 from proteins in food. The vitamin then binds to the intrinsic factor that enables B12 to be absorbed into our bloodstream. You can develop a B12 deficiency if your stomach produces an insufficient amount of hydrochloric acid, a condition common in older adults. But some people inherit a defective gene for intrinsic factor. They don't produce this necessary factor required for B12 to enter the bloodstream, which leads to a deficiency of the vitamin.

Vitamin B12 is found exclusively in animal foods. If you eat meat, poultry and dairy products on a regular basis you're probably okay for B12. The recommended intake for adults is 2.4 micrograms per day.

For strict vegetarians who eat no animal products and don't drink a fortified soy beverage, I strongly recommend a B12 supplement. As a matter of fact, anyone over the age of 50 should be getting their B12 from supplements or fortified foods. That's because up to one-third of older adults produce inadequate amounts of stomach acid and have lost the ability to properly absorb B12 from food. In this case, I recommend a good multivitamin and mineral supplement or a B complex supplement that contains the whole family of B vitamins.

Folate

If you drink alcohol you might consider getting more folate in your diet. A recent Harvard study found that, among women who consumed 15 grams of alcohol per day (about 1-1/2 glasses of beer or wine), those with the highest daily intake of folate (600 micrograms/day) had a 45 percent lower risk for breast cancer compared with women with the lowest folate intake (150–299 micrograms/day).[19] It's thought that alcohol interferes with the transport and metabolism of folate, and may deprive body tissues of this B vitamin, which is essential to DNA synthesis.

To help you meet the recommended daily intake of 400 micrograms a day, practice the following:

- Eat spinach, asparagus and artichokes more often. These vegetables have the most folate, with spinach leading the pack.

- Drink a glass of orange juice with your morning meal.

- Use lentils and other legumes in pasta sauces, chilies and tacos.

- Most often, choose whole-grain breads and cereals.

- Take a multivitamin and mineral supplement or a B complex supplement to ensure you're meeting your needs.

- If you take separate folic acid supplements, be sure to buy one that has vitamin B12 added (folic acid is the synthetic form of folate found in vitamin pills and fortified foods; folate refers to the vitamin as it occurs naturally in foods).

- Refer to my list of folate-rich foods on page 7 in chapter 1.

THE BOTTOM LINE...
Leslie's recommendations for preventing breast cancer

1. Reduce your intake of saturated fat, especially from meat:
   - Eat no more than 3 ounces (80 grams) of meat each day.
   - For protein, choose lean poultry, fish, beans and soy foods most often.
   - When you do eat meat, avoid cooking it well-done.
   - To help you eat an overall low-fat diet, choose 1% or skim milk, yogurt with 1% milkfat (MF) or less and cheese with 15% MF content or less.

2. To get more omega-3 polyunsaturated fat, eat fish three times a week.

3. Eat one soy food each day to boost your intake of soy protein and isoflavones. Encourage your daughters to incorporate these foods into their diet, since researchers believe that it is a lifetime intake that offers protection from breast cancer.

4. To get plant estrogens called lignans, add 1 or 2 tablespoons of ground flaxseed to your foods and recipes.

5. Eat at least five to ten servings of fruits and vegetables every single day.
   - Make sure five of these servings are foods brimming with carotenoid compounds.
   - To boost your intake of vitamin C, get one or two foods packed with this vitamin.

6. Gradually increase your dietary fiber intake to 25 grams each day. To help lower blood levels of your body's own estrogen, focus on foods rich in wheat bran, such as whole-grain breads, 100 percent bran cereals and whole-wheat pasta.

7. Include one probiotic food, such as yogurt or kefir, in your diet each day to get more friendly bacteria in your intestinal tract. If you don't eat these foods, consider taking a probiotic supplement once a day with a meal.

8. Drink more green and black tea to get a source of catechins, natural antioxidant compounds found in tea leaves.

9. Avoid alcoholic beverages. If you do drink, consume no more than one drink each day.

10. Manage your weight before and after menopause.

11. Get more B vitamins into your diet every day, especially folate and vitamin B12. If you drink alcoholic beverages, be sure to boost your intake of folate. To ensure you are meeting your needs, take a multivitamin and mineral supplement every day.

9

Fibrocystic Breast Conditions

Formerly called fibrocystic breast disease, this disorder affects about one-half of all women. If you have ever felt a lump in your breast, you know how frightening the experience can be—it's only natural to worry that the lump could be a sign of breast cancer. Fortunately, most breast lumps are not cancer. Many women live a normal, active life with breasts that are tender and lumpy.

Fibrocystic breast conditions may include breast nodules, breast swelling, tenderness and pain. A woman may experience breast pain only, lumpiness only, or both. Although these breast conditions can be painful, and suspicious lumps can cause anxiety, most do not increase a woman's risk of breast cancer.

The main symptoms of fibrocystic breast conditions are swelling and pain in the breasts, which waxes and wanes with the menstrual cycle. However, women who are severely affected by this condition complain of continuous discomfort. And up to 50 percent of women with breast pain report that it interferes with their sex life and physical activity. Occasionally, a woman may develop breast cysts that require medical attention.

What Causes Fibrocystic Breast Conditions?

The exact cause of this disorder is not known. Most women eventually develop some lumpiness in their breasts. Breast changes usually appear during the years a woman menstruates, and regress with the onset of menopause. In most cases, the small, round lumps appear in the breasts because of hormonal changes associated with menstruation. The hormones estrogen and progesterone that control your menstrual cycle trigger physical responses that make your breasts become lumpy, or fibrocystic, and painful. It's thought that a deficiency of progesterone and an excess of estrogen in the last 14 days of a woman's menstrual cycle are responsible for breast changes.

These symptoms are collectively referred to as fibrocystic breast conditions. You may also hear breast pain and tenderness called cyclic mastalagia or mastitis. Because fibrocystic breast conditions are influenced by hormonal cycles, a woman will find that her breasts become increasingly tender and painful as her body prepares for menstruation. The discomfort normally subsides once her period starts. Over time, breast lumps may develop into cysts, which fill with fluid, causing swelling and pain. Up to 20 percent of women with fibrocystic breast conditions say that their symptoms spontaneously improve over time.

Fibrocystic breast conditions are often associated with the symptoms of premenstrual syndrome (PMS). Some researchers believe that hormonelike compounds called prostaglandins are responsible for causing breast changes. A handful of studies indicate that the development of lumpy breasts may also be stimulated by a diet that includes higher levels of caffeine and dietary fat. Despite these other theories, most of the clues about the cause of fibrocystic breast conditions suggest that estrogen is the key.

Symptoms

Breast lumpiness is one of the main characteristics of fibrocystic breast conditions. A woman may discover only one lump, but it is more common to have multiple lumps. The lumps are tender, come in different sizes and usually move freely within the breast tissue. A woman may also experience some breast pain and swelling, which will become worse just before her menstrual period.

Who's at Risk?

Fibrocystic breast conditions can affect women from puberty to old age. However, this condition affects approximately 50 percent of women between the ages of 30 to 50 years. Breast symptoms usually disappear with menopause, and it is quite rare to find the disorder in postmenopausal women unless they are taking hormone replacement therapy.

Diagnosis

Up to 85 percent of breast lumps are found by patients through breast self-examination. The American Cancer Society recommends that all American women over the age of 20 should be examining their breasts regularly every month. (Go to **www.cancer.org** for a detailed guide to breast self-examination.) The self-examination should be done five to ten days after menstruation, at the same time each month. Using the pads of your fingers, you should examine all of your breast tissue and the tissue under your armpits. You should also examine your breasts visually, looking for physical changes or differences between your breasts. This practice should be continued even when you no longer menstruate. It's also recommended that once a woman turns 40, she have a mammogram (specialized breast x-ray) once every two years to determine overall breast health.

Fibrocystic breast conditions can sometimes imitate the symptoms of true breast cancer or can hide the presence of cancerous growths. Fibrocystic breast lumps and cysts normally feel soft or slightly firm, tender and painful. This distinguishes them from cancerous growths, which tend to be hard and don't usually cause tenderness and pain. However, if a woman's fibrocystic breast condition becomes more advanced, chronic inflammation may cause the soft, fluid-filled cysts to harden and thicken. When this happens, it becomes increasingly difficult to tell the difference between non-cancerous and cancerous growths.

To distinguish hardened cysts from breast cancer, your doctor may order some specific diagnostic tests. He or she will begin by taking a medical history and conducting a physical examination. Your doctor may then order radiological tests, such as a mammogram or an ultrasound (sound wave picture), which are useful in identifying breast cysts. Or your doctor may perform a simple procedure called a needle aspiration. In this test, fluid is removed from the lump using a small, hollow needle. Needle aspiration is also used to drain the contents of large, fluid-filled cysts, in an attempt to relieve pressure on surrounding breast tissue.

In some cases, your doctor may feel that a biopsy is necessary. A small piece of tissue from the lump will be surgically removed and sent to a laboratory for microscopic examination. This procedure will determine if the cells in the lump are benign (non-cancerous) or malignant (cancerous).

❧

Conventional Treatment

If you are suffering from painful breasts at certain times during the month, you may find that putting cold compresses on the tender areas and wearing a well-fitting, supportive bra both day and night will relieve some of your discomfort. Your doctor may recommend pain relievers to treat the aches and pains. If fibrocystic breast conditions are causing you severe pain, you may be treated with medications such as Cyclomen® (danazol), a mild, synthetic male hormone, or tamoxifen, a drug that blocks the action of estrogen. Because these drugs can produce side effects, they should be used for only a short time.

❧

Managing Fibrocystic Breast Conditions

You may have read a number of dietary and nutritional therapies that claim to alleviate your breast symptoms. Based on a review of well-designed studies conducted in women with fibrocystic breast conditions, there is unfortunately little evidence at this time to strongly support many of these popular recommendations. While there is only weak evidence to say that diet may be the cause of fibrocystic breast conditions, what you eat may very well aggravate your symptoms. And since a high level of estrogen, or an increased sensitivity to estrogen, seems to be the dominant theory, any dietary modification that can reduce your circulating level of estrogen may help lessen your symptoms. The first three diet tips—reducing fat, increasing fiber and eating more soy—address this point.

DIETARY STRATEGIES

Dietary Fat

If you have a fibrocystic breast condition, reducing the amount of fat you eat—from the typical North American intake of 35 percent of calories to 15 or 20 percent—may be beneficial. Although studies have not investigated the effect of a low-fat diet on fibrocystic breast conditions per se, there is indirect evidence to support this strategy. Research in women with breast dysplasia (abnormal growth of breast cells) has found a low-fat diet to have a positive effect on the density of breast tissue and the composition of breast fluid.

Eating a high-fat diet is also associated with higher levels of circulating estrogen and cholesterol, a building block of hormones. Studies reveal that when women reduce their fat intake, their blood estrogen levels also decline. The strongest theory for fibrocystic breast conditions is an imbalance between estrogen and progesterone, and excessive levels of estrogen seem to be a key factor. In two small studies, women with fibrocystic breast conditions who followed a 21 percent fat diet for three months experienced a significantly lower level of circulating estrogen and cholesterol.[1] The low-fat diet did not alter progesterone levels.

To understand how dietary fat influences the amount of estrogen that circulates throughout your body, let me take you on a brief course in estrogen metabolism (don't worry, it's very brief!). Your liver attaches estrogen to a molecule of glucaronic acid or a sulfate residue, compounds that make estrogen easier to eliminate from the body. Your liver then puts almost one-half of these estrogen compounds into your bile, a digestive aid that's released into your intestinal tract once you eat a meal. Once in your intestine, bacterial enzymes break the bond between estrogen and glucaronic acid or sulfate residues. Many of these free estrogens are then reabsorbed into your bloodstream.

It seems that a high-fat diet can increase the activity of these bacterial enzymes. That means that more free estrogens will be reabsorbed, increasing the amount of circulating estrogen. Low-fat diets, on the other hand, may slow the action of these intestinal enzymes and reduce the amount of estrogen that re-enters your bloodstream.

Here are a few tips to help you cut back to a 20 percent fat diet:

1. Choose lower-fat animal foods

Instead of...	Choose...
Whole milk	Skim, 1% milk fat (MF)
Yogurt	Products with less than 1.5% MF
Cheese, 31% MF or more	Products with less than 20% MF
Cottage cheese, 2% or 4% MF	Products with 1% MF
Sour cream, 14% MF	Products with 7% MF or less
Cream, 10% or 18% MF	Evaporated 2% or skim milk
Red meat, higher-fat cuts	Flank steak, inside round, sirloin, eye of round, extra lean ground beef, venison
Pork, higher-fat cuts	Center-cut pork chops, pork tenderloin, pork leg (inside round, roast), baked ham, deli ham, back bacon
Poultry, dark meat	Skinless chicken breast, turkey breast, ground turkey
Eggs, whole	Egg whites (2 whites replaces 1 whole)

2. Use added fats and oils sparingly. Replace butter on toast with a sugar-reduced jam; try mustard instead of high-fat spreads on sandwiches; mix tuna with yogurt instead of mayonnaise; top your baked potato with low-fat sour cream instead of butter; order salad dressing on the side. And use oil sparingly in cooking, even if it is olive oil. Invest in a few high-quality non-stick pans. Use

chicken broth or apple juice to prevent sticking in your next stir-fry. I'm sure you are already well versed in low-fat eating, but there are probably a few things you can do to cut back on fat.

3. Read nutrition labels on packaged foods like crackers, frozen entrees, snack foods, cookies and cereals. A lower-fat food will have no more than 3 grams of fat per 100 calories. If you're looking for a food that has 20 percent fat calories or less, make 2 grams of fat per 100 calories your cut-off point.

Dietary Fiber

Just like dietary fat, fiber may influence your circulating estrogen levels. Although most of the research on fiber intake and estrogen levels has focused on breast cancer risk, the findings may be relevant to fibrocystic breast conditions. There have been a few recent studies that show higher-fiber diets reduce estrogen levels in the body. Two studies conducted in premenopausal women suggest that diets high in wheat bran are effective in lowering circulating estrogen. In one study, both a 10- and 20-gram wheat bran supplement significantly lowered estrogen after four weeks.[2] The total fiber intake of these women was between 20 and 32 grams.

Scientists think that fiber may work through its ability to bind estrogen in the intestinal tract, making the hormone less available for absorption into the blood-stream. High-fiber diets cause more estrogen to be excreted. Boosting your fiber intake may also change the acidity of your intestinal tract, slowing the activity of the bacterial enzymes that make estrogen ready for absorption.

Wheat bran belongs to a class of fibers referred to as insoluble. That means they are unable to dissolve in water. They pass through the intestinal tract intact and, in the process, they are able to bind compounds including estrogen. Soluble fibers found in oatmeal, oat bran, dried beans, lentils and psyllium-enriched breakfast cereals also have this ability, even though it has not been specifically studied for its effect on estrogen levels.

It's estimated that Americans eat on average 14 grams of fiber per day—not quite the 20 to 32 grams that may lower estrogen levels. You certainly don't need to rely on a fiber supplement to get more wheat bran into your daily diet. All it takes is a bowl of high-fiber breakfast cereal each morning.

See the Fiber in Foods table on page 29 of chapter 1 for more high-fiber foods. Use the list to gradually add higher-fiber foods to your diet. Too much fiber too soon can cause bloating, gas and diarrhea, so spread fiber-rich foods out over the course of the day. And don't forget that fiber needs fluid to work, so drink at least 8 ounces of fluid with each high-fiber meal and snack.

Soy Isoflavones

As is the case with fat and fiber, the research findings on soy intake and estrogen levels provide indirect evidence that soy foods may possibly be beneficial in preventing fibrocystic breast conditions. Many studies have found that a diet rich in soy foods lowers the level of circulating estrogen in women. Soybeans contain natural chemicals called isoflavones, a class of plant compounds that have weak estrogen activity in the body. One of the main isoflavones in soybeans, called genistein, is able to compete with a woman's own estrogen for binding to estrogen receptors. In so doing, soy isoflavones are able to reduce the amount of estrogen that contacts breast cells.

Most of the studies looking at how soy isoflavones behave in breast cells have been done in the laboratory. And they have been conducted in the hopes of finding a link to preventing breast cancer, not fibrocystic breast conditions. Despite this, the findings do suggest that a regular intake of soy can lower circulating estrogen. And this may help prevent fibrocystic breast symptoms. As you will read throughout this book, soy foods have potential for helping women in a number of ways. Soy may lower blood cholesterol, slow down bone loss, reduce menopausal hot flashes and reduce your risk of breast cancer if you start eating it at a young age. So you can see there are other good reasons to start incorporating this food into your diet. Here are a few ideas to help you get started:

- Pour a calcium-fortified soy beverage on breakfast cereal or in a smoothie, and use in cooking and baking (soups, casseroles, muffins, pancake batters).

- Cube firm tofu and add it to soups—canned or homemade.

- Grill firm tofu on the barbecue. Brush tofu and vegetable kebabs with hoisin sauce or marinate them in teriyaki sauce.

- Substitute firm tofu for ricotta cheese in recipes.

- Use soft tofu in creamy salad dressing or dip recipes.

- Throw canned soybeans in a salad, soup or chili.

- Replace up to one-half of all-purpose flour in a recipe with soy flour.

- Buy roasted soy nuts in health food stores. They come in plain, barbecue, garlic or onion flavors. Enjoy 1/4 cup (60 ml) as a mid-day snack.

- Toss roasted soy nuts in a green salad.

- Replace ground meat with TVP (texturized vegetable protein) in chili, pasta sauce and tacos.

Caffeine

It's long been thought that caffeine plays a role in fibrocystic breast conditions. The interest in caffeine dates back to the late 1970s and early 1980s, when researchers noted higher intakes of caffeine in women with fibrocystic breast conditions. It has been hypothesized that caffeine causes an abnormally high level of energy compounds called cAMP in cells, which may lead to symptoms.

Studies over the past decade have failed to find a relationship between caffeine intake and the development of fibrocystic breast conditions. Drinking coffee may, however, make your symptoms worse. A study from Duke University in Durham, North Carolina, asked 147 women with fibrocystic breast conditions to abstain from caffeine-containing foods, beverages and medication. Among those women who successfully removed caffeine for one year, 69 percent reported a decrease or absence of breast pain.[3]

Cutting back on caffeine certainly can't hurt. In addition to easing breast symptoms, removing caffeine can also help you sleep better (read chapter 6, "Insomnia"). I recommend consuming no more than 400 to 450 milligrams of caffeine a day for good health. While your goal is to get rid of as much caffeine as possible, use this amount as a benchmark to see how much you're consuming now. Eliminate caffeine for three months before you assess its effect on reducing your breast symptoms.

VITAMINS AND MINERALS

Vitamin E

This nutrient has long been promoted to help alleviate fibrocystic breast conditions; its use in treating this disorder dates back to the 1960s. Vitamin E has been claimed to alter blood levels of certain hormones, especially progesterone, but this has not yet been proven. A few small studies from the early 1980s did find that vitamin E was effective in reducing symptoms. However, subsequent well-designed studies that looked at the effect of 150, 300 and 600 international units (IU) of vitamin E in larger numbers of women found no effect on breast pain or lumps.[4] These studies lasted only two or three months, and it is possible that vitamin E might be beneficial if taken for a longer period of time.

While the evidence does not support the use of vitamin E supplements for managing fibrocystic breast conditions, it is certainly worth a try. If you've read my chapter on preventing heart disease, you'll know that I do recommend taking vitamin E for its potential heart benefits. If you decide to give it a try, here's what you need to know:

- Take a supplement that provides 400 IU per day.

- Buy a natural source vitamin E supplement (look for *d-alpha-tocopherol* on the label; synthetic forms are labeled *dl-alpha tocopherol*). Although the body absorbs both synthetic and natural forms equally well, studies suggest that your liver prefers the natural form. It incorporates more natural vitamin E into transport molecules.

- Look for a brand that's labeled "mixed tocopherols" or "mixed vitamin E." Researchers are learning that one form of the vitamin, called gamma tocopherol, may have extra health benefits.

- The daily upper limit for vitamin E is 1000 IU (natural) or 1500 IU (synthetic).

- If you're on blood-thinning medication like Coumadin® (warfarin), don't take vitamin E since it also has slight anti-clotting properties. Talk to your doctor before adding any supplement to your regime.

- Don't forget about food. While dietary sources of vitamin E can't give you 400 IU per day, vitamin-E-rich foods like vegetable oils, nuts, seeds, wheat germ and leafy green vegetables have plenty of other protective nutrients and natural plant compounds.

HERBAL REMEDIES

Evening Primrose Oil (*Oenothera biennis*)

This over-the-counter nutritional supplement is derived from a native North American plant with brightly colored yellow flowers. The oil from evening primrose is a rich source of a fatty acid called gamma linoleic acid (GLA). GLA is an omega-6 fatty acid our bodies produce from linoleic acid, an essential fat found in corn, sunflower and safflower oils.

By providing the body with GLA, evening primrose oil may help ease breast pain and tenderness in two ways. GLA is a polyunsaturated fat, which means it belongs to a class of fats with a different chemical structure than saturated fats (found in meat and dairy products). As a result, they behave differently in the body. Taking evening primrose oil is thought to increase the ratio of polyunsaturated to saturated fats in the body. If saturated fats dominate, some experts believe that this causes your body to be overly sensitive to hormones like estrogen. That's because hormones made from saturated fat are more potent and attach more readily to receptors. What's more, a diet that's high in saturated fat is also believed to impair the conversion of dietary linoleic acid to GLA inside the body. Interestingly, research has found abnormally high levels of saturated fatty acids in women with fibrocystic breast conditions.

Supplementing with evening primrose oil may also alter your body's production of hormonelike compounds called prostaglandins. There are many prostaglandins made in the body. Some are inflammatory and may cause breast pain, and others are considered friendly, as they do not lead to inflammation. GLA produces a special class of friendly prostaglandins called PGE1. These prostaglandins are also thought to reduce the activity of prolactin, a hormone that may be involved in fibrocystic breast conditions.

There is some research to support using evening primrose oil for breast pain and tenderness. Results of studies conducted in 291 women with persistent breast pain have found evening primrose oil to be effective in 45 percent of cases.[5]

Evening primrose oil is very safe; it has been used in many studies without reports of significant side effects. The effective dose is 1.5 to 2 grams taken twice daily. Buy a supplement that is standardized to contain 9 percent GLA. Start by taking three 500 milligram pills at breakfast, and repeat at dinner. Keep in mind that it may take three menstrual cycles before you feel the effects of evening primrose oil, and up to eight months for the supplement to reach its full effect.

Ginkgo Biloba

Besides protecting your brain cells from the hands of time, ginkgo might also help reduce symptoms of fibrocystic breast conditions. French researchers studied 143 women with PMS and found that ginkgo significantly reduced PMS-related breast tenderness, not to mention abdominal bloating, and swollen hands, legs and feet.[6]

The women took ginkgo on day 16 of their cycle and continued until day 5 of their next cycle, at which time they stopped; they resumed taking the herb again on day 16.

The recommended dose of ginkgo is 40 to 80 milligrams, taken three times daily. Start on day 16 (start counting from the first day of your period) and continue until the end of your next period—that means you will take ginkgo for two weeks each month. To buy a high-quality product, make sure the label states it is standardized to contain 24 percent ginkgo flavone glycosides. Ginkgo is very safe but, like most herbal remedies, it may cause mild stomach upset in a small number of women.

One concern is ginkgo's mild blood-thinning effect. It should not be taken with blood-thinning drugs such as Coumadin® (warfarin) or heparin unless your doctor is monitoring you. It is also possible that ginkgo can enhance the effect of other natural health products that also slightly thin the blood (like vitamin E or garlic). Be sure to inform your physician and pharmacist if you are taking a number of these supplements. The herb has not been studied in pregnant or breastfeeding women, so its use is not recommended at these times.

THE BOTTOM LINE...
Leslie's recommendations for fibrocystic breast conditions

1. Eat a low-fat diet. Start by using little or no added fats to foods and in cooking. Read labels on packages of commercial foods—look for no more than 2 grams of fat per 100 calories (this means it has 20 percent fat from calories).

2. Boost your intake of dietary fiber, especially wheat bran. Start by reaching for a bowl of high-fiber breakfast cereal.

3. To help lower the amount of estrogen that comes in contact with your breast cells, consider adding soy foods to your daily diet.

4. If you suffer from breast pain, swelling or lumpiness, eliminate all sources of caffeine from your diet for at least three months.

5. If you're not already taking this supplement, consider adding 400 international units (IU) of vitamin E to your daily nutrition regime. Buy a natural source vitamin E pill. Consider looking for a vitamin E that provides "mixed tocopherols"

or "mixed vitamin E." The daily upper limit for vitamin E is 1000 IU (natural) or 1500 IU (synthetic).

6. If you have cyclic or noncyclic breast pain, take evening primrose oil. Buy a product standardized to contain 9 percent GLA. Take 1.5 grams in the morning and 1.5 grams in the evening for a total of 3 grams per day. Wait at least three menstrual cycles to see if your symptoms improve.

7. If breast swelling is a real problem for you, consider trying ginkgo biloba. Buy a product standardized to 24 percent ginkgo flavone glycosides. Take 40 to 80 milligrams three times daily. Do not use ginkgo if you are pregnant or breast-feeding.

10

Osteoporosis

Osteoporosis can strike women at any age, but it is more prevalent after menopause. It's estimated that more than 8 million American women have osteoporosis, a disease of fragile, brittle bones that are more likely to break. Bone fractures are increasing at a faster rate than ever. By the age of 50, the average Caucasian woman has a 40 percent chance of suffering at least one fracture caused by brittle bones. In fact, the risk of getting a fracture is at least five times the risk of developing breast cancer. You may not realize that more women die each year as a result of fractures from osteoporosis than from breast and ovarian cancer combined.

What Causes Osteoporosis?

Osteoporosis is characterized by low bone mass and deterioration of existing bone tissue. Bones become weaker and more susceptible to fractures. The definition of osteoporosis emphasizes fracture risk, not only low bone density. While many bone fractures are not life threatening, the impact that fractures have on health is underappreciated. For instance, hip fractures lead to death in 20 percent of cases. And close to one-half of elderly women who fracture their hips lose their ability to live independently.

Your bones grow in length and density until your teen years when you finish your growth spurt (between the ages of 11 and 14 years for girls). After this time, your bones continue to increase in density but at a slower rate. Then, sometime in your twenties, your bones achieve what's called their peak mass; once this occurs, they stop building density. This happens between 20 and 30 years of age. At this age you then have all the bone you're ever going to have. Peak bone mass is determined largely by genetics, but nutrition and other lifestyle factors determine whether or not you will achieve your body's genetically programmed peak bone mass.

After you achieve your peak bone mass, natural bone loss begins. Before menopause, women lose bone at a rate of 1 percent per year, the same rate as men. Within the first five years after menopause, women lose bone two to six times faster than premenopausal women do. Then, ten years after menopause, bone loss returns to 1 percent per year. During this ten-year period following menopause, some women have the potential to lose bone very quickly. Others are slow bone losers and won't lose as much bone mass.

Despite its "dead" appearance, bone is very active tissue that contains two types of cells. Osteoclasts are always breaking down the bone in areas where it is not needed. For example, osteoclasts go to work when your diet lacks calcium and they release calcium into the blood for important body functions. Osteoblasts, on the other hand, are responsible for building the support structure of bones as well as adding minerals to strengthen bones.

Your bones are constantly going through a bone remodeling cycle. Osteoclast cells break down bone and osteoblast cells then rebuild. After you've achieved your peak bone mass in your twenties, osteoclast (breakdown) activity wins out.

HORMONES AND BONE HEALTH

Many different hormones influence whether bones are being broken down or rebuilt. They do this by affecting how your body uses calcium. The three main players in calcium and bone metabolism are parathyroid hormone, vitamin D and calcitonin, but steroid drugs and estrogen also play a part.

1. *Parathyroid hormone* (PTH) is secreted by your parathyroid gland. Its job is to keep your blood calcium level stable. Because calcium is critical for blood clotting, muscle contraction and the transmission of nerve impulses, a constant amount of the mineral must be circulated throughout your body at all times. When blood calcium falls too low because you're not consuming enough calcium

in your diet, PTH tells your kidneys to stop excreting calcium. PTH also activates vitamin D in your body, and vitamin D, in turn, causes your intestine to absorb more dietary calcium. And finally, PTH instructs your osteoclasts (bone breakdown cells) to release calcium from your bones into your bloodstream. The net result is bone loss.

2. *Calcitonin* is secreted by your thyroid gland in response to a high calcium level in the bloodstream. This hormone lowers calcium to a normal level by stopping the action of osteoclasts and stimulating the osteoblasts to build new bone. The osteoblasts take calcium from the blood to increase bone density. Calcitonin levels decline with age and with menopause.

3. *Thyroid hormones* can also have an impact on bone loss. Too much of this hormone from an overactive thyroid gland (hyperthyroid) or too much thyroid medication causes a higher rate of bone breakdown. If you take Synthroid® (levothyroxin) for an underactive thyroid gland (hypothyroid), your doctor will check your thyroid hormone levels regularly. If your level is too high, your medication will be adjusted.

4. *Steroid drugs* such as glucocorticoids (e.g., prednisone), used to treat inflammatory conditions like rheumatoid arthritis, lupus and colitis, also increase the rate of bone loss. A side effect of these drugs is their ability to enhance the action of PTH on bone. If you think back to how PTH works, that means your bones will mobilize more calcium into your bloodstream.

5. *Estrogen*, on the other hand, acts to protect bones. This hormone seems to be able to prevent the osteoclasts from releasing calcium from the bone into the bloodstream. Estrogen also causes calcitonin and vitamin D to be released, stimulating new bone growth to occur.

❧

Symptoms

Osteoporosis is a silent disease because bone loss occurs without symptoms. A woman may not know she has the disease until she breaks a bone. The outward signs of osteoporosis are usually not apparent until the disease is quite advanced. Signs that you may have osteoporosis include:

- a broken wrist or rib
- a broken hip
- back pain in the mid to lower spine
- loss of more than 1 inch of height
- a stooped or hunched-over appearance
- a hump forming in the upper back

You may notice that a loss of height and more rounded shoulders influence the way your clothes fit. Clothes that once fit may not fit or hang properly because of a change in your posture.

ॐ

Who's at Risk?

The strength of your bones is determined by 1) their bone mineral density, 2) their rate of self-healing, and 3) the integrity of their support structures. Any factor that jeopardizes these three factors can increase the odds of getting osteoporosis. Here's a list of known risk factors:

- older age
- low bone density
- being female
- slender or petite body structure (you have less bone to start with than does a more heavy-set person)
- deficiency of estrogen (early menopause further increases the risk)
- low calcium and vitamin D intake
- cigarette smoking (enhances the production of inactive estrogens, leading to estrogen deficiency)
- too much alcohol
- excessive caffeine intake

- sedentary lifestyle

- certain medications (e.g., corticosteroids)

- prolonged immobilization (bones need gravity to increase density)

- family history of maternal hip fracture

- previous bone fracture of any type after the age of 50

- certain health conditions (e.g., kidney failure, hyperthyroid, malabsorption states)

♂

Diagnosis

The only way doctors can get a sense of what's happening to your bone is by taking repeated measures of your bone mineral density using a test called the dual-energy-x-ray absorptiometry (DEXA). The DEXA test can detect as little as a 1 percent change in bone density. What this test can't do, however, is detect bone fractures. And it doesn't measure bone density in the upper spine, where a series of small fractures can result in shrinking and dowager's hump, the characteristic hunching of the spine seen in osteoporosis. Doctors use x-rays to detect these types of fractures in your upper spine.

The DEXA test is simple, fast and absolutely painless. You don't even have to undress. To have your lower spine or hip scanned, you lie comfortably on a flat, padded table. Food doesn't interfere with the test results, so you don't have to fast the night before the test. However, you shouldn't take a calcium supplement right before since an undigested pill can be measured as part of your bone density—when you're lying down, your intestines lie on top of your spine.

Once you have the scan, you'll receive a DEXA bone density report. This is a computer-generated image of four vertebrae in your lower spine (L1, L2, L3 and L4). The computer calculates how much bone mineral is present in each single vertebra and then calculates an average bone mineral density (BMD) for three vertebrae: L2, L3 and L4 (L2–L4).

Your DEXA bone density test results are then compared to the bone density of a healthy 30-year-old woman. If your Young Adult Comparison for your lower spine (L2–L4) is 88 percent, this means that your bone density is 88 percent of that of the average 30-year-old woman. In other words, you've lost 12 percent of your bone density. Compared to a woman who still has the bone density of a 30-year-old, your risk of bone fracture doubles for every 10 percent loss of bone density.

Bone density results are also presented as a T score. The T score is the number of levels (standard deviations) your bone density is away from that of a 30-year-old woman. If you are one level away, your T score is 1.0, and you are considered to have osteopenia, or decreased bone mass. If your test comes back saying that your bones are more than 2.5 levels away, you have osteoporosis. If your score is higher still and you have one or more tiny fractures, then you are considered to have severe osteoporosis. If you are over 65 years old, osteopenia doubles your risk for fracture, osteoporosis quadruples it and severe osteoporosis increases the risk of bone fracture twenty-fold.

You'll also notice an Aged Matched Comparison on your report. This compares your bone density to what is expected for your age. If your Aged Matched Comparison is unusually low, your doctor will endeavour to determine what is causing this bone loss.

If you have not yet had a DEXA test, speak to your doctor about having the test if you fall into one of the following categories:

- You're approaching menopause and deciding about hormone replacement therapy (HRT). A bone density test can help you decide whether or not HRT is needed to prevent osteoporosis.

- You have a strong family history of osteoporosis or multiple bone fractures.

- You have premature menopause (less than 45 years old).

- You've been on corticosteroid drugs for a medical condition for three months or longer (e.g., 7.5 milligrams of prednisone).

- You've experienced long-standing malnutrition or malabsorption (e.g., history of anorexia nervosa, celiac disease, Crohn's disease).

- You have a low body weight.

- You have hyperthyroidism.

Your first bone density test serves as a baseline that your future test results will be compared to. If at the age of 50 your first bone density test comes back low (osteopenia), that doesn't mean you have osteoporosis. It may be that you're a slow loser, and later tests will find that your bone mineral content has not changed very much. Bone density tests must be repeated every two years to detect a bone loss of 2 to 3 percent. If future tests show that your bone density has declined rapidly between tests, your doctor will likely recommend drug treatment to slow the rate of bone loss.

❧

Conventional Treatment

ESTROGEN THERAPY

Many studies have shown that hormone replacement therapy protects the bones. Recently the Women's Health Initiative (WHI), one of the largest-ever trials of hormone replacement therapy (HRT), also reported that HRT lowered the risk of osteoporotic bone fractures. Sponsored by the National Institutes of Health, WHI followed more than 27,000 healthy women, aged 50 to 79, taking either combined HRT (estrogen plus progestin) or estrogen only. The goal was to determine whether HRT protected from heart disease and osteoporosis, as well as increased the risk for cancer and blood clots. While there was good news, there was also bad news. Despite the benefits to bone health, combined HRT increased the risk of heart disease, blood clots, stroke and breast cancer.

The study arm investigating combined HRT was halted in July 2002 for public health reasons. While the increased health risks were small, you can imagine that a drug taken by millions of women over many years could result in a large number of women developing breast cancer or heart disease. It was determined that the risks of this hormone regimen outweighed the benefits and HRT is no longer considered the gold standard to prevent osteoporosis and bone fractures.

If you are taking combined HRT solely for the prevention of osteoporosis, consider stopping it. As you will read below, there are many medications that can help lower the odds of osteoporosis and bone fracture with fewer risks. Combined HRT may be appropriate if you are also taking it for the short-term relief of hot flashes and other menopausal symptoms. To decide if HRT is right for you, you must consult with your doctor.

BISPHOSPHONATES

This newer class of non-hormonal drugs offers women with low bone density or osteoporosis an alternative to HRT. Bisphosphonate drugs prevent bone breakdown by binding to the bone surface and inhibiting the activity of the osteoclasts, the cells that strip down old bone. The bisphosphonate drug available in the United States is sold as Fosamax® (aldendronate).

SELECTIVE ESTROGEN RECEPTOR MODULATORS (SERMS)

These so-called designer estrogen drugs offer all the beneficial effects of estrogen (bone protection, cholesterol lowering, hot flash reduction), without any of its negative effects (increased breast cancer risk, endometrial bleeding). A SERM such as Evista® (raloxifene) offers the favorable effects of estrogen on bone and blood cholesterol levels, and it acts as an anti-estrogen in the breast and the uterus. That means it doesn't stimulate the growth of breast or uterine cells. However, unlike estrogen therapy, Evista® does not relieve hot flashes or vaginal dryness.

༄

Managing and Preventing Osteoporosis

Ideally, every woman's goal should be to eat well and exercise regularly in order to: 1) build bone density in her teens and twenties to achieve her peak bone mass, and 2) slow down, as much as possible, age-related bone loss during her thirties, forties and fifties so that bone-sparing medication is not necessary after menopause.

Unfortunately this is not always the case. Some women with low bone density and/or fractures do require drugs to halt bone loss and reduce the risk of bone fracture. Even if you are taking medication for osteoporosis, diet and nutrition can still influence your bone density. Here are some key nutrition strategies to help you delay bone loss. Remember, it's never too late to start paying attention.

DIETARY STRATEGIES

Soy Foods

Soybeans contain naturally occurring compounds called isoflavones, a type of plant estrogen. Genistein and daidzein are the most active isoflavones in soy, and have been the focus of much research. Isoflavones have a chemical structure similar to estrogen and so they are able to bind to estrogen receptors in the body. It is the action of isoflavones on estrogen receptors in the bone that scientists believe may be responsible for soy's potential bone-preserving effect.

The interest in soybeans and osteoporosis began when researchers observed that populations that consume soy foods on a regular basis report much lower rates of hip fracture. Since then, soy foods and their naturally occurring phytoestrogens have been the focus of many studies. While some studies find no effect of soy on bone loss, others show a significant bone-sparing effect.

A three-month study conducted at Iowa State University found that 40 grams of phytoestrogen-rich soy protein powder prevented bone loss in postmenopausal women.[1] Women in this study who were given whey protein powder (a protein made from milk) instead showed significant bone loss in the lower spine. Another study, from Dr. Ken Setchell's group at the Department of Obstetrics and Gynecology, Internal Medicine and Pediatrics at the University of Cincinnati's College of Medicine, found that 60 to 70 milligrams of soy isoflavones, consumed as soy beverage and soy nuts, significantly decreased bone turnover in postmenopausal women.[2] The researchers found that osteoblast activity (bone building) increased by 10.2 percent and osteoclast activity (bone breakdown) decreased by 13.9 percent. Reduced bone turnover was seen after four weeks of eating soy foods.

To reap the potential bone-preserving benefits of soy, aim for a daily intake of at least 50 milligrams of isoflavones. To keep your blood levels of isoflavones up through the day, consume soy foods twice daily. Depending on the food you eat, your blood isoflavone levels will peak four to eight hours later. Twenty-four hours after eating a soy food, your body will have excreted these isoflavones.

Soy foods vary with respect to the amount of isoflavones they contain. Even the same type of food made by different manufacturers can differ in isoflavone content. But here's a general guide to foods and their isoflavone content:

SOY FOOD	SERVING SIZE	ISOFLAVONE CONTENT
Roasted soy nuts	1/4 cup	40–60 milligrams
Green soybeans, uncooked	1/2 cup	70 milligrams
Tempeh, uncooked	3 oz	45 milligrams
Soy flour	1/4 cup	28 milligrams
Tofu, uncooked	4 oz	38 milligrams

Texturized vegetable protein, dry	1/4 cup	15–60 milligrams
Soy beverage, So Nice™ brand	1 cup	60 milligrams
Soy beverage, most brands	1 cup	25 milligrams
Soy protein powder, isolate	2 tbsp	30 milligrams
Soy sauce		none
Soya oil		none

USDA-Iowa State University Database on the Isoflavone Content of Foods.
U.S. Department of Agriculture, Agricultural Research Service, 1999.

Ipriflavone

Ipriflavone is not a food. Rather, it's an isoflavone supplement that's made from daidzein, one of the main phytoestrogens found in soybeans. Since I have just finished discussing soy's potential for maintaining healthy bones, it's a perfect time to discuss ipriflavone. And when it comes to preventing bone loss, this is one supplement you might consider taking.

Research suggests that ipriflavone, taken alone or with calcium, is more effective at maintaining bone density than calcium alone. Studies show that ipriflavone enhances the effects of calcium and vitamin D in preventing osteoporosis when they are taken together. Ipriflavone enhances the action of cells that build bone and inhibits the activity of cells that break down bone.

Based on the positive research findings, you might decide to buy a calcium supplement that has added ipriflavone. Look for a product that contains Ostivone™, a high quality extract of ipriflavone that has been used in scientific research.

The standard dose is 200 milligrams three times daily taken with food. Choose a product that has other nutrients important for bone health, including calcium, vitamin D, magnesium and vitamin C. Such a supplement can replace your standard calcium pill. Brand names of calcium supplements with Ostivone™ added include Rx-Bone Ostivone, Bone Renew, and Bone Protector.

Side effects of ipriflavone are uncommon but may include stomach upset, diarrhea and dizziness. One recent study found that ipriflavone reduced the number of certain white blood cells in some women. So far this side effect was seen in only one study. There have been more than 60 clinical trials that have not shown this effect. Women with hormone-sensitive health conditions such as breast, uterine and ovarian cancer, endometriosis and uterine fibroids should seek the advice of a physician, as ipri-flavone may enhance some effects of estrogen. As with many natural health products, women with liver or kidney disease should use the supplement with caution.

Protein Foods

Eating too much protein may be part of the reason why North American women have high rates of osteoporosis, despite our moderate-to-high calcium intakes. Studies have shown that high levels of dietary protein cause calcium to be excreted by the kidneys. High intakes of animal protein are more detrimental to calcium loss than vegetarian proteins. The effect of eating large quantities of protein is rapid, and it appears that the body doesn't correct for this by absorbing more calcium from food. The protein effect may be very important for people who consume very little calcium or for those who, because of intestinal problems, absorb very little calcium.

While eating very large amounts of protein may not be good for your bones, eating too little isn't healthy either. Protein is an important structural component of bone, and studies have shown that missing out on this important nutrient might actually increase the risk of hip fracture. The Iowa Women's Health Study found that dietary protein protected postmenopausal women from hip fracture. Women who ate the most protein had a 69 percent reduced risk of hip fracture compared to women who ate the least.[3]

Studies have also found that when protein supplements are given to patients with hip fracture, the rate of complications and death is reduced, immediately after surgery and for six months afterwards.[4]

Based on these studies, it seems clear that it's important to be meeting your daily requirement for protein. Women at risk for protein deficiency include

- those who live alone and don't often cook meat, chicken or fish
- those who frequently grab quick meals during the day—bagels, pasta, low-fat frozen dinners
- vegetarians who do not eat animal foods, and do not regularly incorporate high-quality vegetable protein sources into their diet
- those who engage in heavy exercise and fall into any of the above categories

To find out how much protein you need every day, refer to page 33 in chapter 1.

Caffeine

Drinking coffee, tea or colas increases the amount of calcium your kidneys excrete in your urine. This increased calcium excretion continues up to three hours after consuming caffeine. For every 6-ounce cup of coffee you drink, approximately 48 milligrams of calcium is leached from your bones.

The effects of caffeine are likely most detrimental for women who are not meeting their requirements for calcium. One study found that 400 milligrams of caffeine caused calcium loss in women whose daily diet had less than 600 milligrams of calcium.[5] Another study from Tufts University in Boston found that women who consumed less than 800 milligrams of calcium and 450 milligrams of caffeine (about three small cups of coffee) had significantly lower bone densities than women who consumed the same amount of caffeine but more than 800 milligrams of calcium.[6]

Here's what you need to know:

- If you drink coffee, make sure you're meeting your calcium requirements of 1000 to 1500 milligrams a day.
- Add 3 tablespoons of milk (58 mg calcium) or calcium-fortified soy beverage to every cup of coffee you drink.
- Do not consume more than 450 milligrams of caffeine a day. If you have osteoporosis, aim for no more than 200 milligrams (see page 38 in chapter 1 to find out how foods and beverages rate with respect to caffeine).
- If you drink caffeine-containing beverages throughout the day, cut them out after noon. Instead, try water, herbal tea, vegetable juice, milk or a glass of soy beverage.
- Replace coffee with tea, which has substantially less caffeine.
- Instead of plain coffee, try a calcium-rich latte made with milk or fortified soy beverage.

Sodium

Like caffeine, sodium also causes your kidneys to excrete calcium. For every 500-milligram increase in sodium intake, you must eat an additional 40 milligrams of calcium to make up for the increased loss. A study in postmenopausal women determined that a maximum intake of 2000 milligrams of sodium (the amount found in about 3/4 teaspoon of salt) and 1000 milligrams of calcium minimized bone loss.[7]

Although we do need some salt every day, we actually need very little. Salt is a molecule composed of sodium and chloride, both of which are needed to help maintain water balance in our bodies. We continually lose sodium through sweat and urine. The more active we are or the warmer the weather, the more sodium we must replace in the diet. But it takes only about 500 milligrams (1/5 of a teaspoon) of salt to cover the needs of sedentary people in temperate climates. The average American consumes about 2 teaspoons of salt each day, almost 10 times what we need!

To reduce your sodium intake, avoid the salt shaker at the table, minimize the use of salt in cooking and buy commercial food products that are low in added salt. Eating fewer processed foods is one of the best things you can do to cut back on sodium. That's because most of the salt we eat comes from processed and prepared foods. Only one-quarter of our sodium daily intake comes from the salt shaker. You'll find the sodium content of foods listed on page 41 in chapter 1.

VITAMINS AND MINERALS

Calcium

The fact that calcium is the most abundant mineral in the body, and that 99 percent of it is housed within the bones and teeth, underlines the importance of dietary calcium to bone health. During the bone-building process, the osteoblast cells secrete bone mineral consisting of calcium and phosphorus, which strengthens the bone. By providing structural integrity to bones, dietary calcium plays a critical role in preventing osteoporosis.

The remaining 1 percent of your body's calcium circulates in your bloodstream and is vital to your heart, nervous system and muscles. Your body keeps this circulating pool of calcium at a constant level. If your diet lacks calcium and your blood calcium level drops, your parathyroid gland releases parathyroid hormone (PTH), which returns calcium to your blood by taking it from the bones. So when you short-change your diet, you short-change your bones, too.

To see how much calcium you and your female family members need, see the RDA table on page 16 in chapter 1. Many calcium-rich foods provide other important bone-building nutrients like vitamin D, magnesium and potassium. Use the list of calcium-rich foods on page 17 in chapter 1 to help you boost your intake.

Your body does not absorb calcium from all foods equally well. While many plant foods contribute calcium to the diet, some natural compounds in vegetables prevent some of this calcium from being absorbed. Studies show that dairy products contain the most absorbable form of calcium. To enhance the amount of calcium your body absorbs, you should also avoid taking iron supplements with calcium-rich foods. Factors in your diet that hamper your body's ability to absorb calcium include

- large amount of phytates in fiber-rich foods, which can bind with calcium and limit its absorption
- oxalic acid in spinach and some other vegetables (cooking green vegetables boosts their calcium content by releasing some calcium that's bound to oxalic acid)
- too much phosphorus in the diet
- taking iron with calcium-rich foods (iron competes with calcium for absorption)
- drinking tea with a meal rich in calcium (natural compounds in tea, known as tannins, inhibit calcium absorption)
- a lack of vitamin D (as you've read above, vitamin D stimulates the intestine to absorb dietary calcium)

CALCIUM SUPPLEMENTS

Studies do support using calcium supplements to lower your risk of osteoporosis. Researchers at the University of Texas Southwestern Medical Center in Dallas found that a 400-milligram calcium citrate supplement taken twice daily increased bone density in healthy postmenopausal women.[8] In contrast, women in the placebo group experienced a 2.38 percent bone reduction in the lower spine.

Scientists at the University of Massachusetts studied 98 premenopausal women (average age 39 years) and found that those who received 500 milligrams of calcium carbonate increased bone density by 0.3 percent per year.[9] The women in the placebo group lost bone at a rate of 0.4 percent per year in the hip and 0.7 percent in the neck. A number of studies have also shown that older women (and men) who take calcium and vitamin D supplements have a lower incidence of nonvertebral fractures.

If you're thinking you had better take a calcium supplement, you're probably right. Recent surveys have found that many Americans do not get the recommended two to three dairy servings per day. Sure, there's calcium in broccoli and almonds and tofu. But let's be truthful—do you really eat tofu on a daily basis? Are you willing to eat five cups of broccoli to make up for your missing 500 milligrams of calcium? Many women I see in my private practice are not meeting their daily calcium needs and should be taking a calcium supplement. Women may find it difficult to meet their calcium goals if they are lactose intolerant, if they are following a vegetarian diet or if they have poor eating habits. In these cases, supplements are often the only way that I can ensure a client is meeting her calcium needs.

To help you decide if you need a calcium supplement, use my 300 Milligram Rule. One milk serving gives you 300 milligrams of calcium. For every serving you're missing and not replacing with other calcium-rich foods, you need to get 300 milligrams of elemental calcium through a supplement. Here's how to choose a high-quality supplement:

1. Look at the source of calcium. There are many types of calcium supplements on the shelf. Some of the more common types include these:

    *   *Calcium carbonate* is only about 10 to 30 percent absorbed by the body. The amount you absorb depends on how much stomach acid is present. As people age, their stomach produces less hydrochloric acid. Because of this, calcium carbonate is not the best choice for older adults or for people on medications that block acid production. If you do take this form of calcium, take it with meals to increase absorption. Do not take calcium carbonate at bedtime unless you take it with a snack. On the plus side, this is the most inexpensive type of calcium supplement.

    *   *Calcium citrate* is about 30 percent absorbed by the body, so it is a better choice for anyone over the age of 50. Calcium citrate malate is one of the most highly absorbable (and expensive) forms of calcium. Calcium citrate supplements are well absorbed either with meals or on an empty stomach.

    *   *Calcium chelates* (HVP chelate) are supplements that contain calcium bound to an amino acid. In the case of HVP chelate, the amino acid is from vegetable protein. Some manufacturers claim that up to 75 percent of calcium in the chelate form is absorbed by the body.

- *Effervescent calcium supplements* contain calcium carbonate and often other forms of more absorbable calcium. Because they get a head start on disintegrating, they may be absorbed in the intestinal tract more quickly. Dissolve these in water or orange juice.

- *Bone meal* or *dolomite* or *oyster shell* are not recommended, because some products have been found to contain trace amounts of contaminants such as lead and mercury.

2. Know how much elemental calcium each pill gives you. Look on the list of ingredients for this information. The amount of elemental calcium is what you use to calculate your daily intake. Calcium carbonate or calcium chelates may not be 100 percent elemental calcium. The front label may state 500 milligrams, but when you look carefully at the ingredient list you may find the product contains only 350 milligrams of elemental calcium. This will determine how many tablets you need to take to get your recommended dose.

3. Choose a formula with vitamin D and magnesium. These nutrients work in tandem with calcium to promote optimal bone health. For instance, vitamin D increases calcium absorption in your intestine by as much as 30 to 80 percent.

4. Spread larger doses throughout the day. Since all calcium sources (including food sources) are not 100 percent absorbed, it makes sense to split a higher dose over two or three meals. If you've been advised to take 600 milligrams of calcium a day, take a 300-milligram tablet with breakfast and another one at dinner.

5. Take your calcium supplements with a large glass of water.

The daily upper limit for calcium intake is 2500 milligrams from food and supplements. In most healthy people, this amount will not cause any side effects. The major risks from getting too much calcium include kidney stones in people with a history of stones, constipation and gas.

Vitamin D

In addition to getting too little calcium, experts cite a silent epidemic of vitamin D deficiency as a contributing factor to osteoporosis. Most foods have little or no natural vitamin D and only a few foods are actually fortified with the vitamin.

Vitamin D acts like a hormone in your body (a hormone is any compound that's manufactured in one part of the body that affects another part). The active form of vitamin D is made in your liver but it acts on your intestine, your kidneys and your bone. These organs all respond to vitamin D by making calcium available for bone growth. Vitamin D makes calcium and phosphorus available in the blood that bathes the bones, so it can be deposited as bones harden or mineralize. Vitamin D raises blood levels of calcium in three ways—it stimulates your intestine to absorb more dietary calcium, it tells your kidneys to retain calcium and it withdraws calcium from your bones.

As you can see, if you're lacking vitamin D, you are not getting enough calcium into your body to meet your needs, regardless of how much calcium you consume. A vitamin D deficiency will speed up bone loss and increase the risk of fracture at a younger age.

Vitamin D is different from any other nutrient because your body can synthesize it from sunlight. When ultraviolet light hits your skin, a pre-vitamin D is formed. This compound eventually makes its way to your kidneys, where it's transformed into active vitamin D.

In the North, the long winter months result in very little vitamin D being synthesized in the skin. Researchers from Tufts University in Boston have demonstrated that blood levels of vitamin D do indeed fluctuate throughout the year.[10] They are at their lowest point in February-March and they peak in June-July. But even in the summer, you might not be making enough vitamin D, since the sun protection factor (SPF) in your sunscreen blocks the production of vitamin D. When it is sunny, you should expose your hands, face and arms without sunscreen for 10 to 15 minutes, two or three times a week to help you meet your vitamin D needs.

See the RDA table on page 13 in chapter 1 to see how much vitamin D you should be getting every day. Vitamin D requirements from diet increase with age. This is due to the fact that as we get older, our skin becomes less efficient at producing vitamin D from sunlight.

Unfortunately, good food sources of vitamin D are few and far between. Take a look at the Vitamin D in Foods table on page 14 in chapter 1 to see how the foods you eat make up your vitamin D intake.

VITAMIN D SUPPLEMENTS

If you're over 50, if you don't drink at least two glasses of a fortified beverage every day or if winter for you means little exposure to sunshine, then you should reach for a good quality multivitamin and mineral supplement. Most products will give you 400 IU of vitamin D. If you take calcium supplements, buy a product with vitamin D added. Fish oil is another way to get your vitamin D, as 1 teaspoon (5 ml) of cod liver oil packs 450 IU. If you take fish oil capsules, make sure you follow the manufacturer's dosage recommendations or, better yet, get advice from a qualified dietitian or nutritionist. Fish liver oil contains vitamins A and D, two fat-soluble vitamins that are stored in your body. When taken in large doses over a period of time, some types of fish oil supplements can lead to vitamin A and D toxicity.

Other Nutrients

While calcium and vitamin D are critical to healthy bones, other nutrients are also important players in bone building. Together with calcium and vitamin D, they compose the nutrient team that orchestrates the continual process of bone building and bone breakdown.

VITAMIN A

One of this vitamin's important jobs is to support growth and development, especially bone development. I told you earlier that in order to build new bone, the osteoclast cells must first undo parts of old bone. To accomplish this task, osteoclasts contain a sac of degradative enzymes. With the help of vitamin A, these enzymes break down old bone. The fact that bone growth relies on vitamin A is witnessed by the fact that children who are deficient in vitamin A fail to grow properly.

Vitamin A is found pre-formed in animal foods such as fortified milk, cheese, butter, eggs and liver. But we also meet our vitamin A needs by eating bright orange and green fruits and vegetables. The beta-carotene in these plant foods is converted to vitamin A in the body. The best sources of beta-carotene include carrots (surprise!), winter squash, sweet potatoes, spinach, broccoli, rapini, romaine lettuce, apricots, peaches, mango, papaya and cantaloupe.

VITAMIN C

A number of studies of postmenopausal women have linked higher intakes of vitamin C with having a higher bone density. One study revealed that women aged 55 to 64 years who had taken vitamin C supplements for at least 10 years had significantly higher bone mass compared to women who did not supplement their diet.[11] Vitamin C is important for the formation of collagen, a tissue that lends support to bones. This vitamin may also protect bones by acting as an antioxidant and modifying the negative effect of cigarette smoking on bones—many studies have shown that cigarette smoking reduces bone density and increases the risk of fracture.

To get more vitamin C in your diet, reach for citrus fruits, cantaloupe, mango, strawberries, broccoli, brussels sprouts, cauliflower, red pepper and tomato juice. The RDA is 75 milligrams for non-smoking women and 110 milligrams for smokers. To put that in perspective, one medium orange gives you 70 milligrams of vitamin C, and 1/2 cup of red pepper packs 95 milligrams. If you don't think you consume enough vitamin C in your diet, take a multivitamin and mineral pill each day. Or you might choose a calcium supplement with added vitamin C.

VITAMIN K

You've probably heard very little about this fat-soluble vitamin. One of the reasons for its low profile is that vitamin K deficiency is hardly ever seen. That's because the millions of bacteria in our intestinal tract synthesize the vitamin. Once we absorb this manufactured vitamin K, it gets stored in the liver. The vitamin is not a part of the bone mineral complex. Instead it helps make a bone protein called osteocalcin. Doctors can measure the amount of osteocalcin in your blood. A high level indicates that your osteoblasts are busy making new bone. Without enough vitamin K, the bones produce an abnormal protein that cannot bind to the minerals that form the bones. The best food sources of vitamin K are leafy green vegetables, cabbage, milk and liver.

When it comes to bone health, the importance of vitamin K should not be underestimated. The famous Nurses' Health Study from Harvard University found that women with the highest intake of vitamin K had a significantly lower rate of hip fracture compared to women who consumed the least.[12] And guess what—eating lettuce was also linked with fewer hip fractures. Lettuce accounted for most of the vitamin K in their diet. Women who ate one or more servings of the leafy green each day (versus one or fewer servings a week) had a 45 percent lower risk of hip fractures.

PHOSPHORUS

This mineral is an important component of the bone mineral complex. In fact, about 85 percent of phosphorus in the body is found in the bone. It appears that both too little dietary phosphorus and too much can result in bone loss. A high level in the blood causes the release of parathyroid hormone (PTH). If you recall, PTH turns off vitamin D production and, as a result, your intestine absorbs less calcium. Scientists believe that a long-standing imbalance of phosphorus and calcium, caused by too much dietary phosphorus and too little dietary calcium, may contribute to bone breakdown.

On the other hand, if your diet lacks phosphorus and your blood levels become low, your body will release the mineral from your bones in an effort to keep your blood level constant, the same way that calcium blood levels remain stable at the expense of your bone. One of the symptoms of a phosphorus deficiency is bone pain. A low blood phosphorus level can result from poor eating habits, excessive use of phosphorus-binding antacids and intestinal malabsorption.

The daily recommended intake of phosphorus is 700 milligrams. Most of the phosphorus in our diet comes from additives in cheese, bakery products, processed meats and soft drinks. Other food sources include wheat bran, milk, fish, eggs, poultry, beef and pork. As you can probably guess, most people don't have a problem getting enough phosphorus. Just make sure you meet your calcium requirements so that you keep these two minerals in balance.

MAGNESIUM

One-half of the body's magnesium stores are in the bone. But before I continue, I'd like to clear up one piece of misinformation—magnesium does *not* help your body absorb calcium! I can't begin to count the number of times I have heard that it does; on occasion, I've even seen it written in books. Without magnesium, you absorb calcium just fine, but you don't form healthy bones. The mineral helps make PTH, an important regulator of bone building. Animal studies show that a lack of dietary magnesium causes increased bone breakdown and decreased bone synthesis.

It's difficult to say to what extent magnesium plays a role in osteoporosis, since very few studies have actually looked at the effect of dietary magnesium and bone loss. Most of the studies that support the use of magnesium supplements have found that osteoporosis is more common in people who have other health problems that cause a magnesium deficiency, like alcoholism and hyperthyroidism. Interestingly, scientists have found that magnesium levels in bone are actually higher, not lower, in people with osteoporosis.

Magnesium is an important nutrient for bone health, as well as many other processes in the body. The recommended daily intake for women is 320 milligrams. The best food sources are wheat bran, whole-grain breads, cereals and pasta, legumes, nuts, seeds and leafy green vegetables. There's no question in my mind that most people need to step up their magnesium intake. Switching from refined starches like white bread and white pasta to whole-grain products is a good place to start. So many of my clients are lacking magnesium in their diets that I recommend buying a calcium supplement with magnesium. But too much supplemental magnesium can cause diarrhea. For this reason, I suggest you buy a calcium supplement with magnesium in a 2:1 ratio (two parts calcium to one part magnesium).

BORON
While there's no daily recommended intake for boron, studies suggest that a higher intake of this trace mineral may slow down loss of calcium, magnesium and phosphorus through the urine. And that's not all. Boosting your boron intake may also increase your blood estrogen level. Scientists aren't exactly sure how boron keeps calcium in balance, but they think that boron is needed for activation of vitamin D.

A daily intake of 1.5 to 3 milligrams of boron is probably more than adequate to meet your requirements for bone growth and development. The main food sources are fruits and vegetables, but boron content will depend on how much of the mineral is in the soil. If you want to take a supplement, 3 to 9 milligrams per day is a very safe amount. Intakes greater than 500 milligrams a day can cause nausea, vomiting and diarrhea. Your best bet is to strive for at least five servings of fruits and vegetables each day.

MANGANESE, ZINC AND COPPER
These are important helpers (cofactors) for enzymes that are essential to making bone tissue. The impact of these nutrients on bone loss has been studied in postmenopausal women. The women who received a daily supplement of calcium, manganese, copper and zinc did not experience any bone loss of the spine at the end of the two-year study.[13] The placebo group, on the other hand, lost 3.5 percent of their bone mass. Manganese is widely available in foods, and deficiencies have not been seen in humans. Meat and drinking water are your best bets for copper. When it comes to zinc, reach for wheat bran, wheat germ, oysters, seafood, lean red meat and milk.

LIFESTYLE FACTORS

Exercise

Until the age of 30, regular exercise helps women get a head start on building peak bone mass. In fact, studies have found that children who spend the most time being physically active have stronger bones than those who are sedentary. But the effect of exercise doesn't stop once you've achieved your peak mass. Bone cells are constantly active, tearing up old bone and laying down new bone. Participating in weight-bearing activities like brisk walking or stair climbing stimulates bones to increase in strength and density during the pre- and postmenopausal years. One study found that postmenopausal women who worked out three times a week for nine months actually increased their bone mass by 5.2 percent.[14]

If your exercise routine includes weight training there's no need to put away your dumbbells. Researchers have learned that this type of exercise also has a protective effect on bone density in women. Women who worked out with weights for one hour three times a week gained 1.6 percent bone mass; non-exercisers actually lost 3.6 percent of bone in their spine.

If you have osteoporosis, a safe exercise program can help you slow bone loss, improve posture and balance, and build muscle strength and tone. The benefits of exercise can reduce your risk of falling and fracturing a bone.

Your best bet is to incorporate a mix of activities in your week. Aim to get four weight-bearing activities each week and two or three weight workouts. If you have never used weights before, be sure to consult a certified personal trainer. Personal trainers work in fitness clubs and many will come to your home. They'll design a safe and effective program for you. And don't worry, you don't need a basement full of exercise equipment. Some of the best trainers I know teach women creative ways of building muscle strength without using weights.

THE BOTTOM LINE...
Leslie's recommendations for preventing osteoporosis and bone fracture

1. If you're approaching menopause, get your bone density measured to help you and your doctor determine if medication is required to prevent osteoporosis.

2. If you're already a fan of soy foods, consider boosting your intake to achieve a daily intake of at least 50 milligrams of isoflavones.

3. To strengthen your bones, make sure you're eating enough protein-rich foods like fish, poultry, lean meat, legumes, tofu and dairy products. But don't go overboard—some studies suggest that very high intakes of protein cause your kidneys to excrete calcium.

4. To prevent too much calcium from being lost from your body, keep your caffeine intake to a daily maximum of 450 milligrams (no more than three small cups of coffee). If you have osteoporosis, keep this to no more than 200 milligrams. And be sure you're meeting your calcium requirements.

5. Go easy on sodium from processed foods and the salt shaker. For every 500 milligrams (1/5 teaspoon) of additional sodium you consume, you need to consume an extra 40 milligrams of calcium.

6. Depending on your age and your risk for osteoporosis, get 1000 to 1500 milligrams of calcium each day.

   • For every 300-milligram portion of calcium your diet lacks, take a 300-milligram calcium supplement with vitamin D and magnesium added.

   • If you're using a calcium carbonate supplement, be sure to take it with food, since it needs plenty of stomach acid to make it ready for absorption.

   • If you're over 50, or produce less stomach acid because of a medication, buy a supplement made from calcium citrate or calcium chelate.

7. To help you absorb the calcium in your diet, make sure you get 200 to 600 international units of vitamin D each day.

   • Make a real effort to boost your vitamin D intake in the winter, when your body's natural production of the vitamin is reduced by a lack of sunlight.

   • To help you meet your daily needs, take a multivitamin and mineral supplement with 400 IU of vitamin D.

   • If you take calcium supplements, buy one with vitamin D added.

8. Buy a calcium supplement that contains ipriflavone, a synthetic isoflavone manufactured from a natural compound found in soybeans. Take 150 to 200 milligrams three times daily.

9. Other nutrients that help build bone density include vitamin A, vitamin C, vitamin K, magnesium, phosphorus, boron, manganese, zinc and copper. Take a look at the food sources I've outlined to see if your diet is lacking any.

10. If you don't work out now, add regular exercise to your life.

11

Heart Disease and High Cholesterol

Heart disease is a serious health problem faced by postmenopausal women. Heart disease and stroke account for 43 percent of all deaths among American women, representing the top two killers. With the loss of estrogen, a woman's risk of getting heart disease increases four-fold and continues to rise with age.

Compared to men, women are more likely to die in the year following their heart attack. This is largely due to the fact that women get heart disease when they are older and they have more advanced heart disease by the time they are diagnosed. Symptoms like chest pain tend to be ignored or overlooked in women. Both women and their doctors may attribute these symptoms to indigestion, stress or gallbladder problems. As well, women tend to get to a hospital much later after having a heart attack than do men, and they also tend to receive less aggressive therapy.

❧

What Causes Heart Disease?

"Heart disease" is a general term that includes coronary heart disease, congenital heart disease (the kind you're born with), congestive heart failure and malfunctioning heart valves. We'll discuss only coronary heart disease, a disease that affects the blood vessels that feed the heart. Coronary heart disease is caused by atherosclerosis, a gradual process that narrows the heart's arteries and leads to a heart attack.

Atherosclerosis can begin in adolescence when fatty streaks, which may one day cause heart disease, can appear on the lining of arteries as cholesterol sticks to the arteries. The next stage of atherosclerosis is an injury to the lining of an artery. An infection or virus, high blood pressure, cigarette smoke or diabetes may cause this damage. Your body attempts to heal itself, just like it would with any wound. Immune cells are attracted to the injured artery wall and accumulate. Over time, the fatty streaks enlarge and become hardened with minerals, tissue, fat and cells, forming plaques. As plaques form beneath the artery wall, they stiffen arteries and narrow the passage through them. Most people have well-developed plaques by the time they are 30 years old. If atherosclerosis progresses, it can restrict blood flow to the heart.

Blood cells called platelets respond to damaged spots on blood vessels by forming clots. A clot may stick to a plaque and gradually enlarge until it blocks blood flow to an area of the heart. That portion of the heart may die slowly and form scar tissue. But a clot can also break loose, and circulate in the blood until it reaches an artery too small to pass through. When a clot that's wedged in a vessel cuts off the supply of oxygen and nutrients to a part of the heart muscle, a heart attack results.

Who's at Risk?

Risk factors for heart disease are usually classified as either modifiable or non-modifiable. Non-modifiable factors—like getting older or having a strong family history of early heart attacks—are risk factors that you can't change. But you can reduce your risk by changing modifiable risk factors. You can change your diet, exercise more or quit smoking. You can even control risk factors such as high blood pressure or diabetes. Here's a glance at the factors that put you at risk for heart disease (the more risk factors you have, the greater your risk):

Non-modifiable Risk Factors

- You're over 40. As you get older your body becomes less efficient at clearing cholesterol from the bloodstream. With advancing age, many women develop high blood pressure and diabetes, two other risk factors for heart disease.

- You're at or past menopause. Both natural and surgical menopause are associated with an increased risk. Before menopause, estrogen protects the heart by keeping cholesterol levels in check and blood vessels more flexible.

- You have a family history of heart attack prior to age 60. Your risk is even greater if you have a female relative who suffered heart disease.

Modifiable Risk Factors

- You have high blood cholesterol or you don't know.

- You have high blood triglycerides or you don't know.

- You have low HDL cholesterol or you don't know.

- You have high blood pressure or you don't know.

- You smoke cigarettes. Smoking is a more important predictor of heart attack in middle-aged women than it is in men. Women who use oral contraceptives and smoke cigarettes have an even higher risk. Smoking damages the lining of the arteries, increasing the likelihood of plaque formation. Inhaling cigarette smoke also produces free radicals in the body, which then damage LDL cholesterol, making it stick to the artery walls. Finally, smoking increases blood pressure and makes blood clot formation more likely.

- You have a poor diet.

- You don't exercise regularly. Regular exercise helps you maintain a healthy weight. It lowers LDL cholesterol and raises HDL cholesterol, and it strengthens the heart and blood vessels.

- You have diabetes. A woman with diabetes is three times more likely to experience heart disease than a non-diabetic woman. In diabetes, fatty plaques develop and progress much more rapidly.

- Your BMI is more than 25 (see page 45 in chapter 2 to determine your BMI). Carrying extra weight puts stress on your heart and circulatory system. Being overweight can also lead to high blood pressure and elevated blood cholesterol. Excess weight around the waist is much more dangerous to your heart than excess lower body fat.

CHOLESTEROL LEVELS

There are two different kinds of cholesterol. Dietary cholesterol is found in foods and blood cholesterol is made by your liver. For most people, the two are unrelated. That means that dietary cholesterol has little or no effect on the amount of cholesterol in the blood. Cholesterol and fat are transported in your bloodstream on carrier molecules called lipoproteins. The lipoproteins that have received the most attention are low-density lipoproteins (LDL), high-density lipoproteins (HDL) and triglycerides. If you know your cholesterol levels, use the following reference guide to determine if your level is healthy, or if it puts you at higher risk for heart disease.

BLOOD LIPID	DESIRABLE	BORDERLINE RISK	AT RISK
Total cholesterol	<200	200–239	≥240
LDL cholesterol	<130	130–159	≥160
HDL cholesterol	50–60	N/A	<40
Triglycerides	<150	150–199	≥200

Blood lipids are measured in milligrams per deciliter (mg/dl).

Circulating cholesterol contributes to heart disease by becoming part of the fatty plaques that build up on artery walls. The more LDL cholesterol there is in the blood, the more cholesterol there is available to attach to artery walls. The longer you have high LDL levels, the greater the chance more cholesterol has built up in your arteries. While LDL is considered bad, oxidized LDL cholesterol is deemed even worse. Once LDL cholesterol becomes oxidized or damaged by harmful free radical molecules, it then is much more likely to accumulate in your arteries. You'll read below how dietary antioxidants may help prevent such damage to LDL cholesterol particles.

Blood cholesterol levels rise quickly in women after menopause. By the age of 55, women have higher cholesterol levels than men. Having high total cholesterol does not pose as much risk for women as it does for men. What does increase your risk for heart disease is having both a *low HDL cholesterol* and a *high triglyceride level*. It's estimated that this combination increases a woman's risk of heart disease ten-fold. In order to get a more accurate picture of your risk for heart disease, it's important to get *all* types of cholesterol measured, not just your total number. For instance, if your total cholesterol is 250, but your HDL is high, then your risk for heart disease is less.

Your ratio of total cholesterol to HDL cholesterol is considered a better predictor of heart disease risk than LDL or HDL values alone. This score is referred to as your risk ratio—your total cholesterol divided by your HDL cholesterol. Here's a reference guide for women:

Total/HDL Cholesterol (Risk Ratio)

Below average risk	<3.5
Average risk	3.5–5.0
Above average risk	5–10
Much above average risk	>10

HIGH BLOOD PRESSURE

The higher your blood pressure is above normal, the greater your risk for heart disease. Arteries that are stiff from atherosclerosis strain as blood pulses through them. And if you have high blood pressure as well, your arteries are put under much greater stress. Stressed and strained arteries develop more lesions, and fatty plaques grow more frequently.

Blood pressure results from the pressure generated by your heart as it pushes blood through your arteries. When your heart beats, the blood pressure in your arteries rises. When the heart relaxes between beats, blood pressure falls. Your blood pressure is taken as two measures, a systolic and diastolic pressure. A healthy blood pressure in adults is 120/80 (systolic/diastolic). Doctors interpret the bottom number, the diastolic blood pressure, to determine if you have hypertension. Here are the standards used:

Diastolic Blood Pressure

Normal	<85
High-normal	80–89
Mild hypertension	90–99
Moderate hypertension	100–109
Severe hypertension	110–119
Very severe hypertension	>120

Hypertension is more common in women over the age of 55 than it is in men of the same age. High blood pressure has no symptoms. The only way you can detect it is by having it checked regularly. Your blood pressure should be taken when you are relaxed, not stressed. When you're anxious your blood pressure rises, but when you relax it returns to normal. High blood pressure is treated by weight loss, dietary modifications and often medication.

HOMOCYSTEINE

Today many studies are focusing on a compound called homocysteine. Homocysteine is an amino acid that our body produces during cellular metabolism. Normally we convert homocysteine to other harmless amino acids with the help of B vitamins. When this conversion doesn't occur, homocysteine can accumulate in the blood and damage vessel walls, promoting the build-up of cholesterol. Homocysteine levels can accumulate as a result of an inherited genetic defect or a deficiency of B vitamins.

A number of studies have discovered that people with high homocysteine levels have a much higher risk of heart disease. Researchers from Boston found that, among 28,263 postmenopausal women, those with the highest levels of homocysteine had more than twice the risk of heart attack or stroke compared to women with the lowest levels.[1]

At this time, there is no clear definition of normal or healthy levels. But as you'll read below, there are some simple dietary modifications to help prevent homocysteine from accumulating in your bloodstream.

Preventing Heart Disease

Many of the risk factors for heart disease are influenced by what you eat. Here are a few strategies that can reduce your chances of getting heart disease. My nutrition and herbal recommendations will 1) keep your blood lipids at a healthy level, 2) prevent damage or oxidation to your LDL cholesterol, 3) lower blood pressure and 4) promote a little weight loss.

DIETARY STRATEGIES

Dietary Fat

One of the most important strategies for keeping your total and LDL cholesterol levels within the healthy range is to reduce your fat intake to no more than 30 percent of your total calorie intake. If you eat 2000 calories per day, that means consuming no more than 65 grams of fat. If you follow a 1200-calorie weight-loss diet, you should be striving for no more than 40 grams of fat per day. But not all types of dietary fat affect your blood cholesterol the same way. Some fats have a strong impact on your risk for heart disease, whereas others are neutral and don't affect your risk.

1. *Saturated Fat* Dietary fats are named according to their chemical structure. Saturated fats are solid at room temperature. This is the type of fat that's found in animal foods—meat, poultry, eggs and dairy products. Diets high in saturated fat raise your risk for heart disease by increasing the level of blood cholesterol. Saturated fat seems to inhibit the activity of LDL receptors on cells so that this type of cholesterol accumulates in the bloodstream.

   There are many different types of saturated fats in foods and not all of them influence blood cholesterol levels to the same degree. For instance, the saturated fat in dairy products is more cholesterol-raising than the saturated fat in meat. And the type of saturated fat in chocolate does not raise blood cholesterol levels. You certainly don't need to learn the different types of saturated fats in foods. What's most important is to eat less saturated fat, period. Saturated fat should account for less than 10 percent of your daily calories.

FOOD	LOWER-FAT CHOICES OR SUBSTITUTES
Milk	Skim, 1% milkfat (MF)
Yogurt	Products with less than 1.5% MF
Cheese	Products with less than 20% MF
Cottage cheese	Products with 1% MF
Sour cream	Products with 7% MF or less
Cream	Evaporated 2% or skim milk

Red meat	Flank steak, inside round, sirloin, eye of round, extra lean ground beef, venison
Pork	Center-cut pork chops, pork tenderloin, pork leg (inside round, roast), baked ham, deli ham, back bacon
Poultry	Skinless chicken breast, turkey breast, ground turkey
Eggs	Egg whites; 2 whites replace 1 whole egg (you can buy these right beside the fresh eggs in your grocery store)

Making lower-fat choices will help you eat less saturated fat. But pay attention to portion sizes too. When you eat lean meat, your portion size should not exceed 3 ounces (90 grams).

Where does butter fit in? It's true that butter is a concentrated source of saturated fat. But if your blood cholesterol levels are normal, there is no reason why you can't include butter in your diet; just use it sparingly. Even if your blood cholesterol levels are high, you can still use a little butter. Many people have made the switch to margarine because, unlike butter, margarine is made from a vegetable oil that doesn't contain saturated fat. If you do like margarine, be sure you're using a healthy product.

2. *Trans Fat* If you are unfamiliar with this term, you may have heard about hydrogenated fat instead. Hydrogenation is a chemical process that adds hydrogen atoms to liquid vegetable oils. This makes vegetable fats more solid and more useful to food manufacturers. Packaged foods like cookies, crackers and baked goods made with hydrogenated vegetable oils are more palatable and have a longer shelf life. Margarines made by hydrogenating a vegetable oil are firm like butter.

When a vegetable oil is hydrogenated, it becomes saturated *and* it forms a new type of fat called trans fat. Trans fat increases the LDL cholesterol and decreases the HDL cholesterol. Many researchers believe that trans fat is worse for our cholesterol levels than saturated fat. The Harvard Nurses' Health Study revealed that women who had the highest intake of trans fat had a 50 percent higher risk of heart disease compared to women who ate the least.[2] Foods that contributed to their trans fat intake were margarine, cookies, cake and white bread.

The easiest way to reduce your intake of trans fat is to start reading food labels and ingredient lists. Look for the words "partially hydrogenated vegetable oils" and eat foods that contain them less often. As much as 40 percent of the fat in foods like french fries, fast food, doughnuts, pastries, snack foods and commercial cookies is trans fat. If you eat margarine, choose one that's made with non-hydrogenated fat—many brands state this right on the label.

It is anticipated that pre-packaged foods will soon list the grams of trans fat on the Nutrition Facts panel. At the time of writing, the U.S. FDA is moving quickly to require trans fat on nutrition labels after a report from the Institute of Medicine found there is no safe level in people's diets. Eating some trans fat may be unavoidable, but you should limit your intake as much as possible to lower your risk for heart disease. Until the new labeling becomes law, check ingredient lists for the terms *hydrogenated, partially hydrogenated* or *shortening.*

3. *Polyunsaturated Fat* This type of dietary fat is liquid at room temperature. Omega-6 polyunsaturated fats are found in all vegetable oils including canola, sunflower, safflower, corn, sesame and flaxseed. Omega-3 polyunsaturated fats are found in fish and seafood and in certain vegetable oils. Replacing foods that provide mostly saturated fat with those rich in polyunsaturated fats can help you lower your cholesterol level. As I mentioned above, eating less saturated fat is an important way to lower high blood cholesterol levels. A good start would be to eat fish more often than meat or poultry.

But the omega-3 fats found in fish can do more than just help you eat less animal fat. This special class of polyunsaturated fats can lower high levels of blood triglycerides and reduce the stickiness of platelets, the cells that form blood clots in arteries. Omega-3 fats may also increase the flexibility of red blood cells so they can pass more readily through tiny blood vessels. Many studies have found that populations that consume fish a few times each week have lower rates of heart disease.

The American Heart Association recommends we eat fish at least twice weekly to reap its heart-healthy benefits. I recommend, however, that my clients eat fish three times a week. Choose oilier fish for a boost of omega-3—salmon, trout, sardines, herring, mackerel, sea bass and fresh tuna are good choices (canned tuna has very little omega-3 fat).

4. *Monounsaturated Fat* These fats turn semi-solid when you store them in the fridge and are liquid at room temperature. Monounsaturated fats found in olive,

canola and peanut oils are considered to be neutral because they don't influence blood cholesterol levels on their own. Don't eliminate them from your diet just because they won't help lower your cholesterol level. Research suggests that extra-virgin olive oil helps prevent blood clots from forming and acts as an antioxidant to help protect from heart disease. Extra-virgin olive oil has been processed the least and has a darker color.

Dietary Cholesterol

This waxlike fatty substance is found in meat, poultry, eggs, dairy products, fish and seafood. It's particularly plentiful in shrimp, liver and egg yolks. While high-cholesterol diets cause high blood cholesterol in animals, this is not the case in humans. Dietary cholesterol has little or no effect on most people's blood cholesterol. One reason for this is that our intestines absorb only half the cholesterol we eat. If your blood test results reveal that your cholesterol level is too high, you don't have to give up eggs or seafood. A study from Harvard University did not find any significant association between egg intake and risk of heart disease or stroke on healthy men and women.[3] You're safe to enjoy five or six eggs a week, as this will not affect your risk for heart disease.

However, too much dietary cholesterol can raise levels of LDL cholesterol in some people, especially people with hereditary forms of high cholesterol. The American Heart Association recommends that we consume no more than 300 milligrams of cholesterol each day. Choosing animal foods that are lower in saturated fat also helps to cut down on dietary cholesterol. Here's a look at foods that might be contributing to your intake of cholesterol:

FOOD	CHOLESTEROL (MILLIGRAMS)
1 egg, whole	212 mg
1 egg, white only	0 mg
Beef sirloin, lean only, 3 oz (90 g)	64 mg
Calf liver, fried, 3 oz (90 g)	416 mg
Pork loin, lean only, 3 oz (90 g)	71 mg

Chicken breast, no skin, 3 oz (90 g)	73 mg
Salmon, 3 oz (90 g)	54 mg
Shrimp, 3 oz (90 g)	135 mg
Milk, 2% MF, 1 cup (250 ml)	19 mg
Milk, skim, 1 cup (250 ml)	5 mg
Cheese, cheddar, 31% MF, 1 oz (30 g)	31 mg
Cheese, mozzarella, part skim, 1 oz (30 g)	18 mg
Cream, half and half, 12% MF, 2 tbsp (30 ml)	12 mg
Yogurt, 1.5% MF, 3/4 cup (175 ml)	11 mg
Butter, 2 tsp (10 ml)	10 mg

Soy Foods

In the fall of 1999 the U.S. Food and Drug Administration passed a regulation allowing manufacturers of soy foods to add a health claim on the label. Labels on cartons of tofu, soy beverages, veggie dogs and veggie burgers now tell shoppers that eating a low-fat diet containing 25 grams of soy protein a day lowers the risk for heart disease.

In 1995, the soy-and-heart-disease link became popular when researchers from Lexington, Kentucky, published a report in the *New England Journal of Medicine* that analyzed 38 studies on soy and cholesterol.[4] The researchers determined that eating soy protein instead of animal protein significantly lowered high levels of LDL cholesterol and triglycerides. Since then, a number of other studies have confirmed soy's cholesterol-lowering ability.

It appears that soy does more than lower high LDL cholesterol levels. A regular intake of soy may raise your HDL cholesterol, lower high blood pressure and keep blood vessels healthy. Natural compounds in soybeans appear to also act as an antioxidant, preventing oxygen damage to LDL cholesterol (since LDL cholesterol damaged by oxygen free radicals sticks more readily to artery walls).

Soybean's heart-healthy attributes are credited to its protein and isoflavone (phytoestrogens) content. When it comes to lowering cholesterol levels, you need both components. Supplements containing purified isoflavones will not lower your cholesterol levels. If you want to keep your LDL cholesterol levels healthy, add 25 grams of soy protein to your low-fat diet each day. Use the following guide:

SOY FOOD	SOY PROTEIN (GRAMS)
Soy beverage, 1 cup (250 ml)	9 g
Soybeans, canned, 1/2 cup (125 ml)	14 g
Soy nuts, 1/4 cup (60 ml)	14 g
Soy flour, defatted, 1/4 cup (60 ml)	13 g
Soy protein powder, isolate, 1 scoop	25 g
Tempeh, 1/2 cup (125 ml)	19 g
Tofu, regular, 1/2 cup (125 ml)	10 g
Veggie burger, Yves Veggie Cuisine	11 g
Veggie dog, small, Yves Veggie Cuisine	11 g

Soluble Fiber

Plant foods contain a mix of two types of fiber, soluble and insoluble, but they will contain more of one than the other. It's soluble fiber—which dissolves or swells in water—that has been shown to lower high blood cholesterol levels. The best food sources of these fibers include oats and oat bran, psyllium-enriched breakfast cereals, legumes and certain fruits and vegetables.

Adding soluble fiber to a low-fat diet can significantly lower elevated cholesterol levels. Studies show that adding oats and beans to your diet can lower cholesterol by up to 16 percent. And eating a psyllium-enriched breakfast cereal has been shown to lower LDL cholesterol by 9 percent.[5]

There are two ways in which soluble fiber exerts a cholesterol-lowering effect. When this fiber reaches your intestine, it attaches to bile and causes it to be excreted in the stool. Bile is a digestive aid that's released into your intestine after you eat. Your liver makes bile from cholesterol and sends it to your gall bladder to be stored until it's needed. Since soluble fiber causes your body to excrete bile, your liver has to make more of it from cholesterol. The end result is a lower blood cholesterol level. When unabsorbed fiber reaches your colon, bacteria degrade it and form compounds called short-chain fatty acids. These fatty acids may hamper your liver's ability to produce cholesterol.

Here's a list of foods rich in soluble fiber—start adding a few to your daily diet:

BREAKFAST CEREALS	LEGUMES	FRUITS	VEGETABLES
Oatmeal	Kidney beans	Orange	Carrots
Oat bran	Black beans	Grapefruit	Potatoes
Kellogg's All-Bran Buds	Chickpeas	Apple	Sweet potatoes
Psyllium-enriched cereals	Lentils	Strawberries	Green peas
	Soybeans	Pears	
	Navy beans	Cantaloupe	

If you've decided to try a psyllium-rich breakfast cereal, start with a small portion. Too much can cause bloating and gas if you're not used to it. It usually takes two weeks for the bacteria that reside in your intestine to adjust to a higher fiber intake. Start by adding 1/4 to 1/2 cup (60–125 ml) of Kellogg's All-Bran Buds to your usual breakfast cereal. Over the course of two or three weeks, increase your portion. Be sure to increase your water intake as you consume more fiber, as soluble fiber needs fluid in order to work.

Whole Grains

In addition to fiber, whole-grain foods like whole-wheat bread, whole-grain breakfast cereals and oats have other protective ingredients that might help lower the risk of heart disease. Harvard researchers learned from the Nurses' Health Study that women who had the highest intake of whole grains had a 33 percent lower risk of heart disease compared to women who consumed the least.[6] The Iowa Women's Health Study also found a link between whole-grain intake and heart health. In this study of almost 35,000 postmenopausal women, those who ate two servings of whole grains each day had the lowest rates of heart disease.[7]

The heart-protective effects of whole grains may be due to a number of natural compounds. Whole grains are important sources of vitamin E, zinc, selenium, copper, iron and manganese, and special phytochemicals (from plants) called phenols. All of these natural compounds have antioxidant properties and may offer protection from heart disease.

A food made from whole grains means that it contains *all* parts of the grain—the outer bran layer where most of the fiber is, the germ layer that's rich in nutrients like vitamin E and the endosperm that contains the starch. When whole grains are processed into flakes, puffs or white flour, all that's left is the starchy endosperm. Refined grains offer significantly less vitamin E, B6, magnesium, potassium, zinc and fiber. Use the following guide to help you get more whole grains in your diet.

WHOLE GRAIN	REFINED GRAIN
Barley	Cornmeal
Brown rice	Pearled barley
Bulgur	Unbleached flour
Flaxseed	Pasta
Kamut	White rice
Oatmeal	
Oat bran	
Quinoa	
Whole-wheat bread*	
Whole-rye bread	
Spelt	

When buying bread, look for the words "whole-wheat flour" or "whole-rye flour" on the list of ingredients. Wheat flour and unbleached wheat flour mean it's refined.

Nuts

Adding a handful of nuts to your diet may also improve your odds against developing heart disease. Populations that include nuts as a regular part of their diet have lower rates of heart disease. The large Nurses' Health Study discovered that women who ate 5 ounces of nuts each week had a 35 percent lower risk of heart attack and death from heart disease, compared to women who never ate nuts or ate them less than once a month.[8]

Nuts and seeds are rich sources of vitamin E and many important minerals. And nuts are good sources of essential fatty acids (alpha linolenic acid and linoleic acid) as well as dietary fiber. Add a 1/4 cup (60 ml) portion of nuts to your diet five times a week. Try the following:

- Add peanuts to an Asian-style stir-fry.
- Stir-fry collard greens with cashews and a teaspoon of sesame oil.
- Add walnuts to your tossed green salad.
- Try walnut oil in your next salad dressing (use half olive oil and half walnut oil).
- Mix sunflower or pumpkin seeds into a bowl of hot cereal or yogurt.
- Snack on a mix of almonds and dried apricots.
- Sprinkle your casserole with a handful of mixed nuts.

Tea and Flavonoids

According to researchers, natural antioxidants found in green and black tea may protect your heart. For instance, a study looked at the effect of tea, coffee and decaffeinated coffee in 340 people who had had a heart attack. Compared to non-tea-drinkers, those who enjoyed at least one cup a day had a 44 percent lower risk of heart attack.[9]

Tea leaves contain compounds called flavonoids. Literally hundreds of different flavonoids have been identified in plants, and the ones in tea are called catechins. You'll find catechins in green tea, black tea and oolong tea, but not in herbal teas. If you've read chapter 8, "Breast Cancer," you already know that catechins in tea may also help protect from this disease. To incorporate tea into your diet, replace coffee and soft drinks with your favorite type of tea, be it Earl Grey, orange-spice, apricot, raspberry or black currant. In the summer, make your own iced tea from freshly brewed tea and lemons.

Alcohol

If you're in the habit of having a glass of wine with your dinner, you might be doing your heart a favor. Many studies have found that a moderate intake of alcohol reduces the risk of heart disease. The Nurses' Health Study, for example, determined women who consumed one to six drinks a week had a 12 to 17 percent lower risk of dying from heart disease compared to women who abstained from alcohol.[10]

Drinking alcohol, whether it's wine, beer or liquor, raises the level of HDL cholesterol, and it may reduce blood clotting. There is also evidence that antioxidants in wine, especially red wine, may keep LDL cholesterol healthy. Keep in mind that the protective effects of alcohol are most apparent in people over the age of 50 and in those with more than one risk factor for heart disease. If you're a healthy premenopausal woman, a drink a day probably won't do much for your heart.

Health authorities do not advise that you drink a couple of glasses of wine a day. That's because there are too many negative health effects associated with a moderate intake of one or two drinks a day, including increasing your risk for breast cancer.

If you do drink alcohol, keep your intake down to no more than one or two drinks a day. If you are a non-drinker, don't start now. There are plenty of other nutrition strategies you can put in place to reduce the odds of heart disease.

VITAMINS AND MINERALS

B Vitamins

These nutrients won't lower your cholesterol, but they will help keep your homocysteine at a healthy level; a high level of homocysteine is associated with a higher risk of heart attack. In order to prevent homocysteine from accumulating and damaging blood vessels, the body uses three B vitamins—folate, B6 and B12—to convert it into other harmless compounds.

One simple strategy to lower elevated homocysteine levels is to boost your intake of these three B vitamins. Harvard researchers proved this point when they studied 80,000 women for 14 years and found that those who consumed the most folate and vitamin B6 had a 45 percent lower risk of heart disease compared to women who consumed the least.[11] Among those women who got plenty of B vitamins in their diet, the risk of heart disease was also lower if they regularly took a multivitamin and mineral supplement, a major source of folate and B6. See the B vitamin table on page 4 in chapter 1 to see how to get more B's into your daily diet.

If you have difficulty eating a varied diet, I recommend taking a good quality multivitamin and mineral supplement to ensure you're getting your daily B vitamins. If you're over 50, you should be getting your B12 from a supplement anyway. That's because as we age, we become less efficient at producing stomach acid, a necessary aid for B12 absorption from food. Look for a supplement that offers 0.4 to 1.0 milligrams of folic acid, the supplement form of folate.

If you're looking for more B vitamins than a regular multi gives you, choose a "high potency" or "super" formula that contains 30 to 75 milligrams of B vitamins (or 1000 micrograms in the case of folic acid). One word of caution: the B vitamin niacin may cause flushing of the face and chest when it's taken in doses greater than 35 milligrams—this is easily avoided if you take your supplement just after eating a meal. This symptom is harmless and goes away within 20 minutes, but some people find it uncomfortable. To avoid flushing, look for a formula that contains niacinamide, a non-flushing form of niacin, instead.

Vitamin C

Many studies have reported a link between high dietary intakes and high blood levels of vitamin C and a lower risk of heart disease. American researchers observed that rates of heart disease were 27 percent lower in the men and women with the highest vitamin C levels compared to those with the lowest.[12] The level of vitamin C in your bloodstream is a good indicator of the amount of vitamin C in your diet. One Portuguese study conducted among 194 adults determined that, compared to those individuals with marginal vitamin C intakes, those who consumed the most vitamin C had an 80 percent lower risk of heart attack.[13]

Vitamin C may protect from heart disease by acting as an antioxidant. The vitamin is able to neutralize harmful free radical molecules that damage your LDL cholesterol. That means that your LDL cholesterol is less likely to accumulate on artery walls. Studies also suggest vitamin C may inhibit the formation of blood clots by reducing the stickiness of platelets.

The daily recommended intake for vitamin C is 75 milligrams (smokers need 110 milligrams). You can meet your vitamin C requirements fairly easily from food—check out the Vitamin C in Foods table on page 12 in chapter 1.

Vitamin C Supplements

For those of you who don't eat at least two vitamin-C-rich foods each day, a supplement is a good idea. If you're looking for the most C for your money, choose a supplement labeled "Ester C." Studies in the lab have found this form of vitamin C to be more available to the body. If you prefer a chewable supplement, make sure it contains calcium ascorbate or sodium ascorbate, since these forms of vitamin C are less acidic and less harmful to the enamel of your teeth. Take a 500-milligram supplement once or twice a day. There's little point in swallowing much more than that, since your body can use only about 200 milligrams at one time. If you want to take more, split your dose over the course of the day.

Vitamin E

Many studies have shown that vitamin E supplements prevent heart attacks in healthy men and women who don't have existing heart disease. A large study of U.S. nurses, published in the *New England Journal of Medicine*, found that women who took supplemental vitamin E—100 international units or IU—for two years had a 41 percent lower risk of heart attack compared to non-users of supplements.[14] Studies have also found that vitamin E protects against heart disease in men.

This vitamin is a potent antioxidant. Once consumed from the diet or a supplement, vitamin E makes its way to the liver where it is incorporated into the lipoproteins that transport cholesterol. It is here that vitamin E works to protect these compounds from oxygen damage caused by free radicals. Vitamin E may also inhibit blood clot formation and preserve the health of blood vessels that feed the heart.

See the RDA table on page 15 in chapter 1 to see how much vitamin E you need each day. The daily upper limit for vitamin E is 1500 IU of natural vitamin E or 2200 IU of the synthetic form. The best food sources of vitamin E include wheat germ, nuts, seeds, vegetable oils, whole grains and kale.

Vitamin E Supplements

Even if you boost your daily intake of vitamin-E-rich foods, you still won't come close to getting 100 IU, the amount deemed to offer protection in the U.S. Nurses' Health Study. For this reason, you must rely on a supplement. Here's what you need to know about vitamin E supplements:

- Take 100 to 400 IU per day. If you're healthy, there's no evidence to warrant taking more.

- Buy a natural source vitamin E supplement (or look for *d-alpha-tocopherol* on the label; synthetic forms are labeled *dl-alpha tocopherol*). Although the body absorbs both synthetic and natural forms equally well, your liver prefers the natural form. It incorporates more natural vitamin E into carrier molecules.

- Consider choosing a vitamin E supplement that is labeled "mixed tocopherols." Preliminary research shows that one form of vitamin E called gamma-tocopherol has potent anti-inflammatory effects in addition to its antioxidant properties. This may play a role in cancer prevention.

- If you're taking a blood-thinning medication like Coumadin® (warfarin), don't take vitamin E without your doctor's approval, since it has slight anti-clotting properties.

Lycopene

Lycopene is a cousin of beta-carotene, the antioxidant nutrient that's plentiful in carrots, but lycopene is twice as potent as an antioxidant. Lycopene is found in red-colored fruits and vegetables. Tomatoes are the richest source of lycopene, but you'll also find some in pink grapefruit, watermelon, guava and apricots.

Researchers have observed a relationship between the amount of lycopene in the blood and in body fat stores and the risk of heart disease. As an antioxidant, lycopene is yet another dietary defense mechanism against free radical damage to LDL cholesterol. Toronto researchers studied the effect of dietary lycopene in 19 healthy adults and found that a diet supplemented with tomato products doubled lycopene blood levels *and* significantly reduced free radical damage to LDL cholesterol.[15] Lycopene may also lower the level of LDL cholesterol by hampering its production in the liver.

While the research on the role of lycopene in heart disease is just beginning, there's no reason why you shouldn't add this antioxidant to your diet. It appears that an intake of 5 to 7 milligrams offers protection.

FOOD	LYCOPENE (MILLIGRAMS)
Tomato, raw, 1 small	0.8–3.8 mg
Tomatoes, cooked, 1 cup (250 ml)	9.25 mg
Tomato sauce, 1/2 cup (125 ml)	3.1 mg
Tomato paste, 2 tbsp (30 ml)	8.0 mg
Tomato juice, 1 cup (250 ml)	23.0 mg
Ketchup, 2 tbsp (30 ml)	3.1–4.2 mg
Apricots, dried, 10 halves	0.3 mg
Grapefruit, pink, half	4.2 mg
Papaya, 1 whole	6.2–16.5 mg
Watermelon, 1 slice (25 cm × 2 cm)	8.5–26.4 mg

Heat-processed tomato products provide a source of lycopene that is much more available to the body. To increase the amount of lycopene you absorb, add a little olive oil to your pasta sauce. Lycopene is a fat-soluble compound and, as such, it is better absorbed along with a little fat.

LYCOPENE SUPPLEMENTS

Lycopene supplements are available in health food stores and drug stores. If you opt for the supplement route, choose a brand that's made with the Lyc-O-Mato™ or LycoRed™ extract. This source of lycopene is derived from whole tomatoes, and it's the source that has been used in clinical studies. Most supplements offer 5 milligrams of lycopene per tablet.

HERBAL REMEDIES

Garlic

Garlic contains many different sulfur compounds, and one in particular, called S-allyl cysteine (SAC), has been shown to lower LDL cholesterol by up to 10 percent.[16] SAC is present in small amounts in raw garlic, but it increases in concentration when garlic ages. The scientific studies that show a cholesterol-lowering effect have used an extract of aged garlic extract (Kyolic® brand).

Aside from its ability to lower blood cholesterol, garlic may protect from heart disease in other ways. Studies have shown the herb can lower blood triglyceride levels and thin the blood by reducing the stickiness of platelets. The sulfur compounds in aged garlic extract also act as an antioxidant and prevent damage to LDL cholesterol. Finally, a daily dose of aged garlic extract may also have a modest blood-pressure-lowering effect.

Many scientists agree that as little as a half clove each day will offer health benefits. And most people can take one or two cloves a day without any problems. Some people experience stomach upset when they eat raw garlic—the oil-soluble compounds in garlic account for its potential to irritate the stomach and to cause odor.

Try to use more raw garlic in cooking. Add it to sauces, soups, casseroles and salad dressings. Although raw garlic contains very little SAC, a recent study from Penn State University found that if you let crushed garlic sit at room temperature for 10 minutes before cooking with it, more of these beneficial sulfur compounds will be formed.[17]

When it comes to garlic supplements, the scientific research points to aged garlic extract as the supplement of choice, because of its higher concentration of SAC. Generally, two to six capsules a day (one or two with meals) are recommended.

THE BOTTOM LINE...

Leslie's recommendations for preventing heart disease

1. To keep your cholesterol levels in the healthy range, reduce your intake of saturated fat.

2. To eat less trans fat, avoid foods that contain partially hydrogenated vegetable oils. If you use margarine, choose one labeled "non-hydrogenated."

3. Be sure to include the heart-healthy omega-3 fats in your diet. Aim to eat fish three times a week.

4. To increase your intake of alpha-linolenic acid, a member of the omega-3 family, use flaxseed oil, walnut oil and/or canola oil. Include 1/4 cup (60 ml) of nuts in your diet up to five times a week.

5. If you use olive oil, buy the extra-virgin type. It's been processed the least and contains the most antioxidant compounds.

6. If your cholesterol levels are in the normal range, feel free to enjoy one whole egg up to six times a week.

7. If your cholesterol levels are high, add 25 grams of soy protein to your diet each day.

8. Include a source of soluble fiber in your daily diet. Foods like psyllium-enriched breakfast cereals, oatmeal and oat bran can lower elevated cholesterol levels in conjunction with a low-fat diet.

9. When it comes to buying breads, cereals, rice and pasta, always choose whole grain.

10. Drink a cup or more of tea each day as a source of catechins, antioxidant compounds that protect your LDL cholesterol.

11. If you drink alcohol, limit your intake to no more than one alcoholic beverage per day.

12. Boost your intake of B vitamins to help keep your homocysteine levels down. To ensure you are meeting your needs, take a daily multivitamin and mineral supplement, or try a B complex supplement.

13. Eat at least one vitamin-C-rich food each day. If you're concerned that you are not getting enough, add a 500- or 600-milligram supplement of Ester C.

14. For even more antioxidant protection, add vitamin E to your daily diet. To get the amount of vitamin E found protective in the research, take a daily vitamin E supplement (100 to 400 IU).

15. Each day include a source of lycopene in your diet. Heat-processed tomato products are the best food sources. If you choose to take a lycopene supplement, buy a brand that contains the Lyc-O-Mato™ or LycoRed™ extract.

16. To get more heart-protective sulfur compounds, increase your intake of garlic, both raw and cooked. Use 1/2 to 1 clove a day in cooking. If your cholesterol levels are high, consider taking aged garlic extract (it's odorless too!). Take one to two capsules up to three times daily with meals. If you are on blood-thinning medication, check with your physician or pharmacist for possible side effects or interactions.

Part 4

Emotional Health

12

Depression

It is estimated that 20 million adult Americans experience depression every day.[1] Study after study has indicated that women suffer depression twice as often as men.

Rates of depression have been increasing in every generation since 1915. Ongoing scientific research continues to explore the causes of this pervasive condition.

And yet, much of the research on mental illness has been conducted on men, using male standards. As a result, women suffering from mood disorders often do not receive the diagnosis or treatment that is appropriate to their needs. Researchers are only just beginning to understand the factors that contribute to gender-based differences in mental illness.

❧

What Causes Depression?

When faced with the stresses and losses of life, the natural response is sadness and grief. Everyone experiences emotional highs and lows in life and it's very normal to suffer through a bout of the blues once in a while. But depressive illness goes beyond these reactions. Depression is a prolonged emotional response that significantly interferes with the ability to cope with daily living. It may cause profound lifestyle changes and, without treatment, symptoms may linger for months or even years.

There are three types of depression:

1. *Unipolar major depression (clinical depression)* The diagnosis for this condition is made if symptoms of deep despair persist and consistently interfere with normal functioning during a two-week period.

2. *Dysthymia* A milder form of depression, dysthymia is a chronic mood disorder that lasts for at least two years.

3. *Manic depression (bipolar illness)* Less common than the other forms of depression, manic depression involves disruptive cycles of elation or euphoria, alternating with depressive episodes, irritable excitement and mania.

The actual causes of depression are not fully understood. It's thought to result from a combination of factors that include environmental and hereditary conditions, lifestyle choices, stress level and body chemistry. Modern brain imaging technologies reveal that specific neural circuits in the brain do not function properly during depression, impairing the performance of crucial brain chemicals called neurotransmitters. Another theory holds that depression is caused by an imbalance in the body's response to stress, which results in an overactive hormonal system. Some studies also suggest that low levels of certain brain chemicals, known as amines, may slow down the nervous system and impair brain function enough to cause depression.

In women, there is evidence that the hormonal fluctuations of menstruation and pregnancy can trigger mental disorders.

Symptoms

Symptoms of depression develop gradually, over a period of days or weeks. People with depression often appear slow and sad or irritable and anxious. They may be preoccupied with intense feelings of guilt and may have difficulty sleeping, concentrating or experiencing normal emotions. As the depression progresses, they may feel more and more helpless and hopeless and may even have thoughts of suicide and death.

Not everyone with depression experiences a full range of symptoms, and the severity of the symptoms can vary from person to person. To be diagnosed with depression, you must be experiencing at least four of the following indicators consistently over a period of at least two weeks:

- general sluggishness or agitation
- loss of interest in daily activities
- withdrawal
- acute sadness or feeling of emptiness
- demoralization, despair, feelings of worthlessness and hopelessness
- anxiety
- frequent outbursts of anger and rage
- difficulty concentrating, memory loss, unusual indecisiveness
- self-criticism, self-deprecation
- changes in eating habits
- sleep disorders (insomnia, frequent awakening)
- chronic fatigue, lack of energy
- physical discomfort, such as constipation, headaches

In dysthymia, these symptoms are present in a milder form. This illness begins early in life and may last for years, even decades. People with dysthymic depression are pessimistic, humorless, introverted, lethargic and often self-critical. They are preoccupied with inadequacy, failure and negative events.

People with manic depression often appear elated, uncontrollably enthusiastic and intrusively friendly. But they may just as easily become irritable or hostile. As the condition progresses, mental activity speeds up and the need for sleep decreases. A manic person is easily distracted, shifting constantly from one task or project to another, may indulge in inappropriate sexual or personal behaviors or may have delusions of power and wealth. People suffering from mania often do not recognize their own condition and may put themselves at risk in many ways, without ever realizing they are in danger.

A typical depression can last for six to nine months and episodes may recur several times over a lifetime. Symptoms rarely go away on their own, but with professional diagnosis and treatment, depression can be managed and controlled very successfully.

༄

Who's at Risk?

Depression can affect anyone, at any time. The illness is a complicated process and is rarely due to a single event or condition. Some of the main risk factors associated with depression include the following:

1. *Family history* If you have an immediate family member with depression, your risk is much higher. Family environment may also play a role, as children growing up with a depressed person may learn inappropriate ways of handling stress.

2. *Traumatic life events* Early childhood events, such as the loss of a parent, sexual abuse or divorce, increase the risk of adult depression.

3. *Stress* Work-related pressures or negative life events such as the loss of a loved one, a divorce, financial problems or a move to a new location might trigger depression.

4. *Marital and work status* Depression is highest among divorced, separated or widowed people and among those living alone. Unemployment lasting more than six months is also a factor.

5. *Physical illness* Cancer, heart disease, AIDS/HIV, hormonal disorders and thyroid conditions are associated with depression.

6. *Medications* Many medications, including sedatives and pain medications, produce mood disorders as a side effect.

7. *Gender and age* Women suffer from depression and attempt suicide more often than men. Children, adolescents and the elderly experience stressful life events that may predispose them to depression.

8. *Ethnicity* Depression occurs in every culture and ethnic group. However, cultural and ethnic differences do affect the symptoms and treatment of this condition.

9. *Alcohol, drugs and tobacco* Many people who are depressed suffer from alcoholism, too. Alcohol is a depressive drug and will aggravate the symptoms of depression. Some people turn to mood-altering drugs for relief of symptoms, but this type of drug tends to complicate depression and interfere with its treatment. Depression is also associated with an increased frequency of cigarette smoking.

WOMEN AND DEPRESSION

The higher incidence of depression in women begins in adolescence. Teenage girls react to the stresses of forming an identity, confronting sexuality and pursuing independence much differently than boys, and it's here that the seeds of depressive tendencies are sown.

There appears to be a strong relationship between the biology of a woman's body and the incidence of mood disorders. Fluctuations in the level of estrogen can create mood changes shortly before menstruation and after pregnancy. These hormonal fluctuations are also associated with the use of oral contraceptives and with hormone replacement therapy during menopause. Research has confirmed that hormones do indeed affect the brain chemistry that controls our emotions and mood.

The fact that women suffer depression more often than men may be related to the fact that women synthesize serotonin, a brain chemical that carries messages between brain cells, at a lower rate than men. Melatonin, a chemical involved in regulating certain bodily functions, is also produced at different levels in women and men. Both differences may predispose women to become depressed with a lack of sunlight, a condition known as Seasonal Affective Disorder (SAD).

Because of our unique biology, women also suffer from different forms of depression. Between 20 and 40 percent of women experience Premenstrual Syndrome (PMS). PMS can cause mood swings that may interfere with family life and work performance. It is an abnormal response to normal hormone changes and may be associated with malfunctions in brain serotonin levels.

Postpartum depression is a condition experienced by women shortly after pregnancy. Once the baby is born, women may have a bout of the "baby blues," which is a fairly typical reaction to normal hormonal shifts and the pressures of a new role in life. However, in some women, the reaction is more extreme and may involve many of the symptoms of a major depression. If a woman has one episode of postpartum depression, she has a 50 percent chance of developing it again during subsequent pregnancies.

Eating disorders, anxiety disorders and perimenopausal depression are other depressive illnesses that affect women more seriously than men. Women also seem to be more vulnerable to stress, often as a result of poverty, single parenthood, caring for aging parents or exposure to domestic violence and sexual abuse.

ॐ

Diagnosis

Your doctor will usually be able to diagnose depression from its signs and symptoms. A family history of depression may help to confirm the diagnosis. Laboratory tests, especially blood tests, may be used to identify the cause of some depressions. This approach is especially useful in diagnosing women, who may be experiencing hormonal factors that are influencing their condition.

ॐ

Conventional Treatment

Depression is one of the most common and treatable mental disorders. It is usually treated without hospitalization, using a combination of medications and psychotherapy. Even severe depression can be highly responsive to treatment. The earlier treatment begins, the more effective it is and the more likely it will prevent serious recurrences. However, even when treatment is successful, depression may recur. Results of any treatment should be apparent within two to three months.

Several different types of antidepressant drugs are available today and they all provide effective treatment for depression. They work by influencing the activity of brain neurotransmitters, primarily serotonin, norepinephrine and dopamine, and must be taken for several weeks before they begin to work.

1. *Selective serotonin reuptake inhibitors (SSRIs)*—Prozac®, Effexor®, Paxil®, Zoloft®, Serzone®. These drugs raise serotonin levels in the brain. SSRIs have fewer side effects and are often the first choice of treatment for depression. They may cause mild nausea, diarrhea and headaches that usually subside over time. The biggest

disadvantage of SSRIs is the fact that they commonly cause sexual dysfunction (read the section on ginkgo on page 223).

2. *Monoamine oxidase inhibitors (MAOIs)*—Nardil®, Parnate®. These drugs cause an increase in the levels of various brain chemicals, including amines—low amine levels are considered to be one of the causes of depression. MAOIs are rarely used today because they have serious interactions with other medications and with foods that contain tyramine, such as red wine, aged cheeses, soy sauce and yeast extracts.

3. *Tricyclic antidepressants*—Elavil®, Tofranil®, Norpramin®. These are useful in treating depression, but they bring with them a host of unpleasant side effects, such as weight gain, drowsiness, dizziness and an increased heart rate. They are not normally used to treat mild to moderate depression, because the side effects are often worse than the disease.

4. *Psychotherapy*—Individual and group therapy can help to gradually change hope-less and negative attitudes, and can provide guidance in adjusting to the normal pressures of life. It is often used in conjunction with antidepressant drugs.

5. *Electroconvulsive therapy (ECT)*—This treatment is normally used for severe cases of depression. An electric current is applied to the head to induce a seizure in the brain. For reasons not completely understood, the seizure will quickly and very effectively alleviate depression. Occasionally, there may be some temporary memory loss from this treatment.

৵

Managing Depression

DIETARY STRATEGIES

Carbohydrate-Rich Foods

Carbohydrate has been one of the most widely studied nutrients with respect to mood. High-carbohydrate meals have been associated with a calming, relaxing effect and even drowsiness. A meal like pasta allows an amino acid called tryptophan to get into the brain, which is then used to make the neurotransmitter serotonin. Numerous studies have linked high serotonin levels with happier moods and low levels with mild depression. Most of this research has been done in women with PMS. These studies find that mood can be improved within 30 to 90 minutes of consuming a carbohydrate-rich food or beverage.

If you're feeling depressed, try a high-carbohydrate meal that contains very little protein. Protein foods like chicken, meat or fish provide many different amino acids that compete with tryptophan for entry into the brain. That means that less serotonin will be produced. Try pasta with tomato sauce, a toasted whole-grain bagel with jam or a bowl of whole-grain cereal with low-fat milk. You might also try high-carbohydrate beverages like unsweetened fruit juice, a sports recovery drink or even milk.

Omega-3 Fats

Scientists have learned that levels of omega-3 fatty acids, special fats that are plentiful in fish, are lower in people who are depressed. These fatty acids are important components of nerve and brain cell membranes, where they help cells communicate messages effectively. Fish contains two special omega-3 fats called DHA and EPA. It's a lack of DHA that seems to be an important factor in depression. DHA may work to ease depression by altering the structure of cell membranes in the brain, making them more responsive to the effects of serotonin. It's also thought that DHA has anti-inflammatory effects in the brain, which can also influence mood. Some research suggests that fish oil supplements can improve symptoms in patients with clinical depression.

The best sources of omega-3 oils are cold-water fish such as salmon, trout, mackerel, herring, sardines and fresh tuna. If you don't like fish, or you're not prepared to eat it on a frequent basis, there are other ways to get more DHA into your cell membranes. Your body uses food rich in the essential fatty acid *alpha-linolenic acid* to make some DHA. The body cannot make essential fatty acids, so they must be consumed in the diet. If you don't get enough of this fatty acid, your body can't make DHA. With today's emphasis on low-fat and fat-free products, many experts fear we're not getting enough alpha-linolenic acid. Flaxseed oil, canola oil, walnut oil, Omega-3 eggs, soybeans and green leafy vegetables all contain alpha-linolenic acid.

Make an effort to add more omega-3 fats to your diet. Get the majority of your added fats and oils from omega-3 sources. Aim to eat fish at least three times a week. Use flaxseed oil in salad dressings and canola oil in baking and cooking. Store flaxseed and walnut oils in the fridge and don't use them in cooking, as heat and oxygen can easily destroy these fats. It's also important to minimize your intake of animal fat and packaged foods that contain hydrogenated vegetable oils—these fats compete with omega-3 fats in your body, so a diet that favors these fats can deprive your cells of omega-3.

If you have clinical depression, you might be wondering about fish oil supplements. If you decide to go this route, buy a product that offers a combination of EPA and DHA. A good quality fish oil supplement should also contain vitamin E, which is added to help stabilize the oils. Avoid fish *liver* oil capsules. Supplements made from fish livers are a concentrated source of vitamins A and D, and too much of these vitamins can be toxic when taken in large amounts for long periods of time.

The precise dose for treating depression is not yet known. Some experts recommend getting anywhere from 5 to 15 grams of omega-3 fats three times daily. That can amount to a lot of capsules, and there are a few downsides: they can repeat on you, leaving an unpleasant taste in your mouth. But more importantly, fish oil has a blood-thinning effect; if you take other medication that thins the blood, be sure to check with your physician first. *Fish oil supplements should never replace your medication. Always discuss any alternative or complementary treatment with your doctor first.*

VITAMINS AND MINERALS

Vitamin B6

Even marginal deficiencies of the B vitamins have been associated with irritability, depression and mood changes. And if you've suffered from PMS, chances are you've already heard about vitamin B6 (chapter 17, "Premenstrual Syndrome (PMS)" has plenty on this subject). This B vitamin has been the focus of study in more than 900 women suffering from PMS.[2] Based on the evidence available, a daily supplement of B6 seems likely to balance emotions in women suffering from PMS-related depression.

The body uses B6 to form an important enzyme that's needed to convert tryptophan to serotonin, a brain chemical that has a calming and relaxing effect. Healthy women need 1.6 milligrams of the vitamin each day. The best sources of B6 are high-protein foods like meat, fish, and poultry. Other good sources include whole grains, bananas and potatoes. To see how common foods stack up for vitamin B6, see the B6 in Foods table on page 5 in chapter 1.

If you're depressed and you'd like to see if a daily supplement could help, reach for a 50- to 100-milligram pill once a day. Because the eight B vitamins work together,

I recommend a *B complex* supplement that's balanced with all the B's. Taking only one B vitamin in high doses could upset the body's balance. Don't take more than 100 milligrams of B6 each day, since too much can cause irreversible nerve damage.

Folate and Vitamin B12

A number of studies have found that many depressed people are deficient in both of these B vitamins. It has been suggested that lack of these interrelated nutrients may work in a number of ways to cause depression. Both folate and B12 are required in the body for the synthesis of a compound called S-adenosylmethionine or SAMe (read more on this on page 223). SAMe, in turn, is used by the brain to produce neurotransmitters, in particular the amines. So a lack of B12 and/or folate can interfere with this process, resulting in low levels of brain amines that could cause or worsen depression.

A folate deficiency may also impair the brain's ability to synthesize many neurotransmitters including serotonin, the calming chemical you read about earlier. If you are taking any of the serotonin reuptake inhibitor drugs (Prozac®, Effexor®, Paxil®, Zoloft®, Serzone®) for depression, you might be interested to learn that low folate levels in the body are linked with a poorer response to these antidepressant drugs.

While scientists are still unraveling the intricacies involved in B vitamins and mood disorders, it's prudent to make sure your diet is giving you what you need.

1. *Folate* RDA is 400 micrograms (pregnancy 600 mcg; breastfeeding 500 mcg). Best food sources include spinach, artichokes, asparagus, lentils, dried peas and beans, chicken liver, orange juice and wheat germ (turn to page 7 in chapter 1 for a detailed food list). If you supplement, choose a multivitamin and mineral formula with 0.4 to 1 milligrams (400 to 1000 micrograms) of folic acid—the synthetic form of folate—or choose a B complex formula. If you take single supplements of folate, make sure it has B12 added. The daily upper limit for folate is 1000 micrograms.

2. *Vitamin B12* RDA is 2.4 micrograms (pregnancy 2.6 mcg; breastfeeding 2.8 mcg). Best food sources include all animal foods and fortified soy and rice beverages (see page 9 in chapter 1 for a detailed food list). If you are over the age of 50, you should get your B12 from a supplement or fortified foods since we absorb less of this nutrient as we age. Supplement choices include a multivitamin and mineral or a B complex formula. If you are a complete vegetarian and

you do not use fortified soy or rice beverages, take a single B12 supplement providing 500 to 1000 micrograms.

HERBAL REMEDIES

St. John's Wort (*Hypericum perforatum*)

For years this herb has been widely used in Europe to treat both mild depression and Seasonal Affective Disorder. In 1997, British researchers analyzed 26 controlled studies conducted in 1700 patients and concluded that the herb was as effective as certain antidepressant drugs in treating mild to moderate depression.[3]

Many experts believe that St. John's wort works by keeping brain serotonin levels high for a longer period of time, just like the popular antidepressant drugs Paxil®, Zoloft® and Prozac®. It seems the power of St. John's wort lies in two active ingredients, called hypericin and hyperforin. Researchers attribute most of the herb's effectiveness to hyperforin.

When shopping for a St. John's wort product, look for a brand that meets the following criteria:

- It should be standardized to contain hypericin—0.3 percent.
- It should contain a high amount of hyperforin—3 percent. There are some advanced formulas that contain hyperforin, and one manufactured in Europe, called Movana™, has been used in clinical studies.

The effective dosage is one 300-milligram tablet three times a day. The herb is generally well tolerated. When the herb is taken in high doses for a long period of time, it may cause sensitivity to sunlight in very light-skinned individuals. St. John's wort has the potential to interact with a number of medications. Do not take the herb if you are using any of the following drugs: Crixivan® (indinavir), Sandimmune® (cyclosporine), Theo-Dur® (theophylline), Coumadin® (warfarin), birth control pills or Lanoxin® (digoxin). It is not recommended for use during pregnancy and breastfeeding. If you are taking a prescription antidepressant drug, do not take it concurrently with St. John's wort. *Always consult your physician first before stopping any medication.*

Ginkgo Biloba

If you are taking an SSRI drug (Prozac®, Efflexor®, Paxil®, Zoloft®, Serzone®) for your depression and are experiencing side effects that affect your sex life, consider adding ginkgo to your nutrition regime. After a patient taking ginkgo biloba for memory reported improved erections, Californian researchers decided to see if there was something to it. A group of 63 men and women who complained of sexual dysfunction as a result of antidepressant medication were given 60 to 120 milligrams of ginkgo each day. And guess what—a standardized extract of the herb was found to be 84 percent effective in treating sexual dysfunction.[4] And women were more responsive than men with success rates of 91 percent versus 76 percent. A handful of other studies have found similar results.

The active ingredients responsible for ginkgo's beneficial effects are called terpene lactones and ginkgo flavone glycosides. These components act to increase blood flow to the extremities. Guidelines for buying a top quality ginkgo supplement are as follows:

- Choose a product that is standardized to contain 24 percent ginkgo flavone glycosides and 6 percent terpene lactones.
- The EGb 761 extract used in the scientific research is sold as Ginkoba® in the United States.

The recommended dose of ginkgo biloba to reverse sexual dysfunction is 60 milligrams taken twice daily. Start the 120-milligram dose by taking a 40-milligram tablet with each of three meals. On rare occasions ginkgo may cause gastrointestinal upset, headache or an allergic skin reaction in susceptible individuals. The herb should not be used during pregnancy and breastfeeding, and there are no known interactions with other medications.

OTHER NATURAL HEALTH PRODUCTS

SAMe (S-adenosylmethionine)

SAMe is a compound that our body makes naturally from certain amino acids in high-protein foods like fish and meat. The production of SAMe is closely linked with folate and vitamin B12. As you may have read above, deficiencies in these nutrients can lead to depressed levels of SAMe in the brain and nervous system. In the body, SAMe donates a part of itself, a methyl group, to surrounding body tissues, especially the brain. SAMe's role as a methyl donor is what has scientists interested.

SAMe is approved as a prescription drug in 14 countries, and it is available as a dietary supplement in the United States and Canada. European physicians use SAMe to treat patients with depression, and it seems to work. The results of recent well-controlled studies show that SAMe is significantly better than a placebo in treating depression, and it may even be more effective than tricyclic antidepressant medication. These studies show that SAMe works quickly—symptoms improve in as few as four to five days.

Exactly how SAMe works to treat depressive symptoms is not entirely clear. It is associated with higher levels of brain neurotransmitters. But it may also work by favorably changing the composition of cell membranes in the brain, enabling neurotransmitters and cell receptors to work more efficiently.

To treat depression, studies use 800 to 2400 milligrams per day in divided doses. Start with one 400-milligram tablet twice daily, then work up to two tablets three times daily. SAMe is not a very stable molecule; to help it withstand the acidity of your stomach, make sure you buy an enteric-coated product.

The supplement is very well tolerated at the recommended doses, but it may cause nausea and gastrointestinal upset in doses higher than 1600 milligrams. European studies have not found any long-term problems associated with taking SAMe.

If you are currently taking medication for depression and you are thinking about trying SAMe, *do not discontinue your medication without first speaking to your doctor*. When taken with antidepressant drugs, SAMe may have an addictive effect, causing potentially dangerous side effects.

THE BOTTOM LINE...
Leslie's recommendations for managing depression

1. Eat three meals each day plus a mid-day snack to avoid wide fluctuations in blood sugar and neurotransmitter levels.

2. Eat between 5 and 12 servings of grain foods, and 5 to 10 fruits and vegetables each day to ensure you get enough carbohydrates in your diet.

3. Get more omega-3 fats in your diet. If you decide to try fish oil capsules, buy a product that offers both EPA and DHA, and that has added vitamin E to increase its stability.

4. Eliminate alcoholic beverages, which can worsen feelings of depression.

5. Make sure you're getting enough vitamin B6 in your diet.

6. If you suffer from mild depression and you're already taking a multivitamin and mineral pill, try a 50- or 100-milligram B6 supplement every day. If you're not taking a multivitamin and mineral, take a B complex supplement every day (check the ingredients to make sure it gives you 50 to 100 milligrams of B6).

7. Make sure your diet has plenty of folate and vitamin B12.

8. If extra B vitamins do not help your depression, try a standardized extract of St. John's wort. Take 300 milligrams three times a day. Buy a product that is standardized for 0.3 percent hypericin, and that contains a high amount of hyperforin.

9. If you are taking an SSRI drug (Prozac®, Effexor®, Paxil®, Zoloft®, Serzone®) and suffering sexual dysfunction as a side effect, try taking 60 milligrams of ginkgo biloba leaf extract twice daily. Look for an extract that contains 24 percent ginkgo flavone glycosides.

10. Consider taking 800 to 1600 milligrams of SAMe, a dietary supplement that is used to treat depression. Buy an enteric-coated product and take on an empty stomach.

11. If your mood swings do not improve with dietary changes or the recommended supplements, consult your doctor. Serious emotional problems may require medication.

13

Eating Disorders

We live in a society that's dominated by the cult of thinness. Everywhere we look, we're bombarded with the message that thin is beautiful. The waifish looks of ultra-thin models and entertainers have become our ideal—establishing standards of beauty that are not only unattainable, but unhealthy as well. It's no wonder that so many North American women struggle with their body image. By the time they reach adulthood, nearly half of all females have concerns about their weight and many have already begun the vicious cycle of dieting and weight gain. Recent studies show that girls as young as nine years old are preoccupied with their weight.

Some women, especially during their vulnerable teenage years, carry their struggle with body image to the extreme. They become the victims of the complex, chronic illnesses known as eating disorders. Women suffer from these illnesses far more often than men, representing nearly 90 percent of all cases. Among teenage girls, the statistics are even more dramatic. In this age group, eating disorders rank as the third most common cause of chronic illness. Sadly, an increasing number of older women are also seeking treatment for eating disorders.

Anorexia nervosa, bulimia nervosa and *binge eating disorder* are the three main types of eating disorders. Women who suffer from these conditions experience physical, psychological and social symptoms that eventually threaten their well-being, their overall health and even their lives. Eating disorders can be treated with long-term therapy but usually require the intervention of a variety of health professionals, including registered dietitians, physicians and mental-health specialists.

Because the treatment for each type of eating disorder is unique and involves a multidisciplinary approach, it is beyond the scope of this chapter to outline all possible nutrition recommendations. Rather, I have presented important information about each condition to help you better understand the causes, risk factors and symptoms. At the end of the chapter is a list of treatment programs across the United States. If your eating disorder is not serious enough to warrant this type of intervention, I strongly recommend that you seek the advice of a registered dietitian (**www.eatright. org**) to help you develop a plan that will normalize your eating patterns and correct any nutritional deficiencies. This is imperative to prevent long-term health problems associated with eating disorders.

$$\sim$$

Anorexia Nervosa

This eating disorder is characterized by an extreme fear of gaining weight. People with anorexia nervosa are obsessed with being thin and have an unrealistic concept of their body image. Even though they are noticeably underweight, anorexics always believe they're fat. To achieve their goal of weight loss, they eat very little and may exercise excessively. Sometimes they will even engage in self-induced vomiting or they will misuse laxatives or diuretics as part of a binge-purge cycle. Anorexia nervosa is an extremely dangerous and potentially life-threatening condition. People suffering from this eating disorder can literally starve themselves to death.

Anorexia means loss of appetite. Ironically, anorexics are very often hungry. They will become obsessive about food, frequently collecting recipes and making elaborate meals for other people that they will not eat themselves. They ritualize food preparation and will sometimes hide food in special places, but never eat it. They get pleasure from controlling their eating and, as they begin to starve, they may even achieve a sense of euphoria from being so disciplined and successful in achieving their goals.

There is no precise cause of anorexia nervosa but it is thought to be an illness of psychological origin. What begins as a normal desire to lose a few pounds rapidly becomes a compulsive obsession with body image. Anorexia nervosa primarily affects women, particularly young women. Research indicates that these women are responding to societal and cultural pressures that may predispose them to developing an eating disorder.

Often, women with anorexia nervosa have very low self-esteem. They may not feel good about themselves or the way they look. In an attempt to change their self-image, these women may take their interest in dieting and weight loss to an extreme. For some women, anorexia is not an issue of self-confidence but rather a means of taking control of their lives. They may have feelings of powerlessness and of being dominated by outside forces. By taking rigid control of their eating, these women are able to maintain a sense of control over some aspect of their lives. This response is frequently triggered by stress, anxiety or anger toward family members or in other personal relationships.

In many cases, women who suffer from anorexia are perfectionists and over-achievers. In constantly striving to reach perfection, they lay the foundation for failure. They are overly critical of themselves, set unreasonable standards of performance and have a compulsive need to please others. Having low self-confidence and setting unrealistic goals often results in feelings of ineffectiveness that may lead to abnormal eating behaviors.

Studies indicate that there may also be a biochemical explanation behind the psychology of eating disorders. Certain brain chemicals, known as neurotransmitters, are at lower levels in people with anorexia. Reduced levels of serotonin, a powerful neurotransmitter, are known to be associated with depression. There may be a link between anorexia and depression, but further research is needed to confirm the theory. Higher levels of cortisol, a brain hormone released in response to stress, and vasopressin, a brain chemical associated with obsessive-compulsive disorders, have also been identified with anorexia.

SYMPTOMS

The warning signs of anorexia nervosa include

- a preoccupation with food and weight: excessive dieting, counting calories, checking body weight several times a day
- feeling fat, even when weight is below normal; distorted vision of body image
- significant weight loss, with no evidence of related illness
- depression

- denial of hunger, despite an extreme reduction in eating

- strange eating habits: cutting food into small pieces, preferring food of specific texture or color, refusing to eat in front of others

- complaints of feeling cold because loss of body fat leads to dropping body temperatures

- appearance of long, fine hair on the body as a way of conserving body heat after loss of body fat

- brittle hair and nails

- dry, yellow skin

- loss of sex drive

- cessation of menstrual periods

As anorexia progresses, the symptoms of starvation become increasingly evident. Eventually, every major organ in the body will be affected. The heart becomes weaker and pumps less blood through the body. Dehydration sets in and fainting spells are common. Electrolyte imbalances develop, as the body loses potassium, sodium and chloride. This results in fatigue, muscle weakness, irritability, muscle spasms and depression. In severe cases, these physical changes will cause irregular heartbeat, convulsions and death due to kidney or heart failure. Approximately one in ten women suffering from anorexia will die—a death rate that is among the highest for a psychiatric disease.

WHO'S AT RISK?

It's estimated that almost 8 million American women between the ages of 13 and 40 suffer from anorexia nervosa. It is a condition that usually surfaces during the teenage years, when girls are between 14 and 18 years old. Unfortunately, anxiety about weight and body image is beginning at younger and younger ages, with girls as young as nine years old reporting weight concerns. Because adolescence is a time of growth and development, the nutritional disturbances caused by disordered eating can have devastating implications for teenage girls. Adequate energy, protein, vitamins and minerals are all necessary for proper growth. Young girls with eating disorders may lose essential muscle mass, body fat and bone minerals at a crucial point in their development, leaving them at greater risk for osteoporosis, diabetes and high blood pressure in later life.

In many cases, the incidence of anorexia is influenced by social environment. Girls with a peer group or family network that emphasizes physical attractiveness and thinness are more likely to acquire eating disorders. Girls and women with low self-esteem or depressive tendencies are also very susceptible to the condition, especially if they are dealing with high levels of stress or traumatic events such as rape or abuse. There are also indications that anorexia nervosa may run in families.

In our society, there are certain professions or activities that emphasize thinness and appearance to an exceptional degree. People who participate in dancing, gymnastics, wrestling, modeling, acting and long-distance running are likely to be very aware of their weight or body image. They may be particularly susceptible to an eating disorder such as anorexia nervosa.

DIAGNOSIS

Because the eating habits of people with anorexia nervosa are very secretive, the condition can be hard to diagnose. Anorexics typically refuse to admit anything is wrong and may become angry or defensive when family or friends express concern. For this reason, the disorder may go undiagnosed for long periods of time.

Anorexia is usually diagnosed by the appearance of specific symptoms. When a girl loses at least 15 percent of her body weight, there is a good chance that she is anorexic. If she demonstrates a compulsive drive for thinness, coupled with an excessive fear of becoming fat, unhealthy weight-control practices or obsessive thinking about food, weight, body image or exercise, the diagnosis of anorexia is appropriate. In females, anorexia also lowers estrogen production, which causes menstrual cycles to stop. A failure to menstruate for at least three months is another crucial part of the diagnostic puzzle of anorexia.

CONVENTIONAL TREATMENT

Treatment is usually complicated by the fact that most people with the condition deny that they have a problem. They refuse therapy, yet they clearly need help to manage their disorder. Anorexia nervosa rarely goes away on its own.

The goal of therapy for most eating disorders is to restore a normal weight, develop normal eating patterns, overcome unhealthy attitudes about body image and self-worth and provide support to family and friends who may be helping with the recovery process. Because anorexia nervosa has such a widespread influence and affects so many aspects of daily life, effective treatment requires a collaborative effort from a team of health professionals. Often, the team consists of a family physician to manage physical symptoms, a psychiatrist or psychologist to introduce behavioral modification and a nutritionist to establish a healthy diet for recovery.

The sooner anorexia nervosa is identified and treated, the better the eventual outcome. In the early stages, the disorder may be treated without hospitalization. But when weight loss is severe, hospitalization is necessary to restore weight and prevent further physical deterioration. A structured approach that involves careful observation of all eating and elimination—urinating, bowel movements and vomiting—is the first stage of treatment.

When weight is restored and symptoms are stabilized, some type of psychotherapy is required to deal with the underlying emotional issues that trigger the abnormal eating patterns. Family therapy is especially helpful for younger girls, and behavioral or cognitive therapy is also effective in helping replace destructive attitudes with positive ones. A nutritionist will add support by providing advice on proper diet and eating regimens. In some cases, antidepressant medications may be prescribed, but they should not be used as a substitute for appropriate psychological treatment.

Unfortunately, many people with anorexia nervosa have a tendency to relapse and return to dysfunctional eating habits. Long-term therapy and regular health monitoring are essential for a successful result. A strong network of love and support from family and friends is also crucial to the recovery process.

Bulimia Nervosa

Bulimia nervosa is the most common type of eating disorder. You may also hear it referred to as bingeing and purging. A person with this condition will eat large amounts of high-calorie food in a very short period of time, then use vomiting, diuretics or laxatives to eliminate the food before the body can absorb it. Fasting or excessive exercising are other methods that bulimics may use to counteract the weight gain caused by binge eating.

People suffering from bulimia will binge as often as several times a day, sometimes consuming 10,000 calories or more in a matter of minutes or hours. Comfort foods that are sweet, soft and high in calories, such as ice cream, cake or pastry, are favorite choices for bingeing. Immediately after the binge comes the purge, when some bulimics will use as many as 20 or more laxatives a day to rid their bodies of these huge quantities of food.

Just like people with anorexia nervosa, bulimics are extremely afraid of becoming fat and are obsessed with body image. They fear food, and yet they consume vast amounts of it. With anorexia nervosa, the extreme weight loss becomes an obvious signal of the disorder. But people with bulimia usually look quite normal and often show few signs of their condition. Their weight may fluctuate wildly, but usually stays within normal ranges. They may even be slightly heavy. Because bulimics are often very secretive about their abnormal behavior, the presence of bulimia can be hard to identify.

As with most eating disorders, bulimia nervosa is a psychological condition. It may be triggered by elevated stress levels and often affects women who are intelligent and high achievers. In many cases, these women are striving to conform to unrealistic ideals of thinness and beauty, and are using food and weight as a means of controlling their underlying emotional problems. People with bulimia nervosa are very aware of their behavior and feel guilty or remorseful. In this way, they are quite unlike anorexics, who deny the existence of their condition. Nearly half of all people with anorexia go on to develop some symptoms of bulimia.

Studies have shown that bulimics are particularly prone to impulsive behavior. They have difficulty dealing with anxiety, have little self-control and often indulge in drug or alcohol abuse or sexual promiscuity. They are also susceptible to depression, anxiety disorders and social phobias. As with anorexia nervosa, people with bulimia have lower levels of brain neurotransmitters, such as serotonin, which may predispose them to developing these psychological disturbances.

SYMPTOMS

In addition to the preoccupation with food and weight that is characteristic of most eating disorders, symptoms of bulimia may include

- evidence of binge eating, large amounts of food going missing, stealing money or food
- food cravings
- frequent weight fluctuations

- evidence of purging, vomiting, abuse of laxatives or diuretics, frequent fasting or excessive exercising

- swelling of glands under the jaw caused by vomiting

- erosion of tooth enamel and other dental problems caused by vomiting

- feelings of shame, self-reproach and guilt

- emotional changes, depression, irritability, social withdrawal

The purging behavior associated with bulimia can also cause physical complications that are very dangerous to long-term health. Vomiting and purging can lead to imbalances in fluids and electrolytes. When potassium levels fall too low, abnormal heart rhythms develop. Some bulimics use a medication called ipecac to induce vomiting; overuse of this substance has been known to cause sudden death.

WHO'S AT RISK?

Like anorexia, bulimia is primarily a women's disorder. Nearly twice as many women suffer from bulimia as anorexia and, in America, it is estimated that this eating disorder affects up to 2 percent of adolescents and young women. Bulimia tends to develop in later adolescence, often striking young women between the ages of 18 and 20; however, it can appear in earlier adolescence.

As with other eating disorders, bulimia surfaces most often in people who have low self-confidence and are insecure about their appearance. They may be very self-critical and may set unreasonable goals of perfection for themselves. Often, bulimia becomes an issue of control and may be a response to stressful events. Girls reporting sexual or physical abuse are very susceptible to developing an eating disorder such as bulimia. Studies also indicate that the disorder may have a genetic element and may run in families.

DIAGNOSIS

Bulimia is usually suspected in people who are obsessed about weight gain and have wide fluctuations in weight, especially if there is evidence of excessive use of laxatives. Swollen salivary glands and tooth decay are also recognizable signs of the disorder. Blood tests may be necessary to identify dehydration, electrolyte imbalances and nutrient deficiencies.

CONVENTIONAL TREATMENT

In most cases, people with bulimia are treated without hospitalization. Because it is a psychological condition, cognitive and behavioral therapy are necessary to deal with the emotional issues underlying the symptoms of this disorder. As with anorexia nervosa, a multidisciplinary approach to treatment works best. Physicians, nutritionists and mental health professionals will work together to address the many different facets of this eating disorder. In particular, long-term psychotherapy is needed to help reduce destructive tendencies and develop better coping strategies. Antidepressant medication has proven to be an effective psychological intervention.

⁂

Binge Eating Disorder

Binge eating disorder (BED) is a newly recognized condition that has many similarities to bulimia nervosa. People with BED frequently eat huge quantities of food and feel that they have no control over their eating. Unlike bulimics, however, they don't purge afterwards with vomiting or laxatives.

While most of us are guilty of overeating at some time or other, binge eaters have much more serious problems. In most cases, the disorder causes considerable distress to the people who suffer from it and is often accompanied by depression. At this time, scientists are not sure whether depression is a symptom of BED or an underlying cause of the condition. People do report that emotions such as anger, sadness, anxiety or boredom will trigger episodes of binge eating. Studies are currently being done on neurotransmitters and other brain chemicals to determine if they are linked to binge eating disorder.

SYMPTOMS
The symptoms of BED include

- frequently eating an abnormally large amount of food
- feeling unable to control what or how much food is eaten
- eating more rapidly than usual
- eating until uncomfortably full

- eating large amounts of food, even when not hungry
- experiencing feelings of disgust, guilt or depression after overeating
- eating alone because of embarrassment at the quantity of food being eaten

WHO'S AT RISK?

Binge eating disorder occurs most often in people who are overweight and obese—with a BMI greater than 25—and it becomes more prevalent as body weight increases. Obese people with BED become overweight at an earlier age than those without the disorder and may suffer more frequent bouts of losing and regaining weight. However, it is not uncommon for people with normal, healthy weight to suffer from BED. It occurs slightly more often in women than in men and tends to appear in later years, affecting an older population than either anorexia or bulimia nervosa.

DIAGNOSIS

BED can be very difficult to distinguish from other causes of obesity. Because people with the disorder are embarrassed about their behavior, they work very hard to conceal their bingeing tendencies. Right now, there are probably thousands of people suffering from BED who are not properly diagnosed.

Perhaps the most distinctive diagnostic feature of the condition is the depression that accompanies it. Doctors look for overeating habits that establish an "out-of-control" pattern and that are followed by feelings of anxiety, guilt and depression.

CONVENTIONAL TREATMENT

Many of the medical problems related to obesity are also associated with binge eating disorder. Treatment may be necessary for conditions such as high cholesterol, high blood pressure, diabetes, gallbladder disease and heart disease. Other than the appropriate therapies for obesity-related disorders, there are no standard treatments for BED. As with most eating disorders, an approach that involves psychotherapy and antidepressant drugs seems to be most effective. It is essential to deal with the emotional issues of the illness in striving for a successful result. Because people with BED find it very difficult to stay on a treatment regimen and frequently return to inappropriate behavior, long-term therapy is always recommended.

Getting Help for Eating Disorders

The following is a list of selected treatment centers across the United States. The list is intended to aid your research.

Arizona
Rosewood Ranch, Women's Center for Eating Disorders
36075 South Rincon Road
Wickenburg, AZ 85390
Tel: 1-800-845-2211
www.rosewoodranch.com

California
Montecatini
2524 La Costa Avenue
Rancho La Costa, CA 92008
Tel: 760-436-8930
www.montecatinieatingdisorder.com

Rader Programs
Oxnard, CA
1-800-841-1515
www.raderprograms.com

Florida
The Renfrew Center
Miami and Coconut Creek
1-800-736-3739
www.renfrewcenter.com

Illinois
Alexian Brothers Behavorial Health Hospital
1650 Moon Lake Blvd.
Hoffman Estates, IL 60194
Tel: 1-800-432-5005
www.abbhh.org

New York
New York State Psychiatric Institute
Eating Disorders Clinic
Unit 98, 1051 Riverside Drive
New York, NY 10032
Tel: 212-543-5316
www.columbia.edu/~ea12

The Renfrew Center of New York
11 East 36th Street
New York, NY 10016
1-800-736-3739
www.renfrewcenter.com

Washington
The Moore Center for Eating Disorders
1601 114th Avenue S.E., Suite 180
Bellevue, WA 98004
Tel: 425-451-1134
www.moorecenterclinic.com

Part 5

Conception, Pregnancy and Motherhood

14

Infertility

Infertility is a condition that causes couples to be fraught with disappointment, frustration and heartbreak. Defined as the inability to conceive after one year of frequent, unprotected intercourse, infertility affects approximately one in six couples. Throughout North America, infertility is on the rise, possibly due to the increase in sexually transmitted diseases and the decision of a growing number of women to delay having children until later in life.

Once thought to be solely a woman's problem, failure to conceive can be caused by reproductive difficulties in both men and women. Thirty percent of all cases of infertility originate with the woman, 30 percent originate with the man, 30 percent are the result of combined factors and the remaining cases are unexplained.[1]

For women, infertility is often associated with ovarian disorders, and for men it is usually linked to problems with sperm production. Treatment for infertility varies, depending on the reproductive problems involved. Over 80 percent of all infertility cases are treated with either drugs or surgery. In recent years, assisted reproductive technologies (ART), such as *in vitro* fertilization, have been providing effective solutions for many couples struggling with the emotional distress of infertility.

ॐ

What Causes Infertility?

The discovery of infertility usually comes as an unexpected shock, and both partners suffer from the tension, disappointment, anger and grief that accompany a failure to conceive.

CONCEPTION

For a woman, the basis of her future conception is established while she is still in the womb. By the fifth month of her development before birth, a woman's lifetime supply of more than seven million eggs, or ova, has been created and stored in her tiny fetal ovaries. As she grows and matures, millions of these eggs disintegrate, leaving her with about 300,000 eggs available for fertilization by the time she reaches puberty. A woman becomes fertile once her menstrual cycle begins, usually sometime between the ages of nine and sixteen. From this point onwards, an egg will ripen inside her ovaries once every month until she reaches menopause.

Stimulated by a sequence of hormones, the egg matures inside a tiny, saclike structure called a follicle and is released into one of the two fallopian tubes. For conception to take place, a sperm must fertilize the egg as it travels from the ovaries and through the fallopian tubes to reach the uterus.

A man produces sperm in his testicles on a continuous basis throughout his lifetime. Sperm are shaped like tadpoles, carrying genetic material in their "heads" and capable of moving by lashing their "tails" in a swimming motion. During intercourse, a man will ejaculate millions of these sperm into a woman's vagina. Ideally, the sperm will fertilize the egg within 24 hours of ovulation, because both sperm and egg deteriorate fairly quickly. To reach the egg, the sperm must travel through the acidic environment of the vagina into the uterus and up to the fallopian tubes. Although millions of sperm make this difficult journey, only one will penetrate the tough outer membrane of the egg.

Once the first sperm has entered the egg, a chemical reaction takes place, making the egg impenetrable to other sperm. The genetic material in the head of the sperm then combines with the genetic material contained within the egg, completing the process of conception. The fertilized egg travels down through the fallopian tubes into the uterus, where it implants on the thickened lining of the uterine wall, called the endometrium. The woman's body will nurture this tiny collection of cells for nine months within the protective environment of the uterus, as it grows and develops into a fully formed fetus.

FEMALE INFERTILITY

At any stage along the way, from the development of a woman's eggs and ovaries before birth to the migration of a fertilized egg into her uterus, this intricate reproductive process can go astray. Infertility has been linked to many different factors, all of which influence the normal course of conception.

Approximately one-third of female infertility is caused by a failure to ovulate, a condition known as anovulation. Unless ovulation takes place, there is no egg available for the sperm to fertilize. A balance of hormones is necessary for ovulation to occur successfully. Two small glands located in your brain, the hypothalamus and the pituitary gland, regulate most of these hormonal responses.

The hypothalamus secretes gonadotropin-releasing hormone (GnRH), which stimulates the pituitary gland to relay hormonal messages to the ovaries. In response to these messages, the ovaries nurture an egg to maturity and release it into the fallopian tubes, ready to be fertilized. Many factors can interfere with the performance of your hypothalamus, preventing it from sending the correct signals to the pituitary gland. Emotional stress, extreme exercise, dieting, poor nutrition, low body fat, anorexia, medications and environmental toxins can all affect the hypothalamus. When the hypothalamus and the pituitary gland are unable to communicate effectively, conception is disrupted.

The pituitary gland contributes to conception by producing two hormones, follicle-stimulating hormone (FSH) and luteinizing hormone (LH). These hormones stimulate the follicles in the ovaries to grow and release mature eggs. They also tell the ovaries to produce estrogen and progesterone. The pituitary gland may malfunction because of a tumor, an injury, surgical complications or various medical disorders. A defective pituitary gland can over- or under-produce FSH and LH, resulting in ovulation failure.

The pituitary gland also produces prolactin, a hormone involved in the production of breast milk. Prolactin has the effect of suppressing ovulation, acting as a natural form of birth control during pregnancy and breastfeeding. The pituitary gland may secrete too much prolactin due to severe kidney disease, adrenal gland disorders, hypothyroidism and the effect of certain medications. Ten to 20 percent of infertile women have elevated levels of prolactin.

Other glands can affect hormones involved in conception, too. The thyroid gland is one example. This gland establishes your metabolic rate by circulating hormones to control the speed and efficiency of your internal functions. If the thyroid gland becomes overactive (hyperthyroid) or underactive (hypothyroid), it can speed up or slow down your body's ability to use hormones, causing problems with fertility.

Although you may not realize it, every woman has small amounts of male sex hormones, called androgens, circulating through her bloodstream. These hormones are secreted by the adrenal glands and are necessary for normal sexual development. If your adrenal glands malfunction, the elevated levels of male hormones will suppress ovulation. Excessive androgen production is a sign that you may be suffering from a very common disorder known as polycystic ovary syndrome (read chapter 19 for more information), one of the leading causes of female infertility.

There are a variety of ovarian disorders, including cysts, tumors, infections and medical conditions, that can cause infertility. For some women, their ovaries simply fail to function: due to surgery, injury, radiation or chromosomal problems, their ovaries run out of eggs too early, sending them into premature menopause. In rare instances, women are born without ovaries or without a normal supply of eggs, making ovulation impossible.

Several disorders of the uterus can also hamper conception. During the normal reproductive process, progesterone and luteinizing hormone stimulate the uterine lining to thicken into a nourishing bed for the fertilized egg. If the uterus is unable to respond to these hormones, the egg cannot implant properly. The result is usually a spontaneous abortion or miscarriage. Some women find it difficult to carry a fetus to full term because their uterus is structurally abnormal. Others discover that they are infertile because they were born without a uterus.

Infections that affect the reproductive tract are another cause of infertility. Sexually transmitted diseases (STDs) such as gonorrhea, chlamydia and pelvic inflammatory disease are on the rise in North America, and are destroying the fertility of thousands of women every year. These insidious infections can go undetected for long periods of time and, if left untreated, can scar your uterus, block your fallopian tubes and cause the formation of pelvic adhesions. Even frequent yeast infections (vaginitis) can cause tubal damage that is severe enough to prevent the sperm from intercepting the egg. Abdominal or pelvic surgery, appendicitis, endometriosis, ectopic pregnancies or the use of an IUD contraceptive device may also cause uterine or tubal damage. Occasionally, the use of oral contraceptives may delay ovulation for as long as six months, causing temporary infertility.

Many women fail to realize that diet, nutrition and lifestyle can also influence fertility. Excessive exercise, low-calorie diets, eating disorders, obesity, certain medications, elevated stress levels—even the use of vaginal lubricants—are all factors that will interfere with the reproductive process. Fortunately, these are among the easiest fertility problems to correct.

MALE INFERTILITY

Men are considered to be infertile when they don't produce enough sperm or when their sperm are of poor quality. Each time a man ejaculates, he releases approximately 50 million sperm in each milliliter of seminal fluid. If his sperm count drops below 20 million sperm per milliliter of ejaculate, his fertility will be impaired. The quality of the sperm is also important. Normal sperm have oval heads and long tails. Poor quality sperm have large heads and deformed tails. These abnormalities interfere with the motility of the sperm, which means that they are unable to swim to the egg in a vigorous, forward motion. If the sperm cannot reach or penetrate the egg, it is impossible for conception to take place.

Problems with sperm production can result from

- medical illnesses, including mumps and sexually transmitted diseases
- injury to the testicles, an undescended testicle or testicular cancer
- certain drugs, including recreational drugs such as marijuana
- lifestyle factors, such as cigarette smoking or drinking alcohol
- antibodies that are produced by the immune system to attack or disable the sperm
- vasectomy (surgical sterilization)
- overheating the sperm by wearing tight clothes, taking too many long baths or using saunas
- environmental toxins
- defects in the sperm-producing cells

COMBINED INFERTILITY FACTORS

One of the main reasons behind the increased rate of infertility in North America is the age factor. Many couples are waiting until they are well into their thirties or forties before attempting to have children. However, the quality and numbers of both sperm and eggs deteriorate as men and women grow older. By leaving their plans for parenthood until later in life, many couples are putting their chances of conception at risk.

Sometimes infertility arises because the man's sperm is incompatible with the woman's cervical mucous. Normally, the cervix secretes a thick mucous to protect the vagina from foreign invaders, such as bacteria. During ovulation, chemical changes take place to thin out the mucous consistency, allowing the sperm to enter the reproductive tract. For some couples, the chemistry between the sperm and the cervix just isn't right. The mucous remains thick, creating an environment that can block or damage the sperm, preventing conception.

Approximately 10 percent of all infertile couples discover that their infertility has no apparent cause. Both partners appear to be normal, healthy and able to reproduce; however, they simply cannot conceive together. This can be the most frustrating situation of all, as there is no obvious solution.

❧

Symptoms

The main symptom of infertility is the inability to conceive a child after one year of unprotected, frequent intercourse. Each specific medical disorder, hormonal disruption or anatomical abnormality produces additional symptoms in the woman that may indicate infertility. These symptoms may include

- history of recent weight loss or gain
- irregular menstrual periods
- absent menstrual periods (amenorrhea)
- prolonged or heavy periods
- spotting between periods
- abnormal vaginal discharge

- discomfort in the lower abdomen
- pain during sexual intercourse

❧

Who's at Risk?

One in six couples experience infertility problems. Every year, more than one million people in North America consult physicians for diagnosis and treatment of infertility problems.

You may be at increased risk of developing fertility problems if you

- are over 30 years old
- have irregular or absent periods
- have a history or have a partner with a history of sexually transmitted diseases (STDs), pelvic infections or genital infections
- are a woman with excessive hair growth on your face and body (hirsutism)
- have a history of using an intrauterine device (IUD) for birth control
- have had a surgical sterilization reversed or have a partner who has undergone this procedure
- have had abdominal surgery or have a partner who has undergone this type of surgery
- have endometriosis
- have a history of emotional stress

❧

Diagnosis

Because there are so many causes of infertility, an accurate diagnosis requires an extensive period of evaluation. The process will begin with a thorough physical and gynecological examination. Additional tests that may be necessary include the following:

1. *Basal temperature records* There is a slight rise in the body's basal temperature when ovulation occurs. Recording your temperature each morning will help to pinpoint this crucial time in your menstrual cycle. You will be asked to chart your body temperature as soon as you wake up, before you get out of bed.

2. *Cervical mucous tests* The cervical mucous can reveal a great deal of information about the conditions that may be causing your infertility.

   Ferning test   This test determines if your estrogen levels are normal.

   Postcoital test   This test determines if the sperm entering your reproductive tract are healthy and mobile.

3. *Blood tests* Levels of estrogen, progesterone, luteinizing hormone, follicle-stimulating hormone and prolactin are usually measured. Abnormalities in these hormone levels can help explain ovulation difficulties.

4. *X-ray examinations* This test, called a hysterosalpingogram, is used to identify structural abnormalities to your uterus and fallopian tubes, or certain medical conditions that may interfere with fertility.

5. *Laparoscopic surgery* Your uterus, fallopian tubes and ovaries will be examined with a laparoscope, a fiber-optic telescope inserted into your abdomen. This will detect conditions such as scarring in your fallopian tubes, endometriosis and polycystic ovary syndrome.

6. *Semen analysis* This determines the quality, quantity and motility of the sperm, plus the sperm concentration and volume.

৵

Conventional Treatment

Most healthy couples under 35 years of age have a 25 percent chance of becoming pregnant in the first month of trying to conceive. That rate rises to 60 percent after three to six months and reaches 85 percent after one year. For the majority of couples, giving nature enough time is usually the only treatment required for successful conception. That's why most physicians won't evaluate you for infertility until you have tried to become pregnant for at least one year.

In many cases, mis-timed intercourse is the only reason for infertility. Detecting the changes in your body that signal the beginning of ovulation is often the first step towards solving your fertility problems. Your basal temperature chart will help you to pinpoint your most fertile days. A urine test, indicating the presence of luteinizing hormones, is another method of establishing ovulation. By planning intercourse to maximize the chances of a mature egg meeting a viable sperm, your chances of conception may improve considerably.

Since the primary cause of infertility is anovulation, the major objective of most fertility treatments is to stimulate ovulation. The fertility drug Clomid® (clomiphene citrate) triggers ovulation by affecting the release of luteinizing hormone. It has a high success rate but often leads to multiple births. In some women, this drug can cause painful ovarian cysts and may increase the risks of ovarian cancer.

If you are not having success with Clomid®, you may benefit from supplements of the hormones FSH, LH or GnRH. The addition of these hormones should restore a normal menstrual cycle and improve fertility by stimulating egg production.

In some instances, surgery may be necessary to repair damaged reproductive organs. Laparoscopy is performed to open up damaged fallopian tubes or to remove scar tissue resulting from infections or endometriosis. Surgery is also helpful in correcting certain uterine abnormalities and removing polyps and fibroids.

Assisted reproductive technologies (ART) have been available for many years and are proving to be very successful in treating a wide variety of infertility problems. The most well known ART is *in vitro* fertilization. During this fertilization process, fertility drugs are prescribed to stimulate your ovaries to produce many eggs. When they are mature, several eggs are retrieved from your ovaries and fertilized in a laboratory. Between three and five embryos are then implanted into your uterus, in the hope of establishing a successful pregnancy. *In vitro* fertilization is used most frequently for women who have fallopian tube damage, endometriosis, anti-sperm antibodies and unexplained infertility. This technique has a success rate of approximately 25 percent per attempt. There are many other ART techniques that can be discussed with your doctor.

Dealing with infertility is a highly emotional experience for most couples. Fortunately, there is a great deal of research underway in the field of infertility, and treatments are becoming increasingly effective. Continual advances, especially in the area of ART, are offering new hope for couples who dream of the joys of parenthood.

~

Enhancing Female Fertility

DIETARY STRATEGIES

Achieve a Healthy Weight

There's no question that a woman's body weight can affect her chances of becoming pregnant. If you are obese, fat cells can produce enough estrogen to interfere with your ability to conceive. High estrogen levels tell your brain to stop stimulating the development of follicles and as result, ovulation doesn't occur. This is common in women with polycystic ovary syndrome (refer to chapter 19 for more on this disorder). Studies show that losing weight can lead to pregnancy. When obese women lose excess body weight, ovulation resumes, making conception possible.

Weighing too little is not healthy either. Menstruation occurs at a critical level of "fatness." If you lose too much weight, or you are already thin, your body fat diminishes and hormone levels are affected; this, in turn, can lead to the inability to ovulate.

In chapter 2, "Weight Control and Food Sensitivities" I give you tools to assess your body weight. Find out if you are at a healthy weight. If you are overweight and have polycystic ovary syndrome (PCOS), follow my weight loss recommendations and meal plan presented there. Even if you don't have PCOS, these are healthy strategies for any overweight woman.

If you are underweight, read my guidelines for a healthy woman's diet in chapter 1. Incorporate some of these suggestions to make sure you are getting enough calories and nutrients in your daily diet. If you recognize that your low body weight is caused by an eating disorder, read chapter 13, "Eating Disorders," for information on how to begin your recovery process.

Caffeine and Alcohol

If you and your partner have difficulty conceiving, I strongly recommend that you avoid caffeine and alcohol while you try to get pregnant (and of course during your pregnancy, too!). A number of studies have found that consuming more than 300 milligrams of caffeine per day (about 2 cups of coffee) is associated with a delay in conception. A large study from Johns Hopkins University revealed that, compared to women who consumed less than 300 milligrams of caffeine per day, those who consumed more caffeine reduced their chances of conceiving each month by 25 percent.[2] Another study of 104 healthy women found that women who consumed more than the equivalent of 1 cup of coffee per day were half as likely to become pregnant as women who drank less.[3] Other studies find that the relationship between caffeine and fertility is even stronger in women who smoke.[4]

A handful of studies support the notion that drinking alcoholic beverages reduces fertility in women. Women who drink heavily are more likely than non-drinkers to experience infertility problems and spontaneous abortion. A study from the Harvard School of Public Health looked at the effect of alcohol in more than 4000 women. The researchers found that even moderate drinking (two drinks per day) affected the ability to conceive by interfering with ovulation. And the more alcohol consumed, the higher the risk of not conceiving.[5]

VITAMINS AND MINERALS

Vitamin B12

There is some evidence that anemia due to a deficiency of vitamin B12 can cause infertility in women. Two case reports revealed that when women with this nutrient deficiency were given supplemental B12, pregnancy occurred.[6] How a lack of B12 impacts a woman's chances of conceiving is not understood.

Despite the lack of research in this area, it makes sense to ensure you are meeting your needs for this vitamin. Women of childbearing age must consume 2.4 micrograms of B12 every day to cover their needs. B12 is found only in animal foods and in a few products that have been fortified with the vitamin. Take a look at the B12 in Foods table on page 9 of chapter 1 for food sources of this vitamin.

A vitamin B12 deficiency can occur if you don't eat any B12-rich foods (you may be a complete vegetarian), or if your body is incapable of properly absorbing the nutrient. In the latter case, a condition called pernicious anemia results (read more about this in chapter 3, "Anemia"). If you are at risk for developing a B12 deficiency, take a good quality multivitamin and mineral supplement or a B complex formula (it contains the whole family of B vitamins). You'll find guidelines for supplementing with B12 on page 10 in chapter 1.

HERBAL REMEDIES

Chasteberry (*Vitex angus-castus*)

If irregular menstrual periods caused by an imbalance of hormones are interfering with your ability to become pregnant, you might consider trying this herbal remedy. European physicians have used chasteberry since the 1950s to treat menstrual irregularities in women. The herb is believed to work on your pituitary gland, increasing this gland's production of luteinizing hormone (LH). LH in turn boosts the secretion of progesterone during the last 14 days of your menstrual cycle. But it appears that chasteberry also works to keep prolactin levels in check. Its ability to lower excessive levels of prolactin has made it a potential treatment for infertility in some women.

There has been very little published research on the use of this herb for female infertility. In one German study, chasteberry was successful in treating 10 out of 15 women suffering from amenorrhea.[7] In the study, women taking the herb began having regular periods again after six months of treatment. Blood tests revealed an increase in levels of LH and progesterone. A few other European studies suggest that, when taken daily, chasteberry can restore progesterone and prolactin levels to normal and result in pregnancy.

If you decide to try chasteberry, buy a product that is standardized to provide 0.5 percent agnuside and 0.6 percent aucubin, two of the plant's active ingredients. The recommended dose is 175 to 225 milligrams once daily. Keep in mind that this herb does not have an immediate effect. Research and clinical experience suggest that it takes five to seven months to restore regular menstrual periods. And if you have not had a period for more than two years, it can take up to 18 months for chasteberry to kick in.

To date, the herb has a good safety record. In rare cases it may cause gastrointestinal upset and skin rashes. If you become pregnant, stop taking chasteberry as it may stimulate the uterus.

LIFESTYLE FACTORS

Cigarette Smoking

As you'll read in the section on enhancing male fertility, it is quite clear that smoking can negatively affect sperm. But scientists are now learning that smoking can also affect female fertility. According to a recent study from researchers in the U.K., the pregnancy rate among women attending a fertility clinic was significantly lower in smokers compared to non-smokers.[8] Other studies have found that women who smoke while trying to get pregnant experience delayed time to conception compared to both non-smokers and past smokers.[9] Scientists believe that smoking impairs the healthy functioning of a woman's ovaries; it also causes damage to a woman's eggs and the female sex hormone estrogen. If you are planning to start a family and you are a smoker (even a social smoker), I strongly urge you to quit for the benefit of your health and your babies.

❧

Enhancing Male Fertility

VITAMINS AND MINERALS

Antioxidant Nutrients

When it comes to nutrition and fertility, more research has been done in the area of male infertility. It appears that certain vitamins and minerals affect the health and the motility of sperm. Attention has been paid to the antioxidant nutrients, in particular vitamin E, vitamin C and selenium. It is believed that free radicals, dangerous oxygen molecules found in the body, damage sperm. Antioxidants are able to neutralize these harmful chemicals, rendering them inactive in the body.

Two studies have found that vitamin E supplements, taken in doses of 100 and 200 international units (IU), improved sperm activity of infertile men and increased the rate of pregnancy in their partners.[10] Preliminary research suggests that vitamin C may improve sperm count and sperm motility. Studies have also found that, compared to fertile men, infertile men have significantly lower levels of selenium in their semen.[11] This would suggest that selenium plays a role in sperm development. And one Scottish study found that supplemental selenium improved sperm motility in men with low selenium levels.[12]

These studies are far from conclusive. But even if dietary antioxidants don't improve your partner's fertility, they are still important nutrients for you and your partner to be consuming in your diet, and quite possibly taking as supplements. Just read chapter 11, "Heart Disease and High Cholesterol" and you'll understand their significance to health.

Here's what your male partner needs to know:

- *Vitamin C* RDA is 90 milligrams (smokers need 125 milligrams). Best food sources include citrus fruit, citrus juices, cantaloupe, kiwi, mango, strawberries, broccoli, brussels sprouts, cauliflower, red pepper and tomato juice. To supplement, buy a 500- or 600-milligram supplement of Ester C; take once daily. The daily upper limit is 2000 milligrams.

- *Vitamin E* RDA is 15 IU (natural source) and 22 IU (synthetic). Best food sources include wheat germ, nuts, seeds, vegetable oils, whole grains and kale. To supplement, take 100 to 400 IU of natural source vitamin E. Buy a "mixed" vitamin E supplement if possible. The daily upper limit is 1000 IU.

- *Selenium* RDA is 55 micrograms. Best food sources are fish, seafood, chicken, organ meats, whole grains, nuts, onions, garlic and mushrooms. To supplement, take 200 micrograms per day. Check how much your multivitamin and mineral supplement gives you before you buy a separate selenium pill. The daily upper limit is 400 micrograms.

If your partner smokes cigarettes, encourage him to quit (same goes for you). Smoking causes the formation of those nasty free radical compounds that are thought to damage sperm. The damage caused by inhaling cigarette smoke is reflected in the higher recommended intake of vitamin C in smokers.

Vitamin B12

This vitamin may affect your partner's fertility as well as your own. There is some evidence to suggest that a B12 deficiency may lead to lower sperm counts. One study looked at the effects of B12 supplements among infertile men.[13] Supplementing the diet with extra B12 helped only those men with low sperm counts and impaired sperm motility. I realize this is not much to hang your hat on, but have your partner take a look at the B12-rich foods listed on page 10 in chapter 1, and make sure he includes more of them in his diet. Taking a multivitamin and mineral supplement is another simple way to prevent a deficiency.

Zinc

This mineral is essential for growth, sexual development and sperm production. Many studies have found a link between infertility in men and low zinc concentration in seminal fluid. A zinc deficiency may also lead to low testosterone levels. In fact, one small study conducted in men with low testosterone levels found that zinc supplements increased sperm count and the rate of pregnancy in their partners.[14]

The RDA for zinc in men is 11 milligrams per day (women need 8 milligrams). The best food sources include oysters (a whopping 150 milligrams per 3 ounces!), dark turkey meat, lentils, ricotta cheese, tofu, yogurt, lean beef, wheat germ, spinach, broccoli, green beans and tomato juice. If supplements are used, take anywhere from 15 to 30 milligrams (many multivitamin and mineral formulas offer 15 milligrams). Make sure your zinc supplement has 1 milligram of copper since these two minerals work together. Too much zinc has toxic effects, so do not exceed 40 milligrams per day.

L-carnitine

This compound is not considered an essential nutrient because the body makes it in sufficient quantities. Carnitine helps the body generate energy by transporting fat into cells. Most of our body's carnitine is located in our muscles and heart, but a little is also found in the brain, liver and kidneys. It is also present in sperm and seminal fluid. A number of studies have found a positive relationship between sperm count and motility and their concentration of L-carnitine. The higher the concentration of L-carnitine, the higher the sperm count. Researchers have also found that infertile men have much lower levels of L-carnitine in their semen compared to fertile men.[15]

Does that mean that taking L-carnitine can improve male fertility? One Italian study addressed this. The findings revealed that 3 grams per day of L-carnitine taken for three months increased sperm count and sperm motility in 37 out of 47 men.[16]

L-carnitine is found in meat and dairy products. But you won't get 3 grams of this natural compound from diet alone. If your partner decides to try a supplement, the recommended dose is 1 to 3 grams per day. Avoid products that contain D-carnitine or DL-carnitine. These forms compete with L-carnitine in the body and could lead to a deficiency. The supplement is considered safe. Occasional side effects of gastrointestinal upset have been reported.

LIFESTYLE FACTORS

Alcohol, Caffeine and Smoking

Most of the research investigating the effect of alcohol and caffeine on fertility has been done in women. And, as you read earlier, both substances, even in moderation, can reduce a woman's chances of getting pregnant. The effect on male fertility is less clear. Italian researchers found that the risk of having unhealthy sperm increased with the number of cups of coffee per day, compared to the risk in men who had one or fewer cups of coffee daily. The same study showed that alcohol drinkers were at greater risk of having abnormal sperm, and the risk increased with the number of drinks per day.[17]

If your partner is a smoker, one of the most important behavior changes he can make to improve your odds of getting pregnant is to give up cigarettes. Study after study has shown that the harmful chemicals inhaled from cigarettes reduce sperm count, impair the health of sperm and decrease sexual performance. There's little doubt that cigarette smoking increases a man's odds of being infertile. Suggest that your spouse visit his family doctor to learn options available to help him quit smoking.

THE BOTTOM LINE...
Leslie's recommendations for enhancing fertility

1. To ensure an optimal intake of calories, protein, carbohydrates, fat, vitamins and minerals, both you and your partner should follow the healthiest diet possible. Consider consulting a registered dietitian who can assess your diet and develop a customized eating and supplement plan for both of you. Check out **www.eatright .org** to find a professional in your community.

2. Avoid caffeine and alcohol, two beverages that may affect female fertility.

3. Achieve and maintain a healthy body weight.

4. Both you and your partner should make sure you are getting proper amounts of vitamin B12.

5. If you have been experiencing irregular periods, consider the herbal remedy chasteberry (*Vitex angus-castus*). Take 175 to 225 milligrams of an extract standardized to contain 0.5 percent agnuside and 0.6 percent aucubin, once daily.

6. Make sure your male partner consumes plenty of antioxidant nutrients. The ones to pay attention to are vitamin C, vitamin E and selenium.

7. Have your partner assess his intake of zinc from foods.

8. L-carnitine is a natural compound found in animal food and made by the body that may be important for male fertility. If you want to give this a try, your partner should take 1 to 3 grams of L-carnitine daily. Avoid products that contain D-carnitine or DL-carnitine.

15
Pregnancy

Pregnancy is a nine-month continuum that begins with conception and ends with the birth of your new baby. It is a time of tremendous change in your life, often accompanied by feelings of anticipation and fear. It is also a time when maintaining good health is vitally important. From the moment of conception and even before, the choices that you make about diet, exercise and medical care will have a profound effect on the growth and development of your baby. There is no greater gift you can give your child than to live a healthy lifestyle every single day of your pregnancy.

Before you delve into this chapter, I want to let you know that it is not formatted in my usual style. You will not see my recommendations categorized by diet, vitamins/minerals and herbal remedies. Nor do I conclude this chapter with my Bottom Line. Due to the heftiness of this topic, and the fact that nutrition needs and concerns change with each trimester, I have provided nutrition strategies throughout the text. In the latter part of this chapter I sum up by presenting your nutrient and food requirements during all stages of your pregnancy. Therefore, anyone concerned with this topic should read this chapter in its entirety. Enjoy the journey to motherhood!

Confirming Your Pregnancy

The first sign of pregnancy is usually a missed menstrual period. If you're sexually active and your menstrual cycles are quite regular, there's a good chance that you are pregnant if your period is more than a week late. Menstrual cycles usually stop during pregnancy, although some women have been known to have light periods during the entire nine months.

To confirm your pregnancy, you can take a urine test that will detect the presence of pregnancy hormones—HCG (human chorionic gonadotropin)—in your system. You can choose to have the urine test done at your doctor's office or you can do it yourself, using one of the many home pregnancy test kits available in most drugstores. By the second week after conception, home pregnancy tests are 90 percent accurate. As an alternative to the urine test, you can have a blood sample taken at your doctor's office and tested at a laboratory. A blood test can detect pregnancy hormones as early as eight days after conception.

If you wait to confirm your diagnosis until you are four weeks past conception, your doctor will perform an internal examination and physically check for signs of pregnancy. He or she will look for a slight enlargement of your uterus and color changes in your vagina and cervix caused by increased blood flow. This examination is very accurate in determining pregnancy.

A typical pregnancy lasts 39 weeks or nine months from conception. Your expected date of delivery is usually 280 days from the first day of your last menstrual period. However, less than 5 percent of all babies arrive on their due date, so you should anticipate that your baby might arrive earlier or later than expected. Traditionally, pregnancies are divided into three stages or trimesters, each lasting roughly three months. Your body undergoes many changes during these stages and each trimester represents important growth and development milestones. By following a healthy lifestyle and arranging for good prenatal care throughout all the stages of your pregnancy, you can give your baby the very best start in life.

~

The First Trimester

Every pregnancy is unique and the symptoms that you experience may be different from those of other women. By understanding what these symptoms mean and how they affect your body and your baby, you will be better prepared for the many physical and emotional adjustments that lie ahead.

SYMPTOMS

Fatigue

During the early stages of pregnancy, there are profound changes taking place in your body. Your baby, or fetus, is growing rapidly in your uterus and requires many nutrients to build essential structures and systems. Your body produces up to 50 percent more blood to carry these nutrients to the fetus. To handle the increased blood flow, your heart rate speeds up and you breathe faster, which sends more oxygen to the fetus. Your metabolic rate increases and all of your bodily functions are accelerated.

In addition to these physical changes, it's quite natural to feel some emotional stress at this time, even if you're very happy to be pregnant. You may have fears about your baby's health or your ability to be a good mother, or you may worry about work, finances or lifestyle changes. As you adapt to these physical and emotional symptoms, you may find that your energy level drops and you feel much more tired than usual.

Fatigue is a common symptom in the first trimester. This is a time in your pregnancy when you may need to slow down a little, because your body is working hard. Rest as often as you can, take a nap when time allows and go to bed early. Incorporating moderate exercise, such as a 30-minute walk, into your daily routine will increase your energy level and help you combat your feelings of fatigue. Making sure you eat a healthy diet that includes three meals and a mid-day snack will also help you feel more energetic.

Urinary Frequency

It's quite likely that you'll suffer from an increasing need to urinate during these early days of pregnancy. Laughing, sneezing or coughing may cause embarrassing leaking of urine, and you may have to get up more often at night to use the bathroom. Because of the demands of pregnancy, your kidneys are working overtime to filter the larger volume of blood in your system, and this stimulates your body to produce more urine. At the same time, your uterus is growing and putting extra pressure on your bladder. The result is a reduced bladder capacity that keeps you from straying far from a bathroom.

Although you should not be restricting your fluid intake during pregnancy, you may find that avoiding beverages for a few hours before bedtime helps to minimize nighttime interruptions. Wearing panty liners during the day will also help protect you against unexpected leaking.

Morning Sickness

Many women are troubled by nausea and vomiting during the first 14 to 16 weeks of their pregnancies. This is one of the most uncomfortable symptoms of the first trimester and affects nearly 70 percent of all pregnant women. Although it is commonly referred to as morning sickness, nausea is not limited to the morning hours—it can and does occur at any time of the day. Normally, these symptoms will come to an end after the first three to four months but, in some cases, morning sickness will last beyond the first trimester and may even persist throughout the entire pregnancy. Rarely, the vomiting may be so severe that hospitalization is necessary to maintain adequate nutrition and fluid intake.

Nausea and vomiting may be caused by the hormone changes produced by the placenta and the uterus. Increases in the hormone progesterone tend to slow down the gastrointestinal system, allowing food to remain in your stomach for a longer time. This extra digestion time is good for your baby because it helps your body extract additional nutrients from the food you eat. Unfortunately, it may also upset your stomach and add to your feelings of nausea.

STRATEGIES TO REDUCE MORNING SICKNESS
These tips have helped many of my clients.

- *Eat small, frequent meals* every two to three hours, rather than two or three large meals.
- *Avoid hunger;* eat a few crackers before getting out of bed in the morning and don't skip meals.

- *Choose low-fat protein foods* (lean meat, canned tuna, chicken breast, eggs, legumes) *and easily digestible carbohydrates* (fruit, rice, pasta, potatoes, toast, dry cereals).

- *Drink fluids between meals* rather than with meals.

- *Avoid fried foods* or other foods that cause stomach upset, such as gassy vegetables and spicy foods.

- If the smell of hot meals makes you queasy, *try eating cold food.* Try for a sandwich instead of a hot entree.

- To abate nausea, try to *take small sips of fruit juice or a decaffeinated soft drink every 30 minutes.* Some women report that a sports drink like Gatorade or PowerAde provides relief.

- *Have a snack before bed.*

- *Evaluate your surroundings* to find out what could be triggering your nausea. It could be the smell of coffee brewing, the sight of raw food, your perfume, patterned carpets, camera angles on television programs, and so on. It might not always be obvious.

- *Cook with ginger* for relief from nausea and vomiting. Ginger has been scientifically shown to help reduce morning sickness. Research demonstrates that ginger root improves appetite, reduces the stomach's secretion of acid and increases the release of bile, a digestive aid. The active ingredients in the ginger root are known as gingerols and shogaols.

  Buy fresh ginger root and add it to stir-fries and marinades. If you have a juicer, add a thick slice of ginger root to your concoction. You can also prepare ginger tea: steep 0.5 to 1 gram of the dried root in 150 milliliters of boiling water for up to ten minutes and strain; drink one cup three times a day. You can take 250 milligrams of fresh ginger up to four times daily. Ginger extract supplements are available from health food stores or pharmacies. If you take ginger supplements, use them for only a short period of time and do not exceed 1 gram (1000 milligrams) per day. The effects of long-term high doses of ginger on the growing fetus are not known. Adding fresh ginger root to your meals is safe throughout your pregnancy.

Other Symptoms

Your breasts will rapidly increase in size and weight, new milk ducts will grow and breast veins will become more noticeable. You may find that your breasts are tender and sore because of the increased production of estrogen and progesterone hormones. These hormonal changes, as well as the increased blood flow in early pregnancy, may also trigger headaches and dizziness. Stress, fatigue and hunger can make the headaches worse. Warm compresses and relaxation exercises should help ease these mild aches and pains. Painkillers and other medications should be avoided, unless recommended by your doctor.

WEIGHT GAIN

If you are a healthy weight when you become pregnant you should expect to gain between 11 to 16 kilograms (25 to 35 pounds) in total. Here's a look at the recommended weight gain over the course of your pregnancy (see page 45 in chapter 2 to calculate your BMI).

Underweight women (BMI < 20)	28–40 lbs (12.5–18 kg)
Healthy weight women (BMI 20–27)	25–35 lbs (11.5–16 kg)
Overweight women (BMI > 27)	15–25 lbs (7–11.5 kg)
Obese women (BMI > 29)	At least 15 lbs (7 kg)
Twin pregnancy	35–45 lbs (16–20 kg)
Triplets pregnancy	50 lbs (23 kg)

Throughout the first trimester, you should expect to gain only a small amount of extra weight, normally not more than 1.4 to 2.3 kilograms (3 to 5 pounds). Even though your body requires extra nutrients, during the first trimester you need to add only 100 calories to your daily diet to maintain good fetal development.

If you gain too much weight during your pregnancy, you can endanger your own health and that of your baby. Diabetes, high blood pressure and fluid retention are more likely to develop in overweight women. If you gain too much weight, you may also find it difficult to lose the excess pounds after the birth of your baby. You'll find recommended servings and portion sizes from all the food groups later in the chapter.

However, if you are overweight when you become pregnant, you must be careful not to restrict your calorie intake too severely. To nourish your growing baby properly, you must always maintain a balanced diet that provides all the essential nutrients. A low calorie intake during pregnancy can result in the release of ketones into your blood and urine. Chronic ketone production is known to cause mental retardation in infants. If you are underweight when you conceive, or gain too little weight during your pregnancy (less than 9 kilograms, or 20 pounds), you may also be at risk of delivering a baby with low birth weight. Research indicates that the risks of restricting weight gain during pregnancy are potentially more harmful to the fetus than unrestricted weight gain.

FETAL DEVELOPMENT

The first trimester is a very crucial time in your baby's development. During these few weeks, all the essential organs, structures and systems necessary to sustain life are formed. The heart begins beating and the digestive system is developing. The brain, backbone and spinal cord are all growing. Limbs are taking shape and facial features can be seen. Reproductive organs are in place, although they are still too small to indicate the baby's gender. The circulatory and respiratory systems are functioning and so are the liver and kidneys. By the end of the first trimester, the fetus is usually about 7 centimeters (3 inches) long and weighs about 28 grams (1 ounce).

CARE

Once your pregnancy has been confirmed, you should visit your doctor for a complete physical examination. This is usually done during the first six to eight weeks of pregnancy. Your doctor will take a detailed medical history, including chronic medical problems and complications of earlier pregnancies. You will also be given a pelvic and rectal exam to determine the size and position of your uterus. At this stage, routine lab tests will include blood tests for rubella (German measles), hepatitis B, syphilis and other sexually transmitted diseases. Your blood will also be typed and screened for Rh antibodies. HIV testing is recommended, as well as urine tests and a Pap test for cervical cancer. During this appointment, your doctor will also determine the expected date for the delivery of your baby.

After your first visit, you will normally see your doctor once a month for routine examinations, unless there is a medical reason for more frequent appointments. These monthly examinations will continue until the 28th week of pregnancy, when your appointments will increase to once every two weeks. As you approach the end of your pregnancy, your medical visits will be scheduled weekly.

If your doctor suspects that your pregnancy is high-risk for certain medical disorders, he or she may send you for chorionic villi sampling. This is a special test used to identify abnormalities in your fetus that could result in conditions such as cystic fibrosis or Down's syndrome. The chorionic villi are located on the edge of the placenta and are genetically identical to your baby. A small probe is inserted through your vagina and into your uterus, to gather cell samples from the surface of the placenta. By analyzing these cells, a great deal of information can be gathered about the overall health of your baby. The test is usually performed at 10 to 12 weeks and results are available within one or two days. Chorionic villi sampling is similar to amniocentesis, in that both tests identify fetal abnormalities. Chorionic villi sampling gives you results much earlier, although it does carry a slightly higher risk of miscarriage.

The Second Trimester

The second trimester lasts from the 13th to the 28th week of pregnancy. Most women feel their best at this stage, because the discomforts of early pregnancy have subsided and the uncomfortable symptoms of the last trimester are still ahead. At this point you are probably sleeping better and your energy levels are returning to normal.

SYMPTOMS

Aches and Pains
During the second trimester, every organ in your body is busy adapting to the changes of pregnancy. Your growing uterus is the most obvious sign of change, as it begins to protrude out of the abdominal cavity, giving you a much more rounded shape. As the uterus enlarges, it pushes other internal organs out of the way and causes tension in surrounding muscles and ligaments. You may feel pain in your lower abdomen because the structures that support the uterus are stretching and thickening. This type of pain is not severe and it does not pose a threat to your pregnancy. If you are bothered by abdominal pain, try lying down and resting for a short time. Relaxation exercises will help and a warm bath may soothe the aches away.

Back Pain

To allow your baby to pass through your pelvis during birth, the joints in your pelvic area begin to soften and loosen. Sometimes, the panels of muscle running along the front of your abdomen will separate under pressure from your expanding uterus. As well, the growing weight of your fetus changes your center of gravity, causing you to compensate by adjusting your posture. All of these factors may result in back pain during your last two trimesters.

To minimize the discomfort, you should try to maintain a correct posture, with your pelvis tucked in and your shoulders back. Sit with your feet slightly elevated, try not to stand for long periods and sleep on your side with a pillow between your knees and one under your abdomen. Exercises to strengthen your abdominal muscles will also reduce the tension in your back.

Other Symptoms

The hormones that loosen your pelvic joints also affect your intestinal tract, slowing down digestion and causing food to remain longer in your stomach. This allows more time for nutrients to be absorbed into your bloodstream for use by the fetus. Unfortunately, it can also result in nausea, indigestion and bloating. Heartburn is another symptom of this slowdown in digestion. Heartburn develops when the contents of your stomach flow backward into your esophagus. The stomach acids irritate the esophagus, creating the burning sensation that gives heartburn its name. Eating small meals more often during the day can help minimize heartburn. You should also avoid drinking fluids with your meals; instead, have them between meals. Because your intestinal muscles are more relaxed, you may also become constipated, a condition that is aggravated by the pressure of the growing uterus on your rectum.

As you progress through your second trimester, your heart is working twice as fast as it was before you were pregnant, your blood volumes are 50 percent higher and your kidney functions are still accelerated. Skin darkening is a very common symptom at this stage, especially among dark-skinned women. The skin around your nipples, navel and vulva will become a deeper color and you may notice the appearance of a dark line between your navel and your pubic bone. This darkening of the skin usually disappears after pregnancy.

WEIGHT GAIN

Weight gain tends to vary during the second trimester. On average, you should expect to gain about 0.5 kilograms (1 pound) a week after the first three months. You should be striving for a steady, gradual weight gain, without sudden increases or decreases.

FETAL DEVELOPMENT

This is a very exciting time, because you will soon begin to feel your baby move. The kicking and fluttering movements of your growing baby will make the pregnancy feel more emotionally involving and real to you. You can expect to detect some fetal activity by the 20th week of pregnancy.

As you enter your fourth month, most of your baby's bones are formed, facial features are becoming more defined and external genitalia are evident. The brain is growing and the baby's head proportions are more balanced. By the end of the second trimester, your baby's eyes are opening and closing, there is some fat accumulating under the skin and regular intervals of sleeping and waking are beginning. At this stage the baby has grown to 23 centimeters (9 inches) and weighs nearly 670 grams (just over one pound). After 24 to 26 weeks, there is a strong possibility that the baby could survive outside the womb.

CARE

Medical visits during the second trimester focus primarily on tracking the development of the fetus, establishing an accurate due date and monitoring your general health. Your doctor will check your blood pressure and weight, and will discuss any symptoms that you may be experiencing. He or she will also measure the size of your uterus to help determine your baby's true age.

Special tests may be suggested for you during this stage of pregnancy.

1. *Ultrasound exam* This is the safest form of imaging during pregnancy. High-frequency sound waves create images of the fetus that you can see on a monitor. The images are high quality and often show the baby in motion. Many doctors feel that at least one ultrasound should be performed during each pregnancy to make sure that you and your baby are progressing well. Ultrasounds are used to

- record fetal heartbeats and breathing movements

- measure fetal growth

- determine if you are carrying more than one fetus

- find the location of the placenta

- date the pregnancy through fetal measurements

- assess the amount of amniotic fluid

Ultrasound scanning may also be used during the first trimester to confirm evidence of pregnancy and fetal growth. Later in your pregnancy, it may be used to monitor the baby's health or to identify conditions that may cause problems during the pregnancy or delivery.

2. *Alpha-fetoprotein test* Alpha-fetoprotein (AFP) is a substance normally produced by a growing fetus. Between 15 and 18 weeks you may be tested to determine the level of this substance in your blood. A sample of your blood is studied at a laboratory to detect the presence of abnormalities that may cause birth defects such as spina bifida or Down's syndrome.

3. *Amniocentesis* This test involves collecting and analyzing a small sample of the fluid that fills the amniotic sac surrounding the fetus. The amniotic fluid contains skin cells and other genetic material from your developing fetus, so it provides a great deal of valuable information about the health of your baby. The test begins with an ultrasound to locate the position of the baby. Guided by the ultrasound images, a long, thin needle is passed into the uterus to remove a fluid sample. The sample is sent to a laboratory, where it is studied to determine if the fetus has normal chromosomes. Amniocentesis is recommended for women at increased risk for having a baby with a birth defect, especially women who are over 35 years old or who have a family history of birth defects. Amniocentesis is also used to find out if your baby's lungs are mature enough for an early delivery or to follow up on an AFP test that is positive for abnormalities. The procedure is usually performed between 16 and 18 weeks, when there is enough amniotic fluid for an effective sample. There is a 1 in 200 chance of miscarriage after an amniocentesis.

4. *Glucose tolerance testing* This is a test for gestational diabetes. Even if you did not have diabetes before you became pregnant, you may be at risk of developing the disorder during your pregnancy. Changes in hormones and metabolism during pregnancy sometimes affect the ability of your body to produce or use the hormone

insulin. This hormone imbalance creates problems for the health of your baby. To test for gestational diabetes, you will be asked to drink a glucose solution. An hour later, your blood will be tested for abnormal levels of blood glucose. If this test is positive, a follow-up test will be necessary to confirm the diagnosis of gestational diabetes.

5. *Rh factor testing* The Rhesus (Rh) factor is a type of protein that is sometimes present in your blood. If you have it, you are Rh-positive; if you don't, you are Rh-negative. If you and your baby have incompatible Rh factors, your body will produce antibodies that will cause damage or death to your fetus. A sample of your blood will be tested at a laboratory to determine your Rh factor.

6. *Hemoglobin testing* By measuring your hemoglobin levels, your doctor can determine if you have anemia, which is usually caused by an iron deficiency in your blood. Most pregnant women do not absorb enough iron from their food to meet the demands of pregnancy. The condition can be improved with dietary changes and iron supplements.

ॐ

The Third Trimester

The third trimester is a time of conflicting emotions. You will be excited at the prospect of your baby's upcoming birth, yet worried about your baby's health and safety during these crucial last weeks. You'll probably be very tired of being pregnant, yet fear the pain and uncertainty of giving birth. For most women, the final three months of pregnancy is a time of decision-making, planning and great anticipation. This stage lasts from the 28th week of pregnancy until the delivery of your baby.

SYMPTOMS

Sleeping Problems

At the end of your pregnancy, you may have trouble sleeping through the night. By this time, your uterus has undergone enormous change, stretching your abdomen to accommodate the constant growth of the baby, the amniotic fluid and the placenta. As you try to cope with this additional weight and size, it will be more and more difficult for you to find a comfortable sleeping position. To make sleeping easier, you should try to lie on your side, rather than your back, with your legs bent. This takes pressure off the large vein that carries blood from your legs and feet back to your heart, reducing swelling, discomfort and back pain. You may also want to read my recommended dietary approaches in chapter 6, "Insomnia."

Shortness of Breath

In late pregnancy, it is very common for you to feel breathless and tired. Your expanding uterus pushes the diaphragm, a band of muscle underneath your lungs, up higher into your chest. This decreases the capacity of your lungs by just a few centimeters, but that's enough to make you feel short of breath. At the same time, the action of the progesterone in your system causes you to breathe more deeply, increasing the volume of air that you take in with every breath. The result is an enriched oxygen supply that circulates through your bloodstream to meet the demands of your growing fetus. Just before delivery, the pressure on your diaphragm will be relieved when your baby drops farther down into your pelvis. By improving your posture and maintaining a routine of gentle aerobic exercise throughout your pregnancy, you should be able to breathe a little better and increase your lung capacity.

Aches and Pains

You will find that your rapidly growing uterus puts pressure on numerous nerves, muscles and joints, causing you a variety of aches and pains. You can expect to experience at least a few of the following symptoms:

- *Sciatica* This type of low back pain results from pressure on the sciatic nerves that run from your lower back down to your feet.

- *Hip pain* This symptom is caused by hormones that loosen your joints and connective tissue in preparation for delivery.

- *Stretching of the ligaments of your hips and pelvis* Also caused by hormones that loosen connective tissue, this can make walking difficult.

- *Vaginal pain* This symptom may indicate the early stages of dilation in your cervix.

- *Fluid retention* Your hands and feet swell as you retain fluids.

- *Frequent urination* The discomfort that plagued you in the first trimester returns with a vengeance, as the growing fetus squeezes your bladder.

- *Itchy skin* Your skin is stretching and tightening across your abdomen, making it feel dry and itchy.

- *Stretch marks* Reddish or white streaks will develop on your breasts, abdomen and upper thighs.

- *Leaking urine* This symptom is the result of increased pressure on the bladder.

- *Varicose veins* They appear frequently in pregnancy, caused by the pressure of the uterus on the veins in your legs.

Throughout the last trimester of your pregnancy, you will feel uncomfortable and tired much of the time. But your due date is approaching quickly and most of these normal symptoms will subside after delivery. During these last few weeks, rest, gentle exercise and a balanced diet are essential to prepare you for the rigors of delivery and the demands of your newborn infant.

WEIGHT GAIN

Over the course of your third trimester, you will gain approximately 4 kilograms (10 pounds). Your total weight gain during the pregnancy should be in the range of 11 to 16 kilograms (25 to 35 pounds). This includes the 2.5 to 3.5 kilograms (6 to 8 pounds) that your baby weighs, plus the 6 to 11 kilograms (14 to 24 pounds) of amniotic fluid, placenta, uterus and increased breast tissue. These are the ideal targets for an average woman. It is recommended that underweight women gain 5 to 10 pounds more, and overweight women gain 5 to 10 pounds less than these guidelines.

FETAL DEVELOPMENT

In these last weeks of pregnancy, your baby is steadily gaining weight. Fat is building up on your baby's body and a slick, fatty substance called vernix caseosa covers the skin. Thumb sucking may begin and your baby's eyes will open and close. Bones and limbs will elongate and the lungs are maturing. You may notice increased activity, as the baby's movements become more vigorous. When you reach the end of your term, the baby will drop farther down into your abdomen, settling into a position for delivery.

By the 39th week, your baby will weigh approximately 3 kilograms (7 pounds) and have grown to 46 centimeters (18 inches) or more.

CARE

Routine examinations are very important during your last stage of pregnancy. Your doctor will expect to see you every two weeks between your 28th and 36th week, then weekly until delivery. Your weight and blood pressure will be measured regularly and the activity levels of your fetus will be monitored. As your due date approaches, your doctor will check to see if the baby has moved into the proper position for delivery. The baby should be head-down in the uterus, with the head at the top of the birth canal. Some babies are positioned with their feet or buttocks down in a breech presentation.

You can expect to have regular vaginal exams to evaluate the state of your cervix. Your doctor will determine how much the cervix has softened and whether it has begun to efface (thin out) or dilate (open), in preparation for delivery. If your doctor has concerns about your baby's health or you are having a high-risk pregnancy, he or she may perform a non-stress test (NST). This test measures the baby's heart rate when it moves. Using ultrasound techniques, your baby's heart rate will be recorded for 20 minutes. The heartbeat should accelerate as the baby moves. If the acceleration rate is not normal, further tests may be necessary.

∽

Concerns and Complications of Pregnancy

While most women have normal pregnancies and healthy babies, there are some conditions and complications that can create problems for you and your baby. By understanding the concerns and recognizing the symptoms, you will know when to contact your doctor and what the impact will be on the outcome of your pregnancy.

SPOTTING AND BLEEDING

It is not unusual for you to have slight bleeding or spotting during early pregnancy. You may notice a small amount of bleeding about a week or 10 days after conception. This is implantation bleeding and it occurs when the fertilized egg attaches itself to the wall of the uterus. The episode of bleeding should be quite brief. Some women may also have light bleeding at the time of their regular menstrual period throughout the first six months of their pregnancy, or even longer. Most episodes of bleeding are caused by normal events of pregnancy. However, you should always notify your doctor if you have spotting because it can be a warning sign of other problems with your pregnancy.

MISCARRIAGE

If your bleeding is heavy and is accompanied by pain, cramping or fever, or if you notice that you have passed some tissue, you may be experiencing a miscarriage. Also known as a spontaneous abortion, a miscarriage is the loss of a fetus that is less than 28 weeks past conception. It occurs in 15 to 30 percent of all pregnancies, although it often happens so early that many women may not even realize they are pregnant. More than 80 percent of all miscarriages happen in the first 12 weeks of pregnancy.

The most common cause of miscarriage is an abnormality in the fetus's chromosomes. This is an error that occurs as the fertilized egg begins to divide and grow. The abnormality prevents the fetus from implanting or developing properly. Chromosome errors that result in miscarriage do not usually indicate a genetic problem. Other causes of miscarriage include defects in the uterus, hormonal imbalances, viral or bacterial infections or chronic diseases, such as diabetes or high blood pressure. You should be aware that the normal activities of daily life, including exercising, lifting heavy objects or having sex will *not* cause you to miscarry. Nor will a fall or an injury, unless it is very severe.

The main warning sign of a miscarriage is vaginal bleeding. Any type of bleeding may indicate a miscarriage, even if it is quite light, so you should contact your doctor immediately if you begin spotting. Your doctor may suggest bed rest in an attempt to stabilize the pregnancy. However, the miscarriage may continue, despite your best efforts, simply because the fetus does not have the proper chromosomes to survive. During the miscarriage, you will eliminate fetal tissue through your vagina. In some cases, you may need to have a surgical procedure to gently scrape or suction the tissue out of the uterus. If you have a miscarriage, there is very little need to worry about future pregnancies. You have an excellent chance of continuing with other successful pregnancies, even if you have repeated—i.e., more than three—miscarriages.

ECTOPIC PREGNANCY

Vaginal bleeding may also indicate that you are experiencing an ectopic or tubal pregnancy. An ectopic pregnancy occurs when the fertilized egg attaches itself somewhere other than the wall of the uterus. In 95 percent of these cases, the egg becomes stuck inside one of your fallopian tubes, as it travels on its way from the ovary to the uterus. Usually this happens because an infection or inflammation causes the fallopian tube to become partially or completely blocked by scar tissue. In most cases, this type of scarring is the result of pelvic inflammatory disease, a fairly common type of sexually transmitted disease. Because the fallopian tube is not designed to accommodate a growing fetus, the fertilized egg will not develop properly. Eventually, the tube walls will stretch and burst, resulting in a life-threatening loss of blood for you.

At first, you may not be aware that you have an ectopic pregnancy. The first signs are usually sharp, stabbing pain in the pelvis, abdomen, shoulder or neck. Vaginal bleeding and dizziness are other symptoms of this condition. Once your doctor has diagnosed the ectopic pregnancy by sending you for a blood test or ultrasound exam, you will probably require surgery to remove the fetus. Through a small incision in your abdomen, the doctor will insert a long instrument, called a laparoscope, to remove the fetal tissue. Depending on the degree of damage, the fallopian tube will either be repaired or removed. Your chances for a successful pregnancy after an ectopic pregnancy depend on whether the condition was detected early enough to save the fallopian tube. Once you've had one ectopic pregnancy, you are at increased risk of having another one.

VAGINAL YEAST INFECTIONS

It is quite common to have increased vaginal discharge during pregnancy. A normal discharge consists of thin, white mucus and is caused by hormones that stimulate glands in the cervix. However, if you notice a discharge that is green or yellow, strong smelling and accompanied by irritation and itching in your vaginal area, then you may have vaginitis, or a vaginal infection.

A yeast organism called *Candida albicans* often causes vaginal infections. This irritating condition is known as a yeast infection or candidiasis and can be a recurring problem during pregnancy. The *Candida* organism is found in nearly one-quarter of all pregnant women as they approach their due date. Symptoms of a yeast infection include a burning sensation and thick curdlike discharge. It is treated with an anti-fungal drug that is applied in a topical cream or suppository. To prevent these and other vaginal infections, you should keep your vaginal area clean and dry, wear loose-fitting clothing, avoid synthetic materials next to your skin, wear underwear with a cotton insert and avoid douches or feminine hygiene sprays.

Try the following dietary strategies to prevent and treat vaginal yeast infections.

1. *Include fermented milk products in your daily diet.* Foods such as yogurt, kefir (a milk beverage) and sweet acidophilus milk all contain friendly bacteria, known collectively as lactic acid bacteria. You may even know some of their names—*Lactobacillus acidophilus* and bifidobacteria. These bacteria normally live in your intestine where they prevent the growth of infection-causing bacteria and fungi, including yeast. A number of studies have shown that women who consume yogurt or fermented milk beverages each day have a significant reduction in vaginal yeast infections. In fact, one study found that 1 cup of yogurt eaten daily for six months resulted in a three-fold decrease in infection among women experiencing recurrent *Candida* infections. Some studies have found a yogurt douche to be effective against vaginal yeast infections.

   You may already know that these bacteria are available in supplement form. I have often recommended them to clients as a convenient way to get a hefty dose of lactic acid bacteria. However, during pregnancy, I recommend that you stick to eating fermented dairy products as there is very little information on use of supplements at this time. A yogurt a day also gives you close to 300 milligrams of calcium, not to mention protein and some carbohydrate for energy.

2. *Add garlic to your meals.* You may want to use cooked garlic more often than raw, since some women report being sensitive to fresh uncooked garlic during their pregnancy. A daily intake of garlic and its accompanying sulfur compounds has been used to enhance the body's immune system and kill many types of bacteria and fungi. One-half to one clove a day is recommended. You can also buy a liquid extract of aged garlic (Kyolic® brand) that lets you add garlic to foods without peeling, cutting or chopping. If you buy this product from your health food store, add a few drops to your yogurt douche. Garlic has been used alone or in combination with yogurt to treat *Candida* infections.

HEMORRHOIDS

Hemorrhoids are a type of varicose vein that is very common in pregnancy. They are swollen rectal veins that may bleed or protrude through your anus. Hemorrhoids are caused by the increased pressure of your uterus, which interferes with blood flow to the rectal area, causing blood to pool in these veins. Symptoms include bleeding, itching and pain in and around your anus. The best approach is to try to prevent them by avoiding constipation. The straining associated with constipation puts extra pressure on the veins and will aggravate your symptoms. Once hemorrhoids develop, you can minimize the symptoms by keeping your rectal area clean and washing after each bowel movement, soaking in a warm bath, applying cold compresses and avoiding sitting for long periods. Hemorrhoids will usually subside after pregnancy.

Try these strategies to help prevent constipation and hemorrhoids.

1. *Gradually increase your intake of dietary fiber* to 25 grams per day. Foods like wheat bran, whole grains and fruits and vegetables contain insoluble fiber, the type that promotes bowel health. Two of the best ways to boost your fiber intake are to start your day with a bowl of high-fiber breakfast cereal and to include a serving of chickpeas, kidney beans, black beans or lentils in your daily diet. High-fiber cereals are those that have at least 6 grams of fiber per serving, stated on the nutrition panel. If you are constipated, choose a 100 percent bran cereal that gives you 10 to 13 grams of fiber per serving. Mix 1/4 to 1/2 cup (60 to 125 ml) into your usual breakfast cereal. You'll find a list of higher-fiber foods on page 29 in chapter 1. But start slowly—too much fiber too soon can cause bloating and gas, and it may even worsen your constipation.

2. *Drink plenty of water.* Aim for 2 to 3 liters (8 to 12 cups) each day, and more if you exercise. For insoluble fiber to work in your intestinal tract, it needs to absorb water first. By retaining water, fiber acts to increase stool bulk and promote regularity.

3. *Get regular exercise,* such as brisk walking, to help keep your bowel movements regular.

4. *Check the dosage of your iron supplement.* Constipation and nausea may occur when you start taking 120 milligrams of iron or more. These side effects often disappear three to five days after first taking your iron supplement. If they persist, speak to your doctor or dietitian about decreasing the dosage. Many women report they feel better when they take iron in the evening.

ANEMIA

Iron is an essential mineral in the production of red blood cells. During pregnancy, your blood volume increases nearly 50 percent, putting excessive demands on your body's ability to produce vital red blood cells. Your fetus also has specific iron requirements, especially during the last months of pregnancy, when iron stores are building up. When you are not pregnant you need 18 milligrams of iron a day. When you are pregnant, you need 27 milligrams to prevent a deficiency.

If you're not meeting your increased iron needs during pregnancy, your fetus will draw its supply from your iron stores, leaving you anemic and exhausted. Anemia is caused by a decline in the amount of hemoglobin in the blood. Hemoglobin is a protein found in red blood cells and it plays a very important role in carrying oxygen throughout your body. To build up hemoglobin concentrations, you need more iron to help increase the production of red blood cells. Normally, you can meet most of your daily iron needs by following a balanced diet. However, because of the increased demands of pregnancy, it is almost impossible to maintain your iron stores through diet alone. This is why many nutritionists and doctors recommend that women take a special prenatal vitamin supplement throughout their pregnancy. These supplements provide extra iron as well as calcium and folic acid (more on these nutrients later).

If you have anemia, you will feel tired, weak and light-headed. You may also experience shortness of breath and heart palpitations. Anemia develops most often after the 20th week of pregnancy and is identified through blood tests that measure your hemoglobin levels. Your doctor may recommend that you take iron supplements throughout the second half of your pregnancy to avoid developing iron-deficiency anemia.

If you are diagnosed with iron-deficiency anemia, be sure to read chapter 3, "Anemia." In this chapter I discuss your recommended daily intake, the best food sources of iron and how to enhance your body's absorption of this mineral.

RHESUS INCOMPATIBILITY

Fairly early in your pregnancy, your blood will be tested for Rhesus (Rh) factor. Rh factor is a type of protein that is sometimes present on red blood cells. You are Rh-positive if you have the protein and Rh-negative if you don't. Your Rh factor is inherited from your parents and is determined by your genes. If your blood is Rh-positive and your partner's blood is Rh-negative, there is a chance that your baby may inherit Rh-negative genes. When your Rh factor is not compatible with that of your fetus, your immune system will respond by producing antibodies that recognize your baby as a foreign substance in your body. The blood of your first Rh-positive baby will trigger the antibodies. When you become pregnant with a second Rh-negative baby, these antibodies will attack and destroy the fetus's red blood cells, resulting in fatal fetal anemia. To prevent your immune system from producing antibodies, you will be given an injection of Rh immunoglobulin that will destroy the Rh-positive cells in your body. When detected through proper prenatal care, this life-threatening condition is now very rare.

GESTATIONAL DIABETES

Your body normally produces a hormone called insulin that controls the levels of blood sugar or glucose in your blood. If you have diabetes, your body does not produce enough insulin or does not use insulin effectively. During pregnancy, a small number of women develop gestational diabetes, even though they did not have diabetes before they became pregnant. This condition is thought to be caused by elevated hormone levels that produce metabolic changes during pregnancy.

In most cases, gestational diabetes does not cause symptoms and is not a health risk for you. It does, however, create health risks for your baby. If this condition is not treated, your baby is at greater risk of being stillborn or of dying as a newborn. Gestational diabetes also can cause your fetus to have an excessive birth weight. When your baby is very large, you have an increased likelihood of cesarean birth or birth injuries. Babies born to mothers with diabetes are also quite prone to hypoglycemia, or low blood sugar.

The symptoms of gestational diabetes are not very obvious, so the condition must be detected by a glucose tolerance test. It usually develops in the second half of your pregnancy. You may be predisposed to this condition if you are obese, are over 30 years old or have a family history of diabetes. However, nearly half of the women with gestational diabetes have no risk factors at all. To manage this type of diabetes during your pregnancy, you should follow a diet planned for you by a registered dietitian, exercise regularly and have your blood-glucose level tested often. If your condition is severe, you may need insulin injections to control your blood-sugar levels; pregnant women who take daily insulin are three to four times more likely to have a baby with major birth defects.

Gestational diabetes usually disappears immediately after pregnancy, but you are at increased risk of encountering it again in another pregnancy. You are also more prone to developing diabetes in later life. Fortunately, there is no increased risk that your baby will develop diabetes, despite the fact that you had diabetes during pregnancy.

PREECLAMPSIA

Swelling of your ankles and toes is very common and quite normal in pregnancy. This condition is called edema and it indicates that your body is retaining water. But other types of swelling during pregnancy are real causes of concern. Swelling of your face and hands may be a warning sign of preeclampsia.

Preeclampsia is also known as toxemia, and it is a disease characterized by high blood pressure, fluid retention and protein in your urine. It develops in the second half of pregnancy and, if left untreated, can endanger both your life and the life of your baby. Preeclampsia affects nearly 8 percent of all pregnancies and is especially common during first pregnancies. It frequently develops in pregnant teenagers and older women. The exact cause of preeclampsia is not yet known and there is no cure for the condition. It seriously restricts blood flow to the placenta, which may reduce the oxygen and nutrient supply to your fetus. This will retard your baby's growth and cause fetal distress. It can also cause problems for your health by damaging your liver or kidneys, or by causing seizures and bleeding problems.

The first sign of preeclampsia is usually a sudden weight gain of more than 1 kilogram (2 pounds) in a week. This is due to fluid retention, not fat accumulation. You may also develop swelling in your hands and face, headaches and vision problems. The routine blood pressure tests that your doctor performs every month are the best way of detecting this condition in the early stages. A diagnosis of preeclampsia is confirmed if your blood pressure is elevated beyond the normal range or if a urine test indicates the presence of large amounts of protein.

There is no real cure for preeclampsia. In mild cases, your doctor may suggest bed rest. By lying on your side, you will enable blood to flow more freely to the placenta, increasing the nourishment to your fetus. Regular blood pressure, urine and blood tests will be necessary to check on the health of your baby. In more severe cases, you will be hospitalized. Because preeclampsia compromises your baby's supply of nutrients and oxygen, it may be necessary to consider an early delivery. Even though the baby may be at risk because of a premature delivery, the dangerous conditions inside your uterus may create an even greater health risk. A discussion with your doctor will help you make an informed decision regarding the risks and benefits of an early birth. Once the baby is born, your blood pressure usually returns to normal. The condition may recur in later pregnancies, especially if you had a fairly severe case of preeclampsia.

BIRTH DEFECTS

About 3 to 5 percent of all babies are born with birth defects. Statistics indicate that birth defects account for the largest percentage of all infant deaths in North America. Many birth defects are not preventable, because the cause of them is unknown.

Researchers do know, however, that most birth defects occur in the first three months of pregnancy, often before a woman even knows she is pregnant. It is becoming increasingly evident that your state of health at the time of conception is one of the most important factors in protecting your baby from preventable malformations.

Neural Tube Defects

Neural tube defects are congenital malformations that occur during fetal life. They are caused by failure of the neural tube—that eventually forms the body's central nervous system—to close. Neural tube defects are one of the most common congenital malformations seen among live-born infants in North America. The most common neural tube defects are spina bifida and anencephaly.

It's been estimated that approximately 2500 U.S. babies a year are born with neural tube defects, half of whom will have spina bifida, a neural tube defect that prevents the vertebrae of your baby's spine from closing completely. In severe cases, the spinal cord protrudes outside of your baby's body, limiting mobility and causing other neurological dysfunctions. Spina bifida can be surgically corrected, but surgical repair of the lesion is not always associated with improvement in motor function. Children with spina bifida often have long-term problems that require management by a healthcare team.

FOLATE

One nutrient known to prevent birth defects is folate. Folic acid is the synthetic form of folate, the B vitamin necessary for cell division. Making sure you are getting plenty of folate in your diet and taking a folic acid supplement will reduce your chance of having a child with abnormalities of the spine and brain, such as spina bifida.

Folate is needed both before and during the first few weeks of pregnancy to help prevent birth defects. Neural tube defects can occur in a fetus before a woman even realizes she's pregnant. That's why it is so important for all women of childbearing age to pay attention to their folate intake. When you become pregnant, your folate requirements increase from 400 micrograms per day to *600 micrograms*.

See the Folate in Foods table on page 7 in chapter 1 for food sources of folate. Getting your daily 600 micrograms of folic acid from foods is a challenge, even for the healthiest of eaters (unless you're a fan of chicken liver!). It's also known that the synthetic folic acid used in supplements and fortified foods is better absorbed by the body than the B vitamin in foods. For these reasons you are strongly advised to take a folic acid supplement before and during your pregnancy. I recommend that you start taking a prenatal vitamin supplement that offers 400 to 1000 micrograms of folic acid while you are trying to get pregnant and during your pregnancy—most prenatal formulas offer 1000 micrograms of folic acid.

If you take a separate folic acid supplement, be sure to buy one that has vitamin B12 added. High doses of folic acid taken over a period of time can hide a B12 deficiency and result in progressive nerve damage. The upper limit for folic acid intake from a supplement is 1000 micrograms (1 milligram) per day.

Other Causes of Birth Defects

One vitamin you don't want to get too much of during your pregnancy is vitamin A. In fact, if you take a vitamin supplement, make sure it contains no more than 5000 international units (IU) of vitamin A. Most prenatal formulas provide 2500 IU of the vitamin. High intakes of supplemental vitamin A (more than 10,000 IU) are associated with birth defects. You may have read that the nutrient beta-carotene is converted to vitamin A in the body. This is true, but it is not transformed to vitamin A efficiently enough to cause toxicity; don't worry about your beta-carotene intake.

Infectious diseases, such as rubella (German measles) and syphilis can also cause birth defects. Syphilis should be treated with an antibiotic before you become pregnant because it can cause bone and tooth deformities. If you have not had rubella, you should be vaccinated against the disease before you become pregnant. Because the vaccine can also pose problems for a developing fetus, you should wait three months after vaccination before becoming pregnant. A rubella infection in early pregnancy will cause abnormalities in the heart, eyes and ears of your fetus.

MEDICATIONS

Few clinical drug trials involve pregnant women, so the effects of most medications and drugs are still unknown. The same goes for herbal supplements. For this reason, it is sensible for you to avoid all medications throughout your pregnancy, unless prescribed by your doctor. If medications are necessary to manage a health risk, you should always ask for the lowest possible dosage, in order to minimize the impact on your baby. If you have a pre-existing medical condition, such as high blood pressure, diabetes or lupus, you should not discontinue your medication. However, there may be safer drugs that you can take during your pregnancy. Discuss your concerns with your doctor, so that you can weigh the risks and benefits of changing your medication and make an informed decision.

Most medications, even over-the-counter drugs, are particularly dangerous for your fetus during the first trimester. This is the time when vital organs and systems are developing and medications can interfere with normal growth patterns, causing serious health risks and birth defects.

❧

Nutrition Guidelines for a Healthy Pregnancy

Now it's time to look at the whole picture: what and how much you need to eat and what foods and beverages you should avoid during your pregnancy. Let's start by reviewing your nutrient requirements during this exciting time.

Recommended Dietary Allowance (RDA) for Key Nutrients during Pregnancy (Adults and Teens)

NUTRIENT	RDA: NOT PREGNANT	RDA: PREGNANT
Calories	2200 calories/day	1st Trimester: add 100 calories/day 2nd and 3rd Trimesters: add 300 calories/day
Protein	42–45 grams/day	1st Trimester: add 5 grams/day 2nd Trimester: add 20 grams/day 3rd Trimester: add 24 grams/day
Calcium	1000 milligrams/day	Adults: 1000 milligrams/day Teens: 1300 milligrams/day
Vitamin D	200 IU (5 mcg)/day	200 IU (5 mcg)/day
Iron	18 milligrams/day	27 milligrams/day (for entire pregnancy)
Zinc	8 milligrams/day	Adults: 11 milligrams/day Teens: 13 milligrams/day
Folate	400 micrograms/day	600 micrograms/day

A FOOD PLAN FOR PREGNANCY

With a few exceptions—e.g., folate and iron—for which supplements are needed, here's how your nutrient requirements translate into food choices in the following diet. Both pregnant women and teens can use this guide.

FOOD GROUP	FOOD CHOICES	RECOMMENDED DAILY SERVINGS
Grain Foods		5 to 12
(carbohydrates, iron,	Whole-grain bread, 1 slice	
fiber; choose	Bagel, large, 1/4	
whole-grain as	Roll, large, 1/2	
often as possible)	Pita pocket, 1/2	
	Tortilla, 6"	
	Cereal, cold, 3/4 cup (175 ml)	
	Cereal, 100% bran, 1/2 cup (125 ml)	
	Cereal, hot, 1/2 cup (125 ml)	
	Crackers, soda, 6	
	Corn, 1/2 cup (125 ml)	
	Popcorn, plain, 3 cups (750 ml)	
	Grains, cooked, 1/2 cup (125 ml)	
	Pasta, cooked, 1/2 cup (125 ml)	
	Rice, cooked, 1/3 cup (80 ml)	
Vegetables & Fruits		5 to 10
(carbohydrates, fiber,	Vegetables, cooked/raw, 1/2 cup (125 ml)	
vitamins, minerals)	Vegetables, leafy green, 1 cup (250 ml)	
	Fruit, whole, 1 piece	
	Fruit, small (plums, apricots), 4	
	Fruit, cut up, 1 cup (250 ml)	
	Berries, 1 cup (250 ml)	
	Juice, unsweetened, 1/2 to 3/4 cup (125–75 ml)	

Milk & Milk Alternatives		3 to 4
(8 grams protein	Milk, 1 cup (250 ml)	
per serving;	Yogurt, 3/4 cup (175 ml)	
protein, carbohydrates,	Cheese, 1.5 oz (45 g)	
calcium, vitamin D,	Rice beverage, fortified, 1 cup (250 ml)	
vitamin A, zinc)	Soy beverage, fortified, 1 cup (250 ml)	

Meat & Alternatives		6 to 9
(7 grams protein	Fish, lean meat, poultry, 1 oz (30 g)	
per serving;	Egg, whole, 1	
protein, iron, zinc)	Egg whites, 2	
	Legumes (beans, chickpeas, lentils), 1/3 cup (80 ml)	
	Soy nuts, 2 tbsp (30 ml)	
	Tempeh, 1/4 cup (60 ml)	
	Tofu, firm, 1/3 cup (80 ml)	
	Texturized vegetable protein (TVP), 1/3 cup (80 ml)	
	Veggie dog, small, 1	

Fats & Oils*		4 to 6
(essential fatty acids,	Butter, margarine, mayonnaise, 1 tsp (5 ml)	
vitamin E)	Nuts/seeds, 1 tbsp (15 ml)	
	Peanut and nut butters, 1.5 tsp (7 ml)	
	Salad dressing, 2 tsp (10 ml)	
	Vegetable oil, 1 tsp (5 ml)	

Water/Fluid	8 to 12
Water, 1 cup (250 ml)	
Herbal tea**, 1 cup (250 ml)	

All serving sizes are based on measures after cooking.

*To include sources of essential fatty acids choose canola oil, walnut oil, flaxseed oil and nuts and seeds more often as your fat servings.

** Avoid herbal teas listed on page 285.

FOODS TO EAT MORE OF

Omega-3 Fats

As you may already know, fish is an excellent source of a special type of fat called omega-3. Researchers are learning that omega-3 fats may keep us healthy in many ways. Studies suggest that a special omega-3 fat in fish, called docosahexaenoic acid (DHA), may aid in proper brain development during fetal life. Some researchers even hypothesize that a lack of omega-3 fats during your pregnancy can result in learning and behavioral disorders later in a child's life.

Mothers and their growing babies can get DHA in two ways: by eating fish, especially oily varieties like salmon, trout, sardines, herring and mackerel; or by consuming other types of omega-3 fats that the body uses to make DHA.

If you don't like fish, make sure you include the following foods in your diet: canola oil, walnuts and walnut oil, flaxseed and flaxseed oil, Omega-3 eggs, soybeans, tofu and leafy green vegetables. These foods all contain an omega-3 fat called alpha-linolenic acid (ALA) that is essential to the body. Our bodies can't produce ALA and so it must be supplied from food. Once we consume ALA, a small amount is converted into other omega-3 fats, including DHA. Because this essential fat must be part of the diet, your developing baby depends on your intake of both ALA and DHA in fish.

Folate-Rich Foods

I have already emphasized the importance of meeting your folate requirements to prevent a neural tube defect in your newborn. But this issue is so important I want to mention it again. In addition to getting supplemental folic acid from your prenatal multivitamin or a separate folic acid supplement, aim to include at least two good sources of folate in your daily diet. Eat fruits, dark green leafy vegetables, dried peas, beans and lentils, avocado, asparagus and orange juice. Refer to the list on page 4 in chapter 1 to see the best ways to get this important B vitamin in your diet.

FOODS, BEVERAGES AND HERBS TO AVOID

Foods

Some foods have a greater potential for causing food poisoning, and some types of food poisoning are of particular concern during pregnancy. To minimize your risk of food-borne illness, be extra careful to practice safe food handling during your pregnancy. Here's a list of foods to avoid:

TYPE OF FOOD POISONING	RISKY FOODS
Listeriosis can cause miscarriage during the first three months of pregnancy and illness or stillbirth later in pregnancy.	Unpasteurized or raw milk
	Certain soft cheeses
	Some feta cheeses
	Brie, Camembert, blue cheese
	Meat pâtés, processed meats, raw meat and poultry
	Unwashed produce
E. coli infection can cross the placenta and infect your growing baby.	Undercooked beef products
	Unpasteurized milk
	Contaminated water and mayonnaise
	Improperly processed cider

Beverages

COFFEE

The evidence for coffee's ill effect on pregnancy remains unclear at this time. A recent study found that drinking six or more cups of coffee per day was linked to miscarriage.

An analysis of many studies concluded that drinking one to two cups of coffee each day is associated with a very small increase in the risk of both miscarriage and infants with low birth weight. Despite these findings, some studies have found no harmful effects on pregnancy of consuming up to 300 milligrams of caffeine per day (about 2 cups of coffee). To play it safe, I recommend that women avoid coffee during pregnancy and minimize their intake of caffeine from other sources such as colas, tea and dark chocolate.

Caffeine is a stimulant and can cause irritability, nervousness and insomnia. Not only does it cross the placenta and reach the fetus, it also acts as a diuretic, dehydrating your body of valuable fluid. Make the switch to decaf or try herbal teas that are safe to use during pregnancy (see below).

ALCOHOLIC BEVERAGES

There is no question in my mind that use of alcohol should be avoided during pregnancy. Alcohol can cross the placenta and, in the case of heavy drinking (at least four drinks per day), it can cause fetal alcohol syndrome in newborns. Babies born with fetal alcohol syndrome have lower birth weights, smaller heads, abnormal facial features, heart defects and mental retardation. Even occasional, moderate drinking might harm your baby. Fetal alcohol syndrome is seen in 30 to 40 percent of infants whose mothers drank at least 2 ounces of absolute alcohol per day during the first trimester. Mild forms of this disorder have also occurred when women drank 1 ounce of alcohol per day or indulged in binge drinking.

Herbs

At this time there is not enough scientific information about the use of herbal supplements during pregnancy. Very few studies have been done in pregnant women. As a result, most health experts do not recommend that you use herbal remedies during your pregnancy. There are some herbs, however, that are known to cause serious side effects during pregnancy and they should be avoided at all costs; also avoid teas made from these herbs. Herbs to avoid include pennyroyal, comfrey, lobelia, sassafras, barberry, devil's claw root, chamomile, dong quai, goldenseal, lily of the valley, rue, uva ursi, yarrow and coltsfoot. Safe herbal teas include blackberry, citrus peel, ginger, lemon balm, orange peel and rosehip.

16

Breastfeeding

Once again, this chapter is not formatted quite like the others. Because breastfeeding is not a medical condition that requires prevention or management, there is no Bottom Line.

Nature has designed breast milk as the perfect first food for your baby. It is nutritionally superior to all other forms of infant food and is ideally suited to the developmental needs of a newborn human. A growing body of research indicates that breast milk protects babies from illness, provides the basis for good brain growth and promotes early bonding between mother and child. Both the American Academy of Pediatrics and the Canadian Pediatric Society recommend exclusive breastfeeding for at least the first four months of your baby's life. In combination with complementary foods, breastfeeding can be successfully continued until your child is over two years old.

Essentially, your breasts are a network of milk-producing glands called alveoli, supported within an envelope of fibrous and fatty tissue. Each breast contains 15 to 20 glands, connected by milk ducts to your nipple. The alveoli do not mature until they are stimulated by the hormonal surge of estrogen and progesterone that occurs during pregnancy. As these hormone levels increase, small reservoirs of milk develop behind the nipples.

The actual process of breastfeeding or lactation is stimulated by the sucking action of your baby. Nerve endings in the pigmented tissue (areolae) that surrounds the nipple are triggered by the pressure of your baby's tongue. They instantly send a signal to the hypothalamus and pituitary glands in your brain to initiate the flow of milk. These glands release the hormone prolactin to stimulate milk production, and the hormone oxytocin to contract the muscle fibers around the milk glands, which forces the milk into the duct network. The combined action of these two hormones results in the let-down sensation that most women recognize as essential to successful breastfeeding.

Although the composition of breast milk may change as your baby develops, there are only three main types of breast milk:

1. *Colostrum* is produced in the first few days after birth and is released before normal lactation begins. It is the perfect food for newborns and is especially rich in nutrients and antibodies. Appearing as a thin, yellow fluid, colostrum has a very high calorie and protein content and it protects your baby against infection. Because colostrum is so beneficial for your baby, you should consider breastfeeding for the first few days after birth, even if you have decided to bottle feed your baby later.

2. *Foremilk* is a thinner type of milk that is released from your breast at the beginning of a feeding. It is normally lower in fat content and is intended to satisfy your baby's thirst and fluid needs.

3. *Hindmilk* follows foremilk during a feeding. It has a higher fat and calorie content and is important to your baby's growth and overall good health. To ensure that your newborn receives the nutritional benefits of both foremilk and hindmilk, encourage your baby to drain one breast completely before moving on to the other.

Almost every woman can breastfeed. The size and shape of your breasts and nipples do not affect your ability to produce an adequate milk supply for your baby. There are very few medical or environmental reasons why you should not breastfeed. Only if you are taking specific medications or have a serious illness, such as HIV infection, AIDS, tuberculosis, hepatitis or kidney or heart problems, or if your baby has certain medical conditions, would you be advised not to breastfeed.

~

Breast versus Bottle

INFANT BENEFITS OF BREASTFEEDING

Breastfeeding is not the most popular choice among American women. In 1998, only 29 percent of all mothers breastfed at six months postpartum.[1] The Surgeon General's Goal for Healthy People 2010 is that 75 percent of women be breastfeeding at hospital discharge and 50 percent six months thereafter.

When you choose to breastfeed, you are giving your child a significant nutritional advantage from the very first days of life. Human milk contains exactly the right amount of fatty acids, water, lactose (sugar) and amino acids to promote healthy growth, digestion and brain development. The high lactose content of breast milk provides a readily available energy source that is easily digested by your infant. Breast milk also contains vitamin E, a powerful antioxidant that helps to prevent anemia. With a high calcium-to-phosphorous ratio, breast milk will prevent calcium deficiency and will change the pH of your baby's intestinal flora to protect against bacterial diarrheas. In addition to these nutritional benefits, some studies indicate that breastfed babies have a higher intelligence level and are less likely to be overweight in later life. Because breastfed babies tend to consume only as much milk as they need to satisfy their hunger, they are rarely overfed or underfed.

When you breastfeed, you are also choosing to protect your baby against many common illnesses. Approximately 80 percent of the cells in breast milk are macrophages, cells that kill bacteria, fungi and viruses. Breast milk provides antibodies that will give your baby varying degrees of protection against illnesses such as ear infections, pneumonia, bronchitis, diabetes mellitus, German measles and staphylococcal infections. Breastfeeding may also offer a protective effect against Sudden Infant Death Syndrome (SIDS), allergic diseases, and some chronic digestive diseases.

Although breast milk contains more than 100 ingredients that are not found in infant formula, your baby will never develop an allergy to your milk. Occasionally, you may eat something that affects your milk and your baby may react to that particular food. However, if you eliminate that food from your diet, the problem should disappear. Milk that comes directly from your breast is sterile, eliminating the dangers of bacteria in bottles or in water that has not been properly sterilized. As an additional benefit, the exercise of sucking at the breast will strengthen your baby's jaws, promoting good jaw development and straight, healthy teeth.

MATERNAL BENEFITS OF BREASTFEEDING

The benefits of breastfeeding are not limited to your baby. As a mother, you'll find that breastfeeding has many practical advantages. For one thing, it forces you to sit down, rest and relax for a short time every few hours, which helps to restore your energy levels. It's convenient and economical—no bottles to sterilize or formula to buy. The process of lactation helps to stimulate your uterus to contract back to normal size and reduces postpartum bleeding. It may even help you return to pre-pregnancy weight faster by using up extra calories each day. Lactating women also seem to have improved bone remineralization after pregnancy and a decreased risk of ovarian and breast cancer.

Although not always very reliable, breastfeeding is considered to be nature's contraceptive. It suppresses ovulation, reducing your chances of ovulating, menstruating and getting pregnant. However, it is recommended that you use another form of contraceptive while breastfeeding if you want to space out your pregnancies.

DRAWBACKS OF BREASTFEEDING

Despite its many advantages, breastfeeding does have some drawbacks. At times, it can be inconvenient and often requires a complete change in lifestyle, affecting everything from the clothing you wear to the places you go. You are very closely tied to your baby while breastfeeding and, in some cases, your partner may not always be supportive of your decision.

You can overcome some of the inconvenience of breastfeeding by occasionally expressing and storing your breast milk. This will give you the freedom to leave your infant with a babysitter and will allow your partner to share in the feeding routines. Bottles and nipples for storing breast milk should be sterilized and the expressed milk should be refrigerated immediately. It can be stored for up to 48 hours in the fridge or frozen for up to three months. Do not thaw or warm breast milk on the stove or in the microwave, as excessive heat can destroy vital nutrients.

In the early weeks, breastfeeding can be painful. Until your body adjusts to the new demands, your nipples may become cracked and sore and your breasts may become swollen and hard. A warm shower and manual expression of a small amount of excess milk may help to relieve the discomfort of this engorgement. There is also a possibility that you may develop clogged milk ducts, which can lead to a painful infection called mastitis. Most breastfeeding problems can be solved quite easily, although some do require medical attention.

When you decide to stop breastfeeding, or if you choose not to breastfeed at all, your breasts will eventually stop producing milk. Until this happens, though, your breasts may become swollen and painful. A well-fitted bra and ice packs or pain relievers may help ease your discomfort until your milk dries up completely.

PROS AND CONS OF BOTTLE FEEDING

If you are considering an alternative to breastfeeding, or would like to combine breast and bottle feeding, the American Academy of Pediatrics recommends that you use commercial, iron-fortified formulas until your baby is 12 months old. Whole cow's milk may be introduced at that time, but skim milk and partly skimmed milk—1 percent and 2 percent milk fat—are not recommended for the first two years. Soy, rice or other vegetarian beverages are incomplete sources of nutrition and are also not recommended for the first two years. However, you may use soy-based formulas if your child can't have dairy-based products for reasons of health, culture or religion.

Most women choose bottle feeding over breastfeeding because it is convenient and allows for more personal freedom. Your partner can easily share in the feeding responsibilities, and you may feel more comfortable feeding your baby in public with a bottle. When bottle feeding, you should always take care that all bottles and nipples are carefully cleaned and that infant formulas are stored properly.

One of the biggest disadvantages of bottle feeding is the potential for overfeeding. Because there is a predetermined amount of formula in each bottle, you may be tempted to feed your baby more than he or she needs. To avoid this, you should not encourage your child to finish every bottle. Instead, allow your baby to take only as much formula as he or she needs to satisfy hunger. You can offer your baby water between feedings, but try to limit other fluids, such as fruit juice, so that you don't interfere with your baby's intake of nutrient-rich formula.

⁊

Tips for Breastfeeding Success

A recent national survey indicated that over 50 percent of women stop breastfeeding before the recommended six-month minimum time period.[2] The most common reasons given for stopping are inconvenience or a perceived lack of milk supply. Although breastfeeding usually comes naturally to both mother and child, these tips may help you prevent some of the common problems that often contribute to an early decision to stop breastfeeding.

- *Start early* Begin within an hour of delivery, if possible, when your baby's sucking instinct is quite strong.

- *Nurse on demand* Frequent nursing will stimulate your breasts to produce a good milk supply. Crying is considered a late indicator of hunger.

- *No supplements* The more often your baby feeds at your breast, the more milk you will produce. Breast milk satisfies both hunger and thirst, so extra fluids are not usually needed. Don't offer water or formula supplements that might interfere with your baby's appetite.

- *No artificial nipples* The sucking action needed for pacifiers is different from the sucking action of breastfeeding. Don't confuse your baby while he or she is learning to feed. Delay giving a nipple substitute for several weeks.

- *Eat and rest well* To produce enough milk you need to eat a balanced diet, including at least 500 extra calories and 8 to 12 cups (2 to 3 liters) of fluid a day. Rest often to prevent infections, which are aggravated by fatigue.

- *Proper position* To avoid sore nipples, your baby should be encouraged to open the mouth wide and to take your nipple far back into the mouth.

- *Air dry nipples* Until your nipples become accustomed to the sucking action, air dry them or gently blow them dry with a hair dryer after feedings.

- *Natural healing* If your nipples do dry out and crack, coat them with breast milk or natural moisturizers to help healing. Vitamin E or lanolin may also be used to protect your nipples, although your baby may react to these substances.

- *Watch for infection* The signs of infection include fever, breast redness and painful lumps. Make sure you get appropriate medical attention.

჻

Nourishing Your Newborn

Most breastfeeding mothers worry, at one time or another, whether breast milk is really providing their babies with enough nourishment. It's reassuring to know that infants lose as much as 7 percent of their birth weight during the first week of life.

Normally, your baby will start to gain weight within a few days and should regain all of his or her birth weight within ten days. During the first three months of life, your infant will gain approximately 1 kilogram (2 pounds) per month, or an ounce a day. In the third to sixth month, he or she will gain slightly less—about 1/2 ounce each month—and, ideally, your baby should have doubled his or her birth weight by the age of four months.

Healthy newborns should be fed approximately 8 to 12 times every 24 hours, usually spending 10 to 15 minutes on each breast. In the first few weeks after birth, it is not recommended for your baby to go longer than four hours without a feeding.

One of the easiest ways to determine whether your baby is feeding well is to check the number of wet diapers he or she is producing. A normal newborn wets six to eight diapers a day and has two to three bowel movements. A healthy baby should be content after most feedings, and have a vigorous cry, firm skin and a good sucking reflex. While all of these signs indicate successful breastfeeding, it is highly recommended that you and your baby visit a doctor within two to four days of birth for a thorough evaluation. Your doctor will check your baby's growth, monitor his or her fluid intake and ensure that his or her digestive system is working properly. Breastfeeding malnutrition or dehydration is a potentially serious condition that can be easily identified through a routine medical examination.

STRATEGIES FOR BREASTFEEDING

The quality and quantity of breast milk that you produce is primarily dependent on your calorie and fluid intake. Even if your diet is not perfect, you should still be able to produce good quality milk for your baby. Your body adapts to the nutritional demands of your child by drawing on nutrients already in your system. For example, you may actually lose bone mass during breastfeeding because your body will acquire calcium by pulling it out of your bones into your bloodstream. Fortunately, this is a temporary condition and, once you stop breastfeeding or begin to menstruate, your bone mass will start to gradually return to normal.

In order to stay healthy while caring for your baby, you should always eat a balanced diet. To replace the calories lost through breastfeeding, it is necessary to add an extra 500 calories to your daily intake. This should include an extra 20 grams of protein and 100 micrograms of additional folate. The chart below outlines your extra nutrient requirements for breastfeeding and how to meet these needs from your diet.

Recommended Dietary Allowance (RDA) for Key Nutrients during Breastfeeding (Adults and Teens)

NUTRIENT	NOT BREASTFEEDING	BREASTFEEDING
Calories	2200 calories/day	2700 calories/day Do not eat less than 1800 calories/day You may need extra calories if you are • a breastfeeding teenager • a woman breastfeeding more than one infant • underweight or did not gain inadequate weight during your pregnancy • a woman breastfeeding while pregnant
Protein	42–45 grams/day	65 grams/day during first 6 months 62 grams/day during second 6 months If you are breastfeeding more than one baby, you may need extra protein.
Calcium	1000 milligrams/day	Adults: 1000 milligrams/day Teens: 1300 milligrams/day
Vitamin D	200 IU (5 mcg)/day	200 IU (5 mcg)/day
Iron	18 milligrams/day	Adults: 9 milligrams/day Teens: 10 milligrams/day
Zinc	8 milligrams/day	Adults: 12 milligrams/day Teens: 14 milligrams/day
Folate	400 micrograms/day	500 micrograms/day

A FOOD PLAN FOR BREASTFEEDING

Here's how your nutrient requirements translate into food choices. Both breastfeeding women and breastfeeding teens can use this guide.

FOOD GROUP	FOOD CHOICES	RECOMMENDED DAILY SERVINGS
Grain Foods		5 to 12
(carbohydrates, iron, fiber;	Whole-grain bread, 1 slice	
choose whole-grain	Bagel, large, 1/4	
as often as possible)	Roll, large, 1/2	
	Pita pocket, 1/2	
	Tortilla, 6"	
	Cereal, cold, 3/4 cup (175 ml)	
	Cereal, 100% bran, 1/2 cup (125 ml)	
	Cereal, hot, 1/2 cup (125 ml)	
	Crackers, soda, 6	
	Corn, 1/2 cup (125 ml)	
	Popcorn, plain, 3 cups (750 ml)	
	Grains, cooked, 1/2 cup (125 ml)	
	Pasta, cooked, 1/2 cup (125 ml)	
	Rice, cooked, 1/3 cup (80 ml)	
Vegetables & Fruits		5 to 10
(carbohydrates, fiber,	Vegetables, cooked/raw, 1/2 cup (125 ml)	
vitamins, minerals)	Vegetables, leafy green, 1 cup (250 ml)	
	Fruit, whole, 1 piece	
	Fruit, small (plums, apricots), 4	
	Fruit, cut up, 1 cup (250 ml)	
	Berries, 1 cup (250 ml)	
	Juice, unsweetened, 1/2 to 3/4 cup (125–175 ml)	

Milk & Milk Alternatives		3 to 4
(8 grams protein	Milk, 1 cup (250 ml)	
per serving; protein,	Yogurt, 3/4 cup (175 ml)	
carbohydrates,	Cheese, 1.5 oz (45 g)	
calcium, vitamin D,	Rice beverage, fortified, 1 cup (250 ml)	
vitamin A, zinc)	Soy beverage, fortified, 1 cup (250 ml)	

Meat & Alternatives		6 to 9
(7 grams protein	Fish, lean meat, poultry, 1 oz (30 g)	
per serving; protein,	Egg, whole, 1	
iron, zinc)	Egg whites, 2	
	Legumes (beans, chickpeas, lentils), 1/3 cup (80 ml)	
	Soy nuts, 2 tbsp (30 ml)	
	Tempeh, 1/4 cup (60 ml)	
	Tofu, firm, 1/3 cup (75 ml)	
	Texturized vegetable protein (TVP), 1/3 cup (75 ml)	
	Veggie dog, small, 1	

Fats & Oils*		4 to 6
(essential fatty acids,	Butter, margarine, mayonnaise, 1 tsp (5 ml)	
vitamin E)	Nuts/seeds, 1 tbsp (15 ml)	
	Peanut and nut butters, 1.5 tsp (7 ml)	
	Salad dressing, 2 tsp (10 ml)	
	Vegetable oil, 1 tsp (5 ml)	

Water/Fluid		8 to 12
	Water, 1 cup (250 ml)	

All serving sizes are based on measures after cooking.

*More often, include sources of essential fatty acids for optimal brain health of your baby. Choose canola oil, walnut oil, flaxseed oil and nuts and seeds more often as your fat servings. Other good sources are soybeans, tofu and leafy green vegetables.

Foods to Avoid
SPICY FOODS
You may find that certain foods in your diet make your newborn irritable. Foods with a strong or spicy flavor (such as garlic or curry) may alter the flavor of your breast milk, and a sudden change in the taste of your milk may annoy your baby. Some of my clients report that gassy vegetables such as onions, broccoli and cauliflower cause their babies to be fussy during breastfeeding. If you suspect a certain food is causing your infant discomfort, try a dietary challenge: eliminate the food from your diet for three days to see if your baby's reaction subsides, then return the food to your diet and again monitor your infant's reaction. You may have to eliminate certain foods for a period of time. Depending on how long you decide to breastfeed, you may be able to reintroduce this food in your diet without causing upset to your baby.

CAFFEINE
I recommend that you avoid consuming large amounts of caffeine while breastfeeding. Most women can have one or two cups of coffee (up to 350 milligrams of caffeine) without affecting their babies. Amounts greater than this can stimulate your baby, causing irritability and wakefulness. Large doses of caffeine may also interfere with the availability of iron from breast milk and impair your infant's iron stores. Take a moment to review all sources of caffeine in your diet—coffee, tea, iced tea, soft drinks, chocolate and some over-the-counter medications. You'll find a comprehensive list of foods and their caffeine content on page 38 in chapter 1.

ALCOHOL
Alcohol easily enters breast milk. One study found that the alcohol concentration of breast milk peaks within one hour after having a drink. What's more, even small amounts of alcohol—for example, one bottle of beer—may reduce your baby's intake of breast milk. Alcohol may change the flavor of your milk, making it unacceptable to the infant. Because infants metabolize alcohol differently, it may suppress their feeding behavior. And drinking alcohol may even reduce the amount of breast milk you produce.

Despite the claim that a little alcohol facilitates the let-down reflex and allows women to breastfeed more easily, there is no scientific evidence to support this. If you don't want to give up the occasional glass of wine or cocktail, there's no need to worry. A drink once in a while does not appear to affect your ability to produce breast milk, nor does it impair your baby's development. If you have several drinks, however, you should postpone breastfeeding for at least an hour for every drink you consume.

VITAMIN SUPPLEMENTS

If you eat a well-balanced healthy diet, there is little need to take a supplement to meet your nutrient needs for breastfeeding. However, there are circumstances when it might be a good idea:

- You find it difficult to make healthy food choices.
- You are a complete vegetarian (vegan) and you don't use vitamin B12-fortified foods like soy and rice beverages.
- You're concerned about meeting your iron needs because you eat very little red meat and don't choose whole grains very often.
- You avoid dairy products and don't choose calcium-fortified products such as soy and rice beverages or orange juice.
- You're at risk for vitamin D deficiency because you spend very little time in the sun and you don't drink milk or fortified soy/rice milk.

A good quality multivitamin and mineral supplement will help you meet your nutrient needs, with the exception of calcium, during and after breastfeeding. If you are lacking calcium in your diet, I recommend that you take calcium supplements. For every serving of milk or milk alternative you don't get—aim for three a day—take a 300-milligram calcium citrate supplement with vitamin D added. Do not take high-dose single supplements of other nutrients while breastfeeding. Make an effort to choose nutritious, wholesome foods every day.

Weaning to Solids

Nutritionally, your baby will not need solid foods before the age of four to six months. By then, your infant will have established the tongue and mouth movements necessary for swallowing solid foods and will be developmentally ready to try new tastes, textures and methods of feeding. A gradual weaning over weeks or months is the easiest way to introduce solid food. You can begin by replacing one breastfeeding a day with unsweetened fruit juice or formula, offering it in a cup or a bottle. By the time your baby is one year old, he or she should be eating a variety of different foods from the Food Guide Pyramid.

Iron-Fortified Foods

You should be aware that infants are quite susceptible to developing iron-deficiency anemia. For the first four to six months of life, your healthy baby will be protected against iron deficiency by elevated levels of hemoglobin in red blood cells, which will store up to 75 percent of his or her total iron requirements. As growth takes place, those resources will be depleted and you will need to add more iron to your baby's diet.

As I mentioned earlier, an iron-fortified infant formula is recommended for bottle-fed babies because cow's milk does not supply enough iron for your baby's needs. Unfortunately, breast milk doesn't supply enough iron either—it contains only between 0.3 and 0.5 milligrams of iron per liter. To prevent an iron deficiency, the American Academy of Pediatrics recommends a single grain, iron-fortified cereal, such as rice, as your baby's first solid food. This should be introduced at four to six months of age.

When you decide to introduce solid food to your infant, you should offer only one new food at a time. That way, if your baby has an allergic reaction or digestive difficulties, you will know which food caused the problem. To prevent food sensitivities, you should avoid giving your baby cow's milk, wheat, shellfish, egg whites and chocolate until he or she is at least one year old.

Dietary Fat

An infant's calorie and nutrient requirements are higher than those for any other age group. If you restrict the fat in your infant's diet, it may lead to an inadequate energy intake, a deficiency of essential fatty acids and failure to thrive. For this reason, dietary fat should not be restricted in children under the age of two years.

Honey

Do not feed your baby honey or foods that contain honey until he or she is one year of age. This sweetener may contain microbial spores that cause botulism. In infants, but not older children and adults, these spores can germinate in the intestine and produce a toxin which is then absorbed. Symptoms of infant botulism include poor feeding, constipation, loss of tension in the muscles, weakness and difficulty breathing. Spores that cause botulism have also been found in corn syrup; however, no case of infant botulism has ever been linked to corn syrup.

Vitamin D Supplements

The only supplement a breastfed infant may require is vitamin D. This is the case only if your baby is restricted in his or her exposure to sunlight, since ultraviolet rays from the sun cause vitamin D to be produced in the skin. As this may well be the case from November through March in much of northern United States, your pediatrician may recommend a vitamin D supplement for infants from birth to 12 months old. After one year of age, your baby should be consuming food with vitamin D—egg yolks, cow's milk, fish—and supplements may no longer be needed. Ask your pharmacist to recommend a vitamin D supplement for your infant.

Fluoride Supplements

Dental cavities are not a big issue in America, due mainly to the addition of fluoride to our drinking water. What seems to be becoming a problem instead is something called dental fluorosis, a cosmetic condition that shows up on the teeth as white specks, brown-gray stains or pitting. This is the result of increased availability of fluoride in drinking water, foods prepared with fluoridated water, toothpaste, mouthwashes, multivitamin and mineral supplements and so on.

For this reason fluoride supplements are not recommended from birth as they once were. If you live in an area that has little or no fluoride in the water, a supplemental dose of 250 micrograms is recommended from six months to three years of age.

Part 6

Hormonal Health

17

Premenstrual Syndrome (PMS)

Does your life feel out of control for one week out of every month? Does your mood swing from depression to anger at the drop of a hat? Do you feel emotional, tearful and anxious? Do your insatiable cravings for junk food only aggravate the suddenly too-tight fit of your clothes? If you answered yes to one or more of these questions, then you're only too aware that these are symptoms of premenstrual syndrome (PMS). If you suffer from PMS, you're not alone. Countless women all over the world struggle to cope with symptoms like these each day. It's estimated that PMS affects 30 to 40 percent of all women during their childbearing years.

Your Monthly Cycle

Counting the first day of your period as the beginning of your four-week menstrual cycle, the symptoms of PMS appear during the last two weeks. These two weeks are referred to as the luteal phase of your cycle. In fact, there are three distinct phases in each menstrual cycle: the follicular phase, ovulation and the luteal phase. Two areas of the brain, the hypothalamus and the pituitary gland, control all the hormonal changes that regulate each of these distinct stages.

The menstrual cycle begins with the follicular phase of your cycle, which lasts from the first day of your period until the time you ovulate. It begins when the hypothalamus produces gonadotropin-releasing hormones (GnRH). These hormones pass into the pituitary gland and trigger the release of luteinizing hormone (LH) and follicle-stimulating hormone (FSH). Working in combination, these two hormones promote the growth of follicles, tiny saclike structures located in your ovaries, each one surrounding an ovum, or egg. Throughout this time of growth, the follicles produce most of the female sex hormone, estrogen, which circulates in your body. Between 10 and 20 follicles will enlarge, but normally only one egg is released during ovulation.

Ovulation occurs in the middle of your cycle, near day 14. It's at this time that hormone surges trigger one follicle to burst and release its egg. Over the next 36 hours, the egg will travel through your fallopian tubes to reach the uterus.

After ovulation, your body enters the luteal phase. The outer wall of the burst follicle remains in your ovary and transforms into a mass of tissue called the corpus luteum. This tissue begins to secrete the other female sex hormone, progesterone, which prepares your uterus for pregnancy. If the egg is not fertilized and pregnancy doesn't occur, the levels of estrogen and progesterone immediately begin to drop. The lining of the uterus and the unfertilized egg are no longer needed and are eliminated from the body through menstruation. This completes the menstrual cycle and the entire process starts all over again.

What Causes PMS?

Researchers don't know exactly what triggers PMS, but several theories are under investigation. One of the most popular theories suggests that PMS is caused by an imbalance in the levels of estrogen and progesterone. Symptoms may develop because women have too much estrogen and not enough progesterone in their system during the last two weeks of the menstrual cycle. Estrogen affects the kidneys and causes sodium and water retention. Alterations in estrogen and progesterone can also affect the levels of natural brain chemicals called neurotransmitters. It's thought that deficiencies in serotonin and dopamine, two neurotransmitters that affect mood and emotion, may be responsible for the mood swings typical of PMS.

Low levels of progesterone may cause PMS in another way. When progesterone levels drop, so do levels of a related hormone called allopregnanolone. Studies have shown that a deficiency of this hormone may cause anxiety or depression. That's because allopregnanolone appears to influence a neurotransmitter called GABA (gamma-aminobutyric acid), which plays an important role in anxiety.

Excessive levels of a hormone called prolactin may be responsible for breast tenderness and swelling. Prolactin is responsible for stimulating the breast changes and milk production necessary for breastfeeding.

Nutrient deficiencies may also account for certain symptoms of PMS. For instance, breast tenderness may also be caused by a diet lacking in essential fats, which help regulate pain and inflammation. Recent studies have revealed that a deficiency of calcium can cause many PMS symptoms, including agitation, irritability and depression, by stimulating an overproduction of parathyroid hormones. These hormones are believed to influence mood and mental function by interacting with the brain chemical serotonin. PMS may also be related to dietary deficiencies of vitamin B6, magnesium and zinc, or the condition may be triggered by excessive consumption of caffeine, salt, alcohol and red meat.

Finally, it's possible that PMS is associated with medical conditions that have a nutritional component, such as hypoglycemia (low blood sugar) or hypothyroidism (low thyroid hormone level).

ᴈ

Symptoms

PMS is a collection of emotional, psychological and physical symptoms that develop during the 7 to 14 days before the start of your menstrual period. There are more than 150 documented symptoms with the most common being depression. PMS symptoms tend to fall into two main categories:

1. *Physical symptoms* include breast tenderness and swelling, bloating, fluid retention, weight gain, headaches, food cravings (especially for sweet or salty foods), acne, muscle pain, backaches, fatigue, dizziness, sleep disturbances, constipation or diarrhea. Many of these physical symptoms are caused by fluid retention, especially weight gain. In my private practice, women gain an average of 2 to 4

pounds during the premenstrual week. Heavier women may gain as much as 8 pounds. Fluid retention can also cause abdominal bloating. And if you experience constipation it will only add to the misery of bloating and weight gain.

2. *Emotional or psychological symptoms* include mood swings, depression, irritability, aggressiveness or hostility, anxiety, crying spells, changes in sex drive, difficulty concentrating and feelings of low self-esteem.

PMS symptoms vary from woman to woman and they can also be different from one menstrual cycle to the next. In PMS, symptoms get worse as your menstrual cycle progresses and are then relieved when your period begins. When you reach menopause, PMS normally disappears, although the symptoms may recur if you take hormone replacement therapy during your postmenopausal years.

For some women, the physical and emotional changes caused by PMS are so severe that they interfere with their ability to function at work or interact with family and friends. When PMS symptoms seriously undermine quality of life, the condition is called premenstrual dysphoric disorder (PMDD)—a complex medical disorder that has only recently been identified. Thankfully, PMDD affects only a small percentage of women. It's thought to be an excessive reaction to the normal hormonal changes associated with the menstrual cycle.

᠙

Who's at Risk?

Most women suffer from some type of premenstrual discomfort. In fact, 75 to 95 percent of all women experience one or more of the symptoms that are associated with PMS. But research indicates that only 30 to 40 percent of women between the ages of 25 and 50 years report the recurring symptoms indicative of PMS.[1] And only 5 to 10 percent of women develop symptoms severe enough to disrupt lifestyle and daily functioning.

PMS can begin any time after puberty. It's often triggered by a hormonal shock to your system, usually caused by an obstetrical or gynecological event such as pregnancy, tubal ligation or the use of oral contraceptives. Even women who have had hysterectomies can suffer from PMS if their ovaries are left intact after the surgery. Research suggests that you're more susceptible to PMS if you're under a lot of stress, you're under 34 years of age or you drink alcohol. Heredity may also play a role; however, PMS symptoms are not consistent in families and vary considerably among female relatives.

❧

Diagnosis

It can be difficult to diagnose PMS because the symptoms mimic those of many other disorders. Before your doctor can diagnose PMS, he or she must first eliminate the presence of another medical condition such as clinical depression, hypothyroidism, chronic fatigue syndrome, diabetes or irritable bowel syndrome.

The classic indicator of PMS is the timing of your symptoms. Your doctor will try to determine if your symptoms occur consistently around ovulation and continue until the beginning of your period. For the diagnosis of PMS to be correct, there must be a symptom-free interval between menstruation and the next ovulation near day 14 of your cycle. If your symptoms persist during all phases of your menstrual cycle, then you may be suffering from some other medical disorder. To help your doctor with the diagnosis, you may be asked to keep a menstrual diary, where you record your physical and emotional symptoms every day for several months. Because there are no laboratory tests that identify PMS, this diary is one of the most important tools used to assess your condition. To make the diagnosis of PMS, your doctor will look for a pattern of symptoms that occur regularly and have a negative impact on your ability to manage personal relationships and function normally at home and at work.

Your doctor will also review your medical and psychiatric history and conduct a thorough physical examination, including a pelvic exam. In some cases, laboratory tests may be needed to rule out other medical conditions.

❧

Conventional Treatment

Treating PMS can be just as difficult as diagnosing it. That's because the condition affects different women in so many different ways. Most conventional treatment approaches are directed at relieving symptoms and improving the quality of life. Before you embark on a medication to treat a symptom, try implementing the nutritional approaches that follow for three menstrual cycles. If dietary and/or other lifestyle changes don't improve your PMS within three months, your doctor may suggest medications to reduce your symptoms. Keep in mind the drugs below can help alleviate symptoms, but some of them have side effects that may cause problems of their own.

1. *Diuretics* These drugs eliminate excess fluid from your body by increasing urine production; they are often used to treat premenstrual swelling of hands, feet and face.

2. *Analgesics (pain killers)* The most effective of these are the non-steroidal anti-inflammatory medications (NSAIDs) like Anaprox®, which is usually prescribed for headaches, menstrual cramps and pelvic pain.

3. *Antidepressants* These are widely used to treat the depression and mood disorders associated with PMS. They work by increasing the level of natural brain chemicals that are affected by the female sex hormones. Selective serotonin reuptake inhibitors (SSRIs) such as Prozac® and Zoloft® are the most effective in reducing the psychological symptoms of PMS.

4. *Oral contraceptives* These are often prescribed to women to even out hormonal fluctuations. While some women benefit from these pills, others experience no change in their symptoms. Some women find that their symptoms are worsened by birth control pills.

5. *Ovarian suppressors* Drugs such as Danocrine® (a synthetic hormone related to the male sex hormone, testosterone) are sometimes used to stop the menstrual cycle. When the menstrual period stops, studies show that PMS stops, too. While the results of this type of treatment are usually very good, women often do not want to go to such extreme measures to manage their condition. Side effects of ovarian suppressors include the development of menopausal symptoms, such as vaginal dryness and hot flashes.

Managing PMS

Fortunately, there are some fairly simple modifications to your diet and lifestyle that can help you manage this physical and emotional roller coaster. During the worst phases of PMS, drug therapy may be necessary to improve your quality of life.

DIETARY STRATEGIES

Carbohydrates

Many studies have found that high-carbohydrate meals produce a calming, relaxing effect. Carbohydrate-rich foods like whole-grain bread, cereal, rice and pasta allow an amino acid called tryptophan to get into the brain (amino acids are the building blocks of protein and are found in all foods). The brain uses tryptophan to make the neurotransmitter serotonin. Researchers have linked high serotonin levels with happier moods, and low levels with mild depression and irritability in women with PMS. One study found that meals high in carbohydrates improved the mood in young women within 30 minutes of consumption.[2] Another study found that when women with PMS took a high-carbohydrate drink their mood improved within 90 minutes.[3]

If your mood is affected by PMS, eat high-carbohydrate meals that contain very little protein. High-protein foods like chicken, meat or fish supply the body with more amino acids that compete with tryptophan for entry into the brain. Try pasta with tomato sauce, a toasted whole-grain bagel with jam or a bowl of cereal with low-fat milk.

If your mood needs a boost during the day, reach for a high-carbohydrate beverage. Drop by a pharmacy and pick up a liquid dietary supplement called PMS Escape™. It's a flavored, powdered drink mix made from a blend of carbohydrates, vitamins and minerals that's thought to act by boosting the normal level of serotonin in the brain. The product was developed by Dr. Judith Wurtman, a research scientist at Massachusetts Institute of Technology (MIT) and pioneer in the carbohydrate-serotonin connection. You can also try a sports carbohydrate replacement drink available from your local health food or sporting goods store; they're sold as powder mixes or ready-to-drink and come in a variety of flavors.

Meal Timing

Try to eat once every four to five hours. That means eating three meals *and* one or two mid-day snacks. This is important to do every day of the month for improved energy levels, but it becomes even more essential during the premenstrual week. One reason is that the levels of neurotransmitters in your brain are susceptible to fluctuations in the levels of nutrients in your bloodstream. So any drastic change in your normal eating pattern—crash dieting, bingeing, or meal or snack skipping—can alter neurotransmitters in your brain and, as a result, alter your mood. Secondly, the hormonal fluctuations of PMS make you more susceptible to a low blood-sugar level. If you've ever experienced low blood sugar you know that it can cause low energy, increased appetite and hunger, irritability and headaches. So don't forget that mid-afternoon snack. It can prevent you from bingeing on potato chips or chocolate.

Low-Glycemic Carbohydrates

There was a time when nutritionists like myself encouraged people to get the majority of their carbohydrates from starchy foods like bread, pasta and rice, rather than simple sugars in desserts, candy and juice. This was because starchy foods have more nutrients than sugar and we thought that they were digested and absorbed in the bloodstream more slowly, leading to more stable blood-sugar or blood-glucose levels and better energy levels. As research continues, our knowledge about carbohydrates grows. We have learned that all starchy foods are not created equal. For example, the carbohydrates in a bagel are absorbed into your bloodstream at a faster rate than the sugar in a can of pop! It turns out that starchy foods vary widely in how quickly they're converted to blood glucose.

Nutritionists now classify carbohydrate foods according to their glycemic index (GI), or their ability to cause a rise in blood sugar. Foods with a low GI raise your blood sugar more slowly than foods with a high GI. When you eat a food that quickly raises your blood sugar you will get a burst of energy. But this spike in sugar also causes your pancreas to release a large amount of insulin into your bloodstream. Since insulin's job is to lower your blood sugar, your quick energy boost will be followed by a crash. That can lead to increased hunger and carbohydrate cravings.

Foods with a low GI, on the other hand, take longer to digest and lead to a gradual, slow rise in blood glucose. You don't get the insulin surge, and the energy from low GI food lasts longer. The glycemic index of a food depends on cooking time, fiber content, fat content and ripeness.

To satisfy your appetite and keep your blood-sugar levels stable for a longer period of time choose low GI foods at meal and snack times. Here are some examples:

Foods with Low Glycemic Index

Bread, Grains and Cereals

Pumpernickel (whole-grain) bread	Yam
Rye bread, 100%	Red River cereal
Bulgur	Special K
Rice	All-Bran Buds
Pasta	100% Bran cereal
Barley	

Legumes

Baked Beans	Kidney beans
Chickpeas	Soybeans
Lentils	

Fruit

Grapes	Apricots, dried
Orange	Plum
Apple	Cherries
Peach	

Dairy Products

Yogurt	Milk

If you're on the go, throw an energy bar in your bag for a mid-day snack. Choose a bar that contains carbohydrates and about 14 grams of protein—e.g., Genisoy™, SoyOne™, Balance® bar, PR Ironman® bar, Zone Perfect® bar.

Dietary Fat

If there's one more reason to cut back your fat intake, it's to help minimize your PMS symptoms. A few studies have shown that women with PMS who are put on a low-fat diet suffer fewer and less intense PMS symptoms.[4] Researchers have found that diets consisting of 15 to 20 percent calories from fat are associated with less water retention, less weight gain and fewer menstrual cramps.[5] A low-fat diet may affect your PMS symptoms by influencing the levels of hormone, especially estrogen, in your body.

Use the following chart to help you trim excess fat in your diet.

FOOD	LOWER-FAT CHOICE
Dairy Products	
Milk	Skim, 1% milk fat (MF)
Yogurt	Products with less than 1.5% MF
Cheese	Products with less than 20% MF
Cottage cheese	Products with 1% MF
Sour cream	Products with 7% MF or less
Cream	Evaporated 2% or skim milk
Meat, Poultry, Eggs	
Red meat	Flank steak, inside round, sirloin, eye of round, extra lean ground beef, venison
Pork	Center-cut pork chops, pork tenderloin, pork leg (inside round, roast), baked ham, deli ham, back bacon
Poultry	Skinless chicken breast, turkey breast, ground turkey
Eggs	Egg whites (2 whites replace 1 whole egg). You can buy these right beside the fresh eggs in your grocery store.

Choosing lower-fat foods will definitely help you cut back on fat calories. But it's also important to watch your portion size of animal foods, even those that are lower in fat. When eating meat or poultry, aim for no more than a 3 ounce (90 gram) serving, the size of a deck of cards. And watch those added fats and oils—use less oil, margarine, butter, sauces and dressings in cooking. To help you eat a 15 to 20 percent fat diet, aim for no more than 4 teaspoons of added fat each day.

Essential Fats and Evening Primrose Oil (EPO)

Before you cut out too much fat, keep in mind that not all fats are bad for your health. In fact, some types of fat are needed to help you stay healthy. These essential fatty acids (EFAs) cannot be manufactured by the body and must be consumed from food or supplements each day. EFAs perform many functions in the body but, when it comes to PMS, they may play an important role in reducing pain and inflammation.

There are two EFAs found in foods: linoleic acid (found in corn, sunflower and safflower oils) and alpha-linolenic acid (plentiful in flaxseed, canola and walnut oils). Once consumed, these EFAs are transformed into prostaglandins, powerful hormone-like compounds that regulate our blood, immune system and hormones. Prostaglandins can either increase inflammation or decrease it. Manipulating the type of fat you eat can alter levels of prostaglandins in the body: diets that emphasize animal fats favor the production of inflammatory prostaglandins, whereas diets rich in fish, grains and vegetable oils favor the formation of less inflammatory prostaglandins.

Researchers studying women with PMS have focused on a beneficial, less inflammatory prostaglandin called PGE_1. It's been theorized that in PMS there is a reduced ability to make PGE_1 from essential fats in the diet, and this can cause symptoms such as breast pain and tenderness, irritability, depression and headache.

The essential fatty acid linoleic acid gives rise to PGE_1 in the body. With the help of an enzyme, linoleic acid is converted to gamma-linoleic acid (GLA), which is then transformed into PGE_1 and other friendly prostaglandins. Now you can see that it is actually GLA that's needed to produce the beneficial prostaglandins.

There is very little GLA in food and therefore any GLA must be made from linoleic acid in the diet. Some researchers feel that women with PMS may have difficulty carrying out this conversion. What's more, many dietary factors—such as animal fat, alcohol and hydrogenated vegetable oils—can interfere with the conversion of linoleic acid to GLA. The enzyme responsible for this conversion requires zinc, magnesium and vitamins B6 and C to function properly. So a high-fat diet that's missing important vitamins and minerals can hamper GLA production and contribute to low levels of PGE_1. But even if your body has no problem turning linoleic acid from food into GLA, it's thought that the amount of GLA actually made may not be enough to cope with the requirement for prostaglandin formation.

This is where GLA supplements enter the story. You may have heard of evening primrose oil (EPO). Well, evening primrose oil is an excellent source of GLA. Evening primrose is a bright yellow wildflower that's native to North America. The seeds of the plant contain oil that is rich in GLA. Other sources of GLA are borage oil and black currant oil.

A number of studies have investigated the effectiveness of EPO in alleviating PMS symptoms. The results are mixed; unfortunately, I cannot tell you with conviction that EPO will ease your symptoms. A handful of studies in the 1980s did show that daily supplements of evening primrose oil outperformed the placebo pill with respect to improving PMS symptoms of breast tenderness, irritability and depression. In a few studies the difference between EPO and placebos was statistically significant.

But studies performed in the past ten years have not found any beneficial effects of EPO in treating PMS as a whole. Where EPO appears to offer most promise is in treating breast pain and tenderness. Some studies have found the supplement to be as effective as certain drugs used to treat cyclic breast pain. In fact, researchers from the University of Wales in Great Britain concluded that EPO was the best first-line therapy for cyclic breast pain.[6] And when it comes to side effects, EPO was superior to prescription drugs—less than 2 percent of women who took the supplement complained of headache and/or mild stomach upset.

What's my bottom line on EPO? It may not help balance your mood, but it does appear to be effective at relieving the breast tenderness and breast pain associated with PMS. And EPO is very safe. Based on the research, the effective dose is 3 to 4 grams per day, split into two doses. Buy a supplement that is standardized to contain 9 percent GLA; start by taking three 500-milligram pills at breakfast and repeat at dinner. Keep in mind that it may take three menstrual cycles before you feel the effects of EPO, so don't give up. And it can take up to eight months for EPO to reach its full effect.

Sodium

Fluid retention, bloating and weight gain are without a doubt the most common PMS complaints among my clients. High levels of estrogen associated with PMS can cause your kidneys to retain water and sodium. Eliminating table salt and foods high in sodium the week before your period will certainly help prevent swollen hands and feet, not to mention tight waistbands.

Sodium is an essential nutrient that our body needs to maintain its fluid balance, but we actually need only a very tiny amount. For sedentary Americans, all it takes is a mere 500 milligrams (or 1/5 teaspoon) of sodium to cover the body's requirement. If you sweat during exercise you need a little more salt, but not much. You might have already guessed that we're getting much more sodium than we need—10 times more. Each day the average American consumes about two teaspoons of salt.

To help cut back on sodium, avoid the salt shaker at the table, minimize the use of salt in cooking, and buy commercial food products that are low in added salt. Eating fewer processed foods is one of the key strategies to de-salt your diet. Most of the salt we consume every day comes from processed and prepared foods—only one-fourth comes from the salt shaker!

See the list on page 41 of chapter 1 to help you cut down on foods high in sodium. Aim for no more than 2400 milligrams of sodium each day (that's 1 teaspoon of salt). To season your foods without adding salt, use herbs, spices, flavored vinegars and fruit juices. Remember that the sodium content of convenience foods labeled "low sodium" or "reduced salt" can vary, so be sure to check the nutrition information panel. And don't forget to rinse canned vegetables to remove excess salt.

Alcohol and Caffeine

I mentioned earlier that research suggests women with PMS are more likely to drink alcohol. Alcoholic beverages can certainly cause or worsen many PMS symptoms, including fatigue, irritability, depression, bowel irregularities, appetite fluctuation and fluid retention. Alcohol has a dehydrating effect on the body, which can leave you feeling sluggish. But alcohol can also cause fatigue by robbing you of a good night's sleep. Studies show that alcohol interferes with the body's ability to fall into REM (rapid eye movement) sleep, the restorative phase of sleep that leaves you feeling refreshed and energetic. If you suffer from PMS, avoid alcohol completely during the 7 to 14 days before your menstrual period. During the rest of the month, aim for no more than seven drinks per week.

Caffeine can aggravate irritability, anxiety, headaches, diarrhea, fatigue and breast tenderness. Drinking coffee during the day can turn to overstimulation by your fourth or fifth cup, causing irritability, nervousness, anxiety, insomnia and fatigue. As little as two small cups of coffee in the morning can affect your sleep that night by blocking the brain's production of a natural sleep-inducing chemical called adenosine.

How much caffeine is too much? Most experts agree that a daily dose of 400 to 450 milligrams of caffeine does not pose a risk for healthy people. But this recommendation is based on caffeine's effects on blood pressure and other health conditions, not your ability to sleep soundly. If your PMS symptoms include irritability, anxiousness or general fatigue, I recommend consuming no more than 200 milligrams of caffeine daily, and preferably none.

Use the table on page 38 in chapter 1 to assess your daily caffeine intake. If you find you're overdoing it, cut back gradually over a period of several weeks to minimize withdrawal symptoms such as headaches, tiredness or muscle pain. Start by eliminating caffeine from the latter part of your day. Stick to a "no caffeine" rule after noon. Switch to low-caffeine beverages like tea or hot chocolate, or caffeine-free alternatives such as decaf coffee, herbal tea, cereal coffee, juice, milk or water. If you're still hooked on coffee, order a latte or cappuccino to get extra calcium (more on calcium and PMS later—keep reading!).

VITAMINS AND MINERALS

Vitamin B6

When it comes to PMS, this B vitamin is one of the most heavily studied nutrients. The research dates back to 1973 when scientists found that supplemental B6 was useful in treating depression associated with the birth control pill. Further studies have shown that a daily supplement of 50 to 100 milligrams of B6 eases mood swings in women suffering from PMS. In 1999 British researchers analyzed the results from nine clinical trials involving 940 women with PMS.[7] They concluded that B6 was significantly better than the placebo treatment in relieving PMS-related depression. However, since many of these studies were considered to have flaws, it is not possible to say with certainty that the vitamin is an effective treatment for PMS.

The studies do suggest, however, that doses of up to 100 milligrams per day of B6 are likely to benefit women who experience premenstrual depression. A study published in 2000 from the University of Reading in the United Kingdom found that 50 milligrams of B6 combined with 200 milligrams of magnesium had a significant but modest effect of reducing anxiety-related PMS symptoms, including nervous tension, mood swings, irritability and anxiety.[8]

How vitamin B6 works to ease depression is not entirely understood. It is known that B6 is needed for the production of two brain chemicals: serotonin and dopamine. I mentioned earlier in this chapter that brain serotonin levels have a potent effect on mood. Dopamine regulates the secretion of prolactin, a hormone that may be linked to PMS.

You need at least 1.6 milligrams of vitamin B6 to maintain your health and prevent deficiency. If your diet lacks protein foods and whole grains, chances are you're running low. See the B6 in Foods table on page 5 in chapter 1 for foods that will pack more B6 into your diet.

B6 Supplements

If you experience depression before your monthly period, you might give B6 a try. Use the following guide for supplementing safely:

- For maximum effectiveness, take 50 to 100 milligrams of vitamin B6 daily for three days before the expected onset of your symptoms.

- Stop taking B6 one or two days after your period begins (i.e., day 2 or 3 of your menstrual cycle).

- More is not better. Studies have not demonstrated that you get a better effect by taking more B6. Supplementing with too much B6 for a period of time has toxic effects, including irreversible nerve damage.

You don't have to take a supplement that contains only vitamin B6. You might prefer to take a B complex pill that contains the entire B vitamin family or a high-potency multivitamin and mineral supplement. Both of these supplements should contain 50 to 100 milligrams of B6, but check the label to be sure. You might be interested to learn that a few studies have shown that women with PMS who were given a daily multivitamin and mineral pill reported fewer PMS symptoms. Vitamins and minerals work together in the body and many may have a synergistic effect. In my opinion, it makes sense to take a balanced vitamin supplement.

Vitamin E

Three randomized clinical trials revealed that vitamin E supplements improved PMS-related mood swings, anxiety, headache, food cravings and insomnia.[9] In one study, women with PMS were given 150 international units (IU), 300 IU or 600 IU of vitamin E. All doses were more effective at relieving symptoms than the placebo pill.

How vitamin E may work to help your PMS is not understood. However, the vitamin is famous for its role as an antioxidant, a substance that can combat harmful free radicals in the body. Free radicals damage cells and are believed to play a role in the development of heart disease, certain cancers, cataracts and Alzheimer's disease. There is a large body of evidence to suggest that taking a vitamin E supplement each day can lower the risk of heart disease. So if you're not taking vitamin E now, you might want to add it to your daily nutrition regime. It just might help your PMS and protect your heart!

VITAMIN E SUPPLEMENTS

It's impossible to get close to the 150 IU of vitamin E from foods in your daily diet. The richest sources of vitamin E are vegetable oils, nuts, seeds and wheat germ. Leafy green vegetables, especially kale, are also good sources. But if you consider that 1 tablespoon (15 ml) of olive oil provides only 2.6 IU of the vitamin—and even 2 tablespoons (30 ml) of toasted wheat germ gives you a mere 4 IU—you can see why you must rely on a supplement to get 150 to 600 IU.

To help you choose the right vitamin E supplement, consider the following:

- Start taking 200 to 400 IU per day.
- Buy a "natural source" vitamin E supplement (look for *d-alpha-tocopherol* on the label; synthetic forms are labeled *dl-alpha tocopherol*). Although the body absorbs both synthetic and natural forms equally well, your liver prefers the natural form, as it incorporates more natural vitamin E into transport molecules.
- If you're on blood-thinning medication like Coumadin® (warfarin), don't take vitamin E, since it also has slight anti-clotting properties. Talk to your doctor before adding any supplement to your regime.

Calcium

This is one mineral you'll want to get more of if you suffer from PMS. In 1998, a well-designed study of 466 women found that those who took 1200 milligrams of supplemental calcium daily for three months had a significant reduction in PMS symptoms, especially mood swings, low back pain, food cravings and fluid retention.[10] The majority of women experienced a 50 percent reduction in overall symptoms, compared to a 36 percent improvement among women who took the placebo pill. What's more, the strongest improvement was observed during the third menstrual cycle, which implies that the effect of calcium supplements increases with continued use.

We have a few clues as to how calcium may work to alleviate PMS. Many of the symptoms of a calcium deficiency are similar to those of PMS. And there is evidence that blood levels of calcium are low in women with PMS. Low calcium levels cause an overproduction of parathyroid hormone, which interacts with serotonin in the brain to affect mood, so calcium supplements may ease PMS symptoms by replenishing a deficiency. Interestingly, there seems to be a connection between PMS and development of osteoporosis later in life. Perhaps PMS is a monthly reminder that you're lacking adequate amounts of calcium in your diet.

If you're a woman between the ages of 19 and 50, you need 1000 milligrams of calcium each day. For a list of calcium-rich foods, see the Calcium in Foods table on page 17 in chapter 1.

CALCIUM SUPPLEMENTS

In addition to increasing your intake of calcium-rich foods, consider taking a daily calcium supplement to get up to the 1200 milligram target that was found to be effective in the PMS study. To help you determine your need for a calcium supplement, use my 300 Milligram Rule: one milk serving gives you 300 milligrams of calcium, so for every serving you're missing and not replacing with other calcium-rich foods, you need to get 300 milligrams of elemental calcium through a supplement. But before you rush off to the health food store, there are a few things to look for when buying a supplement.

Many of my clients have described their frustration at buying a calcium supplement. Should you choose calcium carbonate or calcium citrate? Is a 600-milligram pill better than two 300-milligram tablets? What about added vitamin D and magnesium? To help make your next calcium shopping experience stress-free, follow these guidelines for choosing a high-quality supplement.

1. *Look at the source of calcium.* There are many types of calcium supplements on the shelf. Here are some of the more common types:
   - *Calcium carbonate* is only about 10 to 30 percent absorbed by the body. The amount you absorb depends on how much stomach acid is present; as people

age their stomachs produce less hydrochloric acid. Always take calcium carbonate supplements with meals to increase their absorption. Do not take calcium carbonate at bedtime, unless you take it with a snack. On the plus side, calcium carbonate is the most inexpensive type of calcium, and you can get 500 milligrams of elemental calcium in one pill.

- *Calcium citrate* is absorbed more effectively than calcium carbonate—it's about 30 percent absorbed. Calcium citrate malate is one of the most highly absorbable and expensive forms of calcium. Calcium citrate supplements are well absorbed, either with meals or on an empty stomach. You won't find more than 300 milligrams of elemental calcium in calcium citrate pills.

- *Calcium chelates (HVP chelate)* are supplements that contain calcium bound to an amino acid. In the case of calcium HVP chelate, the amino acid is from vegetable protein. Some manufacturers claim that up to 75 percent of calcium in the chelate form is absorbed by the body.

- *Effervescent calcium supplements* contain calcium carbonate and often other forms of more absorbable calcium, so they may be better absorbed in some people. And because they get a head start on disintegrating, they may be absorbed in the intestinal tract more quickly. Dissolve these in water or orange juice.

- *Calcium from bone meal* or *dolomite* or *oyster shell* is not recommended, because some products have been found to contain trace quantities of contaminants such as lead and mercury.

2. *Determine how much elemental calcium each pill gives you.* Look on the list of ingredients for this information. The amount of elemental calcium is what you use to calculate your daily intake. Calcium carbonate or calcium chelates may not be 100 percent elemental calcium. The front label may state 500 milligrams, but when you look on the back or side of the bottle at the ingredient list you may find the product contains only 350 milligrams of elemental calcium. This will determine how many tablets you need to take to get your recommended dose.

3. *Choose a formula with vitamin D and magnesium.* These nutrients work in tandem with calcium to promote optimal bone health. For instance, vitamin D increases calcium absorption in your intestine by as much as 30 to 80 percent. As you will read later in this chapter, magnesium may also help ease certain PMS symptoms.

4. *Spread larger doses throughout the day.* Since all calcium sources, including food sources, are not 100 percent absorbed, it makes sense to split a higher dose over two or three meals. If you've been advised to take 600 milligrams of calcium a day, take a 300-milligram tablet with breakfast and another one at dinner.

5. *Take your calcium supplements with a large glass of water.*

The daily upper limit for calcium intake is 2500 milligrams from food and supplements. In most healthy people, this amount will not cause any side effects. The major risks from getting too much calcium include kidney stones, constipation and gas. In people who have a history of kidney stones, excessive intakes of calcium—greater than 2500 milligrams—can increase the risk of stone formation.

Magnesium

According to a handful of studies, boosting your intake of this important mineral may improve symptoms of depression, anxiety, fluid retention and breast tenderness. Research also suggests that magnesium supplements may prevent migraine headaches (the migraine studies were not specifically conducted on women with PMS).

Your body contains about 24 grams of this mineral—half in your bones and half in your tissues. Magnesium is found in all body cells and fluids, where it is needed to maintain fluid balance by pumping sodium and potassium in and out of cells. It's also used by more than 300 enzymes, including those that produce energy. A handful of studies have found lower blood levels of magnesium in women with PMS.

Studies have determined a daily dose of 200 to 360 milligrams of supplemental magnesium to be effective in easing PMS symptoms.[11] The recommended daily allowance (RDA) for magnesium can be found on the RDA table on page 21 in chapter 1.

Research suggests that women may be consuming too little magnesium. One survey of 27,000 Americans revealed that only 25 percent got enough of the mineral each day.[12] The best sources of magnesium are whole foods including unrefined grains, nuts, seeds, legumes, dried fruit and green vegetables.

MAGNESIUM SUPPLEMENTS

By looking at the list on page 21 in chapter 1, you may realize that it can be challenging to eat a magnesium-rich diet. In addition to including these foods in your daily diet, consider taking a magnesium supplement to help you combat PMS symptoms—in particular, fluid retention, mood swings and menstrual migraines (read chapter 7, "Migraines," for more about this). Here's how to supplement safely:

- If you take calcium supplements, buy one with magnesium added. You can choose either a 1:1 ratio supplement, meaning the supplement contains an equal amount of calcium and magnesium, or a 2:1 ratio, in which there is twice as much calcium as magnesium. For instance, a 2:1 calcium citrate supplement will generally give you 300 milligrams of calcium and 150 milligrams of magnesium. Depending on your diet, you might need to take one of these supplements two or three times a day.

- If you don't need supplemental calcium, but you want to try taking magnesium for your PMS, buy a supplement made from magnesium citrate, aspartate, succinate or fumarate. The body absorbs these forms of the mineral more efficiently.

- The daily upper safe limit for magnesium is 350 milligrams per day from a supplement—more than this can cause diarrhea, nausea and stomach cramps.

- Be sure you are meeting your daily requirements for calcium (read the section on page 318) since magnesium supplements may reduce calcium absorption.

HERBAL REMEDIES

Chasteberry (*Vitex angus-castus*)

European physicians have prescribed this herbal remedy for more than 40 years to regulate the menstrual cycle and ease PMS symptoms. One German study, which followed more than 1600 women with PMS for three months, found that 93 percent of women taking chasteberry reported symptom improvement or complete relief.[13] The researchers assessed all PMS symptom categories including mood swings, anxiety, food cravings and fluid retention. While it is true there are a limited number of well-controlled clinical studies assessing the effectiveness of *vitex*, the experience of physicians has long established the practical use of the herb in women with PMS.

The active ingredients in *vitex* are believed to act on the pituitary gland in the brain to cause the release of a neurotransmitter called dopamine. This, in turn, appears to result in an increase in the production of progesterone, leading to a normal balance of estrogen and progesterone. Through its action on dopamine in the brain, studies show that *vitex* also suppresses the release of prolactin, thereby lowering excessive levels that may cause breast tenderness and swelling during the premenstrual week.

The recommended dose of chasteberry is 175 to 225 milligrams once daily. Choose a product that is standardized to contain 0.5 percent agnuside and 0.6 percent aucubin, two of the plant's active ingredients. But don't expect immediate results. It takes at least four weeks for the herb to kick in, and probably months for it to reach its full effect. Side effects are rarely seen in women taking *vitex*. Mild side effects occasionally reported include nausea, headache and skin rash.

Since it inhibits prolactin secretion, and prolactin is necessary for milk production, *vitex* should not be used during breastfeeding. The herb has not been evaluated in pregnant women. If you are on a medication that interacts with the brain chemical dopamine (e.g., the antidepressants Wellbutrin® and Effexor®) be sure to tell your doctor that you are taking *vitex*. He or she should monitor you closely to make sure that the herb doesn't interact with your medication to make it less effective. If you are taking birth control pills or hormone replacement therapy, use caution. Although there have been no case reports, theoretically *vitex* could interfere with the effectiveness of these medications because of its hormone-regulating activity.

Ginkgo Biloba

No doubt you've heard that ginkgo might improve your memory and protect your brain cells from the ravages of aging. Well, it turns out this herbal remedy might also be useful in treating PMS. This finding actually occurred by accident; women who took ginkgo for brain health noticed that fluid retention associated with their menstrual cycle lessened while on the herb. Then, in 1993, researchers from France conducted a formal study of 143 women with PMS.[14] They found ginkgo to be significantly more effective than the placebo in treating PMS-related breast tenderness, abdominal bloating and swollen hands, legs and feet. The women took ginkgo on day 16 of their cycle and continued until day 5 of their next cycle, at which time they stopped; they resumed taking the herbal remedy again on day 16.

The recommended dose of ginkgo biloba is 40 to 80 milligrams three times daily. Start on day 16 and continue until the end of your next period. Essentially, you take ginkgo for two weeks each month. Be sure to buy a product standardized to contain 24 percent ginkgo flavone glycosides. The herb is very safe but, like most herbal remedies, it can cause mild stomach upset in a small number of women.

One concern is ginkgo's mild blood-thinning effect. It should not be taken with blood-thinning drugs such as Coumadin® (warfarin), heparin and Trental® unless your doctor is monitoring you. It is also possible that ginkgo can enhance the effect of other natural health products, such as vitamin E or garlic, that also slightly thin the blood. Be sure to inform your physician and pharmacist if you are taking more than one of these products. Since ginkgo has not been studied in pregnant or breastfeeding women, I don't recommend that you use it at these times.

Feverfew (*Tanacetum parthenium*)

Since the 1970s this herbal remedy has been widely used in Europe to prevent migraine headaches, although it has not been used specifically for PMS headaches. Of the few studies that have been conducted, feverfew has been effective at reducing both the number of migraines and the nausea and vomiting that occur with them. Researchers believe that feverfew reduces the frequency and intensity of migraines by preventing the release of substances that dilate blood vessels and cause inflammation. Studies show that powdered feverfew leaf is effective, but not alcohol extracts made from the herb.

The recommended dose is 80 to 100 milligrams daily of powdered feverfew leaf. You can also try taking the herb at the onset of a migraine to ease the symptoms. Because scientists don't yet know what components of the herb contribute to its effectiveness, an effective standardized extract is not available. Feverfew is deemed to be very safe, as it rarely causes side effects other than mild gastrointestinal upset. The herb may cause an allergic reaction in people sensitive to members of the Asteracease/Compositae plant family: ragweed, daisy, marigold and chrysanthemum. The safety of feverfew has not been studied in pregnant or nursing women or those with liver or kidney disease.

St. John's Wort (*Hypericum perforatum*)

This yellow-flowered plant has long been heralded for its ability to balance emotions. For years, it's been widely used in Europe to treat both mild depression and Seasonal Affective Disorder. An analysis of 26 controlled studies conducted in 1700 patients concluded that the herb was as effective as certain antidepressant drugs in treating mild to moderate depression.[15] Recently a small pilot study found that St. John's wort taken daily for two months yielded significant improvements in PMS-related depression.[16]

Scientists are still trying to determine exactly how this herbal remedy works. Many experts believe it acts by keeping brain serotonin levels high for a longer period of time, just like the popular antidepressant drugs Paxil®, Zoloft® and Prozac®.

The power of St. John's wort lies in two active ingredients, called hypericin and hyperforin. Researchers attribute most of the herb's effectiveness to hyperforin. A large German study found that people who took a St. John's wort extract with a higher amount of hyperforin reported better improvement in symptoms than those who took an extract with a lesser amount. In fact, 70 percent reported their depression was much or very much improved.[17]

If possible, I always recommend herbal extracts that have been backed by scientific study. In the case of St. John's wort, look for a product that meets the following criteria: it should be standardized to contain 0.3 percent hypericin and it should contain a high amount of hyperforin. There are some advanced formulas now on the market, and one in particular, called Movana™, has been used in clinical studies.

The effective dosage is one 300-milligram tablet three times daily. The herb has a strong record of safety; however, in a few cases it has been reported to cause sensitivity to sunlight in very light-skinned individuals. Although St. John's wort may be safe when taken alone for mild depression, it can have a negative effect when taken with medications used to treat AIDS, certain viruses, depression, seizures and organ transplants, and with birth control pills. St. John's wort increases the rate at which some of these medications are broken down by the liver, and as a result the herb may reduce the effectiveness of the drug. If you are taking any prescription medications, be sure to contact your physician before starting on St. John's wort.

Kava Kava (*Piper methysticum*)

You might have heard about using kava to combat the anxiety, apprehension or nervousness associated with PMS. This herb is extracted from the roots of a South Pacific pepper plant. Experts believe that kava's active ingredients, called kavalactones, exert their effect by working on the limbic system of the brain, the center of our emotions. Studies have found kava to be useful in treating anxiety. One double-blind study proved the effectiveness of a standardized kava extract against the Hamilton Anxiety Scale, a scale used by psychiatrists to measure levels of anxiety.[18] Another study found that menopausal women with anxiety disorders obtained significant relief with kava, without the negative side effects of traditional drugs like Valium®.[19]

Buy a product that is standardized to contain 30 percent kavalactones. According to the research, this is the most effective extract. The daily dose of kava used in the studies ranges from 60 to 120 milligrams of kavalactones. For most products, this translates into one to three tablets or capsules daily; start with one standardized tablet. You should notice relief in one week, but it can take up to a month for the herb to reach its full effect. If you find that this dose doesn't help your symptoms, increase the dose. Do not exceed a daily dose of 300 milligrams of kavalactones.

Kava may cause mild side effects, including stomach upset, headaches and dizziness. Until recently, kava was considered a safe herb. However, a growing number of reports from Europe, describing liver damage in people taking kava, have caused concern. If you decide to use kava, *inform your physician first.* The herb should not be used with alcohol, tranquilizers, antidepressants or sedatives. Its safety has not been evaluated in pregnant or nursing women or people with liver or kidney disease.

LIFESTYLE FACTORS

Exercise
Regular exercise is an excellent way to manage your PMS symptoms. Start with a program of regular aerobic exercise for 30 minutes, at least three to four times each week. Activities such as brisk walking, jogging, stair climbing, biking or swimming offer many other health benefits, in addition to reducing your PMS discomfort.

Reduce Stress
There's no question that PMS is closely related to stress. Reducing the stress in your life and promoting more time for relaxation will go a long way towards improving your quality of life and minimizing the effects of PMS. Deep breathing exercises, biofeedback and progressive muscle relaxation techniques can be very effective in helping you control your response to PMS symptoms.

THE BOTTOM LINE...
Leslie's recommendations for managing PMS

1. Eat a high-carbohydrate diet. Carbohydrate-rich foods like whole grains, pasta, cereal, rice and fruit trigger the production of serotonin, a brain neurotransmitter associated with relaxed, happier moods.

2. Eat once every four to five hours to keep your blood-sugar levels stable. Plan for between-meal snacks.

3. Choose low glycemic carbohydrate foods that get digested and converted to blood sugar more slowly than other carbohydrate-containing foods to stabilize your energy levels and keep hunger at bay.

4. Eat a low-fat diet as this may help to reduce the level of circulating estrogen.

5. If you suffer from breast tenderness and breast pain each month, consider trying evening primrose oil. Take three 500-milligram capsules twice daily. Buy a product that is standardized to 9 percent GLA.

6. If fluid retention, swelling, bloating and weight gain plague you, drastically cut back on sodium two weeks before your period (ideally all month long!). Aim for no more than 2400 milligrams of sodium each day.

7. Avoid alcohol for 7 to 14 days before your period since it causes fatigue and may affect your mood.

8. To help reduce irritability, anxiety and general fatigue, aim for no more than 200 milligrams of caffeine per day (preferably none).

9. If your PMS symptoms include depression, boost your intake of vitamin B6. Take 50 to 100 milligrams of B6 from day 16 of one menstrual cycle to day 3 of your next menstrual cycle.

10. Add a daily vitamin E supplement to your nutrition regime. It may help improve mood swings, anxiety, headache, food cravings and insomnia. And it may also protect from heart disease!

11. To help with mood swings, low back pain, food cravings and fluid retention, get 1000 to 1200 milligrams of calcium every day. If you rely on supplements, choose a calcium citrate pill with added vitamin D and magnesium.

12. Add magnesium-rich foods to your diet. Getting more magnesium may help improve mood swings, anxiety, fluid retention and headache. If you take a supplement (whether it's combined with calcium or taken on its own), don't take more than 350 milligrams. Choose a supplement made from magnesium citrate, aspartate, succinate or fumarate.

13. Once your diet and nutritional intake is up to speed, try a standardized extract of chasteberry (*Vitex castus-angus*) for overall PMS relief. Take 175 to 225 milligrams once daily. Buy a product that is standardized to 0.5 percent agnuside.

14. If fluid retention is your only PMS symptom, try 40 to 80 milligrams of ginkgo biloba three times daily. Start this on day 16 of your menstrual cycle and continue until the end of your next period. Buy an extract standardized to contain 24 percent ginkgo flavone glycosides.

15. To help prevent PMS migraine headaches, try 80 to 100 milligrams of powdered feverfew leaf once daily.

16. If vitamin B6 has not helped your monthly depression, try St. John's wort. Take 300 milligrams three times daily. Buy a product standardized to contain 0.3 percent hypericin and a high amount of hyperforin. This herb may interact with a number of prescription medications.

17. Finally, if anxiety is your only PMS complaint, an herbal remedy called kava kava might help. Since kava may cause liver-related side effects, *consult your doctor first.*

18

Perimenopause

If you are a woman in your forties or early fifties, chances are you're experiencing changes in your monthly menstrual cycle, not to mention a myriad of uncomfortable physical symptoms.

The signs and symptoms associated with menopause occur over a period of time called *perimenopause*, which literally means "around menopause." For many women, the first sign of perimenopause is an erratic menstrual cycle—skipped, lighter or shorter periods. The hallmark of this countdown to menopause is a fluctuating level of the female sex hormones, estrogen and progesterone. Estrogen highs can bring on PMS-like symptoms including mood swings, fluid retention and headaches, whereas estrogen lows promise hot flashes, vaginal dryness and forgetfulness.

You're considered to have reached *menopause* when a year has passed since your last period. Although it can vary, the average age at which an American woman hits menopause is 51. It's at this time that women enter *postmenopause*, the phase of life in which the risk for heart disease, osteoporosis and breast cancer increases. I have devoted a separate chapter to deal with each of these health concerns associated with the postmenopausal years.

Your Menstrual Cycle

In order to understand what's happening to your body during menopause, it helps to know how your hormones normally act during the childbearing years. During the early part of your monthly cycle, your ovaries produce estrogen. Your brain responds to this increasing estrogen level by telling your pituitary gland to release follicle stimulating hormone (FSH) and luteinizing hormone (LH). These two hormones, in turn, act on your ovaries. FSH causes egg follicles to develop and release estrogen. When your circulating estrogen rises to a critical level, the pituitary gland releases a surge of LH. This influx of LH causes ovulation by telling the follicle to release a mature egg.

The empty egg follicle turns into something called the corpus luteum, a gland that produces progesterone after ovulation. During the last 14 days of your menstrual cycle, progesterone prepares your body for pregnancy by thickening the lining of your uterus. If conception does not occur, the corpus luteum becomes smaller, estrogen and progesterone levels fall and your uterine lining sheds, resulting in your period. Lower levels of estrogen and progesterone signal your pituitary to release FSH and LH and the cycle continues.

What Causes Perimenopause?

As you get older, your supply of eggs and follicles dwindles. Fewer follicles means that your ovaries are producing less estrogen. Lower levels of estrogen and progesterone tell your pituitary gland that it's time to release FSH and then LH. But now your ovaries are unable to respond to FSH and LH. They can't produce much estrogen and release an egg and, as a result, your brain keeps telling your pituitary gland to make your ovaries ovulate. So your pituitary gland keeps releasing more and more FSH. This constant production of FSH can trigger hot flashes. With no egg being released from your ovary, there's no corpus luteum and consequently no progesterone secretion. Without progesterone your body won't shed its uterine lining and you'll miss a period. With lower levels of hormones, your periods will also become shorter and eventually they will cease.

Symptoms

HOT FLASHES AND NIGHT SWEATS

Hot flashes are, without a doubt, the most commonly reported symptom of menopause; in fact, they occur in 60 to 85 percent of North American women. It's estimated that 10 to 15 percent of women have them severely enough to interfere with their daily life. On average, hot flashes persist for three to five years, but in 50 percent of women they last up to five years.

There is often a warning signal or aura that precedes a hot flash. A hot flash may begin as pressure in the head, a headache or a wave of nausea. A sensation of heat then starts in the head and neck, and spreads to the torso, arms and entire body. Sweating follows and is most intense in the upper body. Clothing may become soaked, particularly if hot flashes occur during sleep—night sweats are another term for hot flashes that occur during sleep. Chills or shakes may follow as a result of a drop in body temperature. The entire event can last a few seconds to several minutes, and it may take an hour for chills to subside.

Scientists believe that when estrogen levels drop, your body's temperature control system malfunctions. It senses that you are too hot, even though your body temperature is normal, and attempts to cool you down by increasing your heartbeat and sending more blood to your skin, especially in your head and neck. Blood vessels in your skin then dilate, which causes heat to escape from your body. As a result, your skin flushes and you sweat. Hot flashes are actually your body's way of cooling you down.

INSOMNIA

Often night sweats cause disrupted sleep. While many women have no difficulty going back to sleep, some simply cannot. Night after night of little sleep will leave you exhausted, and that's when other perimenopausal symptoms can take over your life. Fatigue can lead to irritability, depression and forgetfulness. Many experts believe that there is something else going on to interrupt sleep, something that's not related to hot flashes during sleep.

MOOD SWINGS

Most women describe the mood swings of perimenopause like those of premenstrual syndrome (PMS). They talk about crying at the drop of a hat, or blowing up at a spouse for no good reason. These feelings can be disruptive to both your personal life and work life. Not all women experience mood swings during the transition years. Studies show that if a woman has had a hysterectomy she's more likely to feel depressed. Women who are irritable and cranky during PMS tend to experience those same mood swings during perimenopause.

Mood swings are partly due to a loss of estrogen. Although we don't fully understand what's going on in the body, we do know that natural chemicals in the brain, called neurotransmitters, respond to hormonal fluctuations of the menstrual cycle. Some of these chemicals stimulate nerves that make us more alert. Others interact with nerves to calm us down. The hormonal ups and downs of perimenopause may also make us more sensitive to feelings and emotions. You'll find nutritional strategies that may help you manage mild to moderate depression presented in chapter 12, "Depression."

MEMORY PROBLEMS

We've all had memory lapses at one time or another, but there is definitely a link between brain power and hormonal fluctuations. During perimenopause there are a few things happening to your body that may cause forgetfulness. For one, there's an aging process going on. The older we get the more short-term memory we lose. Other menopausal symptoms such as insomnia and fatigue can cause memory problems.

Evidence also suggests that estrogen affects the brain chemistry and structure that's involved in memory, and that the loss of estrogen associated with menopause may be largely responsible for memory decline. Estrogen may be needed to transfer nerve messages to specific regions in the brain. And the hormone may also be important in preventing blood clots in the brain, which can cause oxygen deprivation and loss of brain tissue.

HEAVY BLEEDING

More than 75 percent of women will experience some change to their monthly cycle. A number of years before her last period, a woman may notice that her cycles become less frequent or closer together. And often a woman's period shortens in duration as estrogen production fluctuates and ovulation occurs less often. While an erratic menstrual cycle can be annoying, what's more distressing is heavy bleeding that can occur with your period.

Heavy bleeding is usually caused by an imbalance of estrogen and progesterone. When ovulation does not occur and your ovaries don't release an egg, progesterone is not produced. This means that estrogen is allowed to continue to build up the uterine lining. The lining becomes very thick and releases a lot of blood when it sheds in response to a drop in your estrogen levels. As your estrogen levels decline with approaching menopause, heavy bleeding will become less of an issue.

In some cases, heavy bleeding can be the sign of something else going on in the uterus: polyps, a fibroid or, less commonly, cancer. You should always alert your gynecologist if your periods last more than seven days, if you bleed between your periods or if your menstrual flow becomes much heavier than usual.

If heavy flow has plagued you for some time and your energy level is dragging, ask your family doctor to measure your iron level. Your *hemoglobin* level measures circulating iron in red blood cells, and your *ferritin* level measures the amount of iron stored in your liver, spleen and bone marrow. A blood test will determine if you have an iron deficiency and may indicate the need for single iron supplements.

꒖

Who's at Risk?

Perimenopausal symptoms can affect women ten years before menopause, when hormonal changes kick in. Today in America almost 30 million women are between the ages of 40 and 54, the phase of life when levels of certain hormones are changing and dwindling. While perimenopause can start in a woman's late thirties, most women begin noticing symptoms in their forties.

Not all women experience uncomfortable symptoms associated with perimenopause. Although research is lacking in this area, there are a few factors that might increase your risk for suffering one or more of the side effects of midlife hormonal fluctuations. Ask yourself the following questions:

- Are you in your mid to late forties?
- Did your mother experience any perimenopausal symptoms?
- Do you suffer from nasty premenstrual symptoms, especially mood swings?
- Do you eat a diet that's high in animal fat and lacking fruits, vegetables and fiber?

- Do you drink too much alcohol and coffee?

- Is your life full of stress and tension?

- Do you lack adequate sleep on a regular basis?

- Do you lack regular exercise?

⁓

Conventional Treatment

Should you take HRT (hormone replacement therapy)? Many women take HRT to get relief from troublesome symptoms such as mood swings or hot flashes. There's no question that short-term estrogen therapy alleviates these symptoms. Other women may have started on HRT after discussing health risks with their family physician.

If you are taking HRT, you may be wondering if you should continue. Today many women are confused about hormones in light of news reports that the risks of combined HRT (estrogen plus progestin) outweigh the benefits. In July 2002, the Women's Health Initiative (WHI) study on combined HRT was abruptly halted. Sponsored by the National Institutes of Health, WHI followed more than 27,000 healthy women, aged 50 to 79, taking either combined HRT or estrogen only. The goal was to determine whether HRT protected from heart disease and osteoporosis, as well as the increased risk for cancer and blood clots.

After a little more than five years of study, the results revealed that women taking *combined HRT* were at increased risk for heart disease, blood clots, stroke and breast cancer. Although the risks were small, it was enough to stop the investigation of combined HRT. The hormone regimen did protect from hip fracture and colon cancer, but more women suffered a serious health event than a positive one. Women in the study taking *estrogen only* were told to continue taking their pills as before, because it remained uncertain whether the benefits outweigh the risks. At the time of writing, no further data had been reported.

This new knowledge about HRT has led the American College of Obstetrics and Gynecologists and the North American Menopause Society to revise guidelines on the appropriate use of combined HRT:

- The number one indication for combined HRT is to treat menopausal symptoms such as hot flashes, night sweats and mood swings in women with a uterus.
- The use of combined HRT and estrogen-only therapy should be used for the shortest duration possible and at lower-than-standard doses. It remains unknown whether patches and creams are any safer than pills.
- Women who have been on HRT for five years or more should talk with their physicians about whether to continue.
- If you decide to discontinue HRT, ask your doctor the best way to do so.
- Combined HRT should not be used to treat heart disease. Your doctor should discuss other options with you.

If you are considering HRT, review with your doctor why you want to take the drug, your personal benefits without HRT and your increased health risks with HRT use.

❧

Managing Perimenopause

Today, more and more American women are seeking alternative approaches to HRT. Whether you are trying to ease hot flashes, manage mood swings or prevent heart disease, changing your diet, adding vitamin and mineral supplements and choosing helpful herbal remedies can make you feel better. While the list below is not all-encompassing, it highlights a few important strategies that can help ease perimenopausal symptoms. If you're looking for a more comprehensive guide to managing perimenopausal symptoms, pick up a copy of my book *The Ultimate Nutrition Guide for Menopause* (John Wiley and Sons, 2003).

DIETARY STRATEGIES

Trigger Foods

Eliminate foods in your diet that can worsen hot flashes, insomnia or mood swings. Caffeine-containing foods and beverages like coffee, tea, dark chocolate, colas, certain orange sodas and root beers affect hot flashes and the quality of your sleep. My first recommendation to clients wanting to cut down is to avoid caffeine in the afternoon.

Replace these beverages with caffeine-free or decaffeinated beverages like herbal tea, mineral water, fruit and vegetable juices or decaf coffee. Keep in mind that certain medications, including Midol®, Excedrin® and Anacin®, can pack a lot of caffeine.

Keep your alcohol intake to no more than one drink a day, preferably none when you're experiencing hot flashes or when you're under stress. Drinking alcoholic beverages can bring on a hot flash, interrupt your sleep and affect mood. To lessen alcohol's effect, try to drink alcohol with a meal. If you drink alcohol on an empty stomach, about 20 percent is absorbed directly across the walls of your stomach and reaches the brain within a minute, but when the stomach is full of food, alcohol has less chance of touching the walls and passing through, so the effect on your brain is delayed. When you're out socializing, drink no more than one drink every hour. Since the liver can't metabolize alcohol any faster than this, drinking slowly will ensure your blood alcohol concentration doesn't rise. To slow your pace, alternate one alcoholic drink with a non-alcoholic drink. One drink is equivalent to 5 ounces of wine, 12 ounces of beer, 10 ounces of wine cooler or 1.5 ounces of liquor.

If you are experiencing hot flashes, stay away from spicy foods. Many women complain that certain spices can trigger a hot flash.

Soy Foods and Isoflavones

Foods made from soybeans are getting plenty of attention these days. Studies have found that soy foods not only have the ability to protect from heart disease (read more about this in chapter 11, "Heart Disease and High Cholesterol"), but they may also help ease menopausal hot flashes. A twelve-week Italian study looked at the effects of soy protein on hot flashes in 104 women aged 48 to 61 years.[1] The study found that, compared to the placebo group, the women who consumed 60 grams of soy protein powder reported a 26 percent reduction in the average number of hot flashes by week three, and a 33 percent reduction by week four.

Soybeans contain naturally occurring compounds called isoflavones, a type of phyto or plant estrogen. Genistein and daidzein are the most active soy isoflavones and have been the focus of much research. Isoflavones have a similar structure to the hormone estrogen and, as a result, they have a weak estrogenic effect in the body. Even though isoflavones in soy are about 50 times less potent than estrogen, they are able to offer women a source of estrogen. When a woman's estrogen levels are low during perimenopause, a regular intake of foods like roasted soy nuts, soy beverages and tofu can help reduce hot flashes.

While it's true that a daily intake of soy has helped a number of my clients ease their hot flashes, studies don't find it to be a stupendously effective remedy. It tends to decrease the frequency and severity of hot flashes by 20 percent, a modest effect at best. Will a 20 percent improvement mean that much to your symptoms? It might and it might not. I meet many women in my practice who tell me that any improvement is welcome.

How much soy should you eat? The precise answer to this question has yet to be answered. Most experts believe that a daily intake of 40 to 80 milligrams of phyto-estrogens is probably needed to help alleviate hot flashes and reduce other health risks. See the Isoflavones in Soy Foods table on page 35 in chapter 1 to see how many phytoestrogens are found in common soy foods.

Wondering how to use soy foods? To get you started, try some of my suggestions below:

- Use a calcium-fortified soy beverage on cereal or in a breakfast smoothie.
- Use a calcium-fortified soy beverage in cooking and baking (e.g., soups, casseroles, muffins, pancake batters).
- Add canned soybeans to chili or soup.
- Cube firm tofu and add to soups—homemade or store bought.
- Grill firm tofu on the barbecue. First marinate tofu in balsamic vinegar or brush with hoisin sauce and then make tofu kebabs with vegetables.
- Substitute firm tofu for ricotta cheese in lasagna and cheesecake recipes.
- Use silken tofu in creamy salad dressing or dip recipes.
- Replace one-quarter of the all-purpose flour in a recipe with soy flour.
- Snack on roasted soy nuts—plain, barbecue, garlic or onion flavored.
- Add roasted soy nuts to a green salad.
- Replace ground meat with TVP (texturized vegetable protein) or veggie ground round in chili, pasta sauce and tacos.
- Try veggie burgers (with soy protein) and veggie dogs on the grill.

If you're having difficulty making soy foods a regular part of your diet, consider using a high-quality soy protein powder. Throw a scoop of soy protein powder into a homemade breakfast smoothie or a glass of orange juice. But keep in mind that soy protein powders vary in quality. Depending on how the manufacturer extracts the protein from the soybean, you can end up with little or a lot of isoflavones. Look for products made with isolated soy protein. Soy protein isolates are the purest form of soy protein—the protein is completely separated, or isolated, from the carbohydrate and fat portion of the soybean. Most are made using a water extraction process, which preserves the naturally occurring isoflavones.

My advice is to buy a product that's made with Supro® brand soy protein isolate. It's manufactured using an isoflavone-friendly process and it's also the soy protein isolate that's used in scientific studies. Products that use Supro® include Genisoy's protein powder, Twin Lab's Vege Fuel®, GNC's Challenge 95% ISP®, GNC's Challenge Soy Solution®, Nutrel's Soy Serenity® and Soy Strategy® and Naturade's Total Soy®.

Carbohydrates

If you're ever told that drinking a glass of warm milk can help you sleep, don't laugh. There is some science to back this home remedy. Carbohydrate-containing foods like milk, cereal or a slice of toast provide the brain with an amino acid called tryptophan. The brain uses tryptophan as a building block to manufacture a neurotransmitter called serotonin. And serotonin has been shown to facilitate sleep, improve mood, diminish pain and even reduce appetite.

Since I don't often recommend snacks after dinner, especially for clients who are trying to lose weight, this recommendation is not intended to make you gain weight. Eat something *small* or drink a glass of low-fat milk or soy beverage. Try it for a week. If your insomnia has not improved, look at other factors that may be disrupting sleep.

If you're feeling depressed or irritable, try a high-carbohydrate meal that contains very little protein. The more protein you eat, whether it's chicken, meat or fish, the more amino acids will be available to compete with tryptophan for entry into the brain. Remember that we want to let tryptophan into the brain so it can be used to produce serotonin. Try pasta with tomato sauce, a toasted whole-grain bagel with jam or a bowl of cereal with low-fat milk.

If you're suffering from fuzzy thinking, make sure your breakfast includes some carbohydrates—be sure to eat breakfast, period. Studies in both children and adults have shown that, compared to breakfast skippers, individuals who eat the morning meal score higher on tests of mental performance that morning. The speed of information retrieval, a component of memory, seems to be most affected by breakfast skipping.

Breakfast foods like cereal, fruit, yogurt and whole-grain toast supply carbohydrates, that, when converted to glucose in the bloodstream, the brain cells use for energy. After a night of sleeping we wake up with low blood-glucose levels that need to be replenished.

VITAMINS AND MINERALS

Vitamin B12 for Insomnia

Many studies have found that vitamin B12 promotes sleep, especially in people with sleep disorders. Researchers in Japan have used 1.5 to 3 milligrams of the vitamin each day to restore normal sleep patterns in patients.[2] Exactly how this B vitamin works is not completely understood. Some researchers believe it acts by working with melatonin, a hormone that's involved in maintaining the body's internal clock. It's thought that B12 may prevent disturbances in melatonin release.

The daily recommended intake for vitamin B12 for healthy women is 2.4 micrograms. Women over the age of 50 should get their B12 mainly by eating foods fortified with the vitamin, or by taking a supplement. This is because up to 30 percent of older adults have lost the ability to properly absorb naturally occurring B12 in foods. Vitamin B12 is found in all animal foods—meat, poultry, fish, eggs and dairy products. If you're eating these foods every day, chances are you are meeting your B12 needs. Foods fortified with the vitamin include soy beverages, rice beverages and breakfast cereals (but check labels to be sure).

If you fall into one of the following categories, I do recommend you take a B12 supplement:

- You're over 50 years of age.

- You're taking antacid medication for reflux or a stomach ulcer.

- You're a strict vegetarian who eats no animal foods.

Vitamin B12 supplements come in 500- or 1000-microgram sizes. To ensure you're meeting your requirements, I recommend 500 micrograms once a day, with a meal. Or you may choose to take a B complex supplement to ensure you are meeting your needs for all eight B vitamins.

Choline for Memory

Although not an official vitamin, choline is a member of the B vitamin family. It's found in egg yolks, organ meats and legumes, and it's used as a building block for a memory neurotransmitter called acetylcholine. Supplements of choline have been shown to enhance memory and reaction time in animals, particularly aging animals. Researchers believe that choline supplements will improve brain tasks only if you're deficient in the nutrient. Stress and aging can deplete choline levels.

While we don't yet know if supplemental choline will improve memory in people who have normal levels of choline, it's still important to get enough of this nutrient in your diet. Choline is needed in the diet because the amount synthesized by our body appears to be insufficient to meet our needs. Healthy women need 425 milligrams of choline each day. The best food sources are egg yolks, liver and other organ meats, brewer's yeast, wheat germ, soybeans, peanuts and green peas.

If you don't eat these foods regularly, you can get choline from lecithin supplements. The maximum safe limit is 3500 milligrams (3.5 grams) of choline a day. High doses of choline can cause low blood pressure and a fishy body odor in some people.

Iron for Heavy Periods

If you're experiencing heavy menstrual flow, it's extremely important to eat an iron-rich diet. Iron is used by red blood cells to form hemoglobin, the molecule that transports oxygen from your lungs to your cells. If your diet falls short on iron, or if your body loses iron faster than your diet can replace it, red blood cell levels drop and less oxygen is delivered to your tissues. Symptoms of iron deficiency include weakness, lethargy and fatigue upon exertion. Iron deficiency is a progressive condition, which means even if your iron stores aren't low enough to diagnose anemia, you can still be deficient and feel the symptoms.

While you're still menstruating, you need 18 milligrams of iron each day. Iron in food comes in two forms—heme iron and nonheme iron. Heme iron is the most efficiently absorbed and is found in red meat, chicken, eggs and fish. Nonheme iron comes from plant foods like whole grains, legumes (lentils, chickpeas, kidney beans), fruits and vegetables. The body has a harder time absorbing nonheme iron from foods. Eating foods rich in vitamin C with sources of nonheme iron will allow your body to absorb much more. If you include a little heme iron (i.e., meat) with your meal you'll also increase the absorption of nonheme iron. The best iron sources are lean beef, tofu, legumes, enriched breakfast cereals, whole-grain breads, raisins, dried apricots, prune juice, spinach and peas.

To help you get your daily 18 milligrams of iron, a multivitamin and mineral supplement is a wise idea. Most formulas provide 10 milligrams of iron, but you can find multivitamins that provide up to 18. If you're experiencing persistent heavy bleeding, the recommended daily intake might not be enough to meet your needs. Sometimes 100-milligram tablets of supplemental iron are recommended to rebuild your iron stores. Because these supplements are toxic in large doses, you should take iron pills only if your doctor has determined you have low iron levels. If you are advised to take an iron pill, take it on an empty stomach to enhance absorption. Take single iron supplements for one to three months and then have your blood retested by your doctor. Once your iron stores are replenished, discontinue your iron supplement. Many people find that taking their iron supplement before bed reduces stomach upset. Iron can be constipating, so I recommend you boost your fiber and water intake at this time.

If iron-deficiency anemia is diagnosed from a blood test, take a 100-milligram iron supplement two or three times a day after meals. After six to eight weeks your doctor will retest your blood to determine iron levels. Once iron supplements are discontinued, return to your multivitamin and mineral supplement.

HERBAL REMEDIES

Black Cohosh Root (*Cimicifuga racemosa*) for Hot Flashes

In Germany, this herb has been used for more than 40 years by more than 1.5 million women. Based on my clinical experience with clients and the findings from controlled scientific studies, black cohosh is definitely the most promising herbal remedy for treating menopausal hot flashes. In fact, many randomized controlled trials have found black cohosh to be just as effective as estrogen therapy at relieving flashes.[3] The advantage black cohosh offers is that it doesn't have the uncomfortable side effects associated with hormone therapy. And studies in the lab have found that black cohosh dramatically inhibits the growth of breast cancer cells, unlike estrogen, which promotes such cell growth.

Exactly how the herb works is currently under scientific debate. Researchers don't believe it acts like estrogen. Instead, black cohosh is thought to exert its effect by interacting with certain brain receptors. Black cohosh contains naturally occurring compounds called triterpene glycosides that are thought to be responsible for the plant's effect.

Buy a product that is standardized to contain 2.5 percent triterpene glycosides. Standardization means that each pill is guaranteed to give you a certain amount of the active ingredient. Take one 40-milligram tablet twice daily. The specific black cohosh that was used in virtually all of the scientific research is sold under the name Remifemin®. This product is sold as a 20-milligram tablet, since a recent study showed that a lower dose of the herb is equally effective. It may take up to four weeks for you to notice an effect. The only potential side effect that's been reported in a small number of women is mild stomach upset and headache. Black cohosh should not be used by pregnant or breastfeeding women.

Today there are many menopausal supplements sold in pharmacies and health food stores. These products combine a number of herbs known to ease a variety of perimenopausal symptoms. You might decide to give one of these products a try instead of taking black cohosh alone. One product relatively new to America is Kyolic® Estro-Logic™. This supplement contains standardized black cohosh, soy isoflavones and a number of other herbs supportive to menopause. A gynecologist, Dr. Kathleen Fry, and a medical herbalist, Claudia Wingo, developed it. The product is currently being studied in a trial of 100 menopausal women. Preliminary findings look promising. The herbal combination appears to be effective at easing a number of common menopausal complaints, including hot flashes. Other brands include Menopause Multiple and Menopause Formula.

Valerian (*Valeriana officinalis*) for Insomnia

This native North American plant acts like a mild sedative on the central nervous system. Valerian root makes getting to sleep easier and it increases deep sleep. Unlike popular prescribed sleeping pills, valerian does not lead to dependence or addiction. Nor does it cause a morning drug hangover. Scientists have learned that valerian promotes sleep by interacting with two brain receptors called GABA receptors and benzodiazepine receptors. Compared to drugs like Valium® and Xanax®, valerian binds very weakly to brain receptors.

In one double-blind study conducted in Germany, 44 percent of patients taking valerian root reported perfect sleep, and 89 percent reported improved sleep, compared to those taking the placebo pill.[4] Another small study found that individuals with mild insomnia who took 450 milligrams of valerian experienced a significant decrease in sleep problems. The same researchers studied 128 individuals and found that, compared to the placebo, 400 milligrams of valerian produced a significant improvement in sleep quality in people who considered themselves poor sleepers.[5]

Many experts attribute the herb's effect to essential oils in the root. Buy a product that is standardized to contain at least 0.5 percent essential oils or 0.8 percent *valerenic acid*. Take 400 to 900 milligrams in capsule or tablet form, 30 minutes to one hour before bedtime. If you wake up feeling groggy, reduce the dose. Don't expect results overnight. The herb works better when used over a period of time.

Do not take valerian with alcohol or sedative medications. The herb is not recommended for use during pregnancy and breastfeeding.

Kava Kava (*Piper methysticum*) for Anxiety

Anxiety is a mood change often reported by many perimenopausal women. It's described as a feeling of apprehension, uncertainty and fear. It's also associated with physical changes—an increased heart rate, sweating and even tremors. Anxiety can also cause insomnia, or make existing sleep problems worse.

Kava kava is a herb that is extracted from the roots of a South Pacific pepper plant. The use of kava dates back to the 18th century, when natives of Polynesia participated in kava drinking ceremonies to produce a soothing, relaxing effect without altering consciousness. Today, this herbal extract is used to calm the nerves without acting as a stimulant. In higher doses it's used as a sleeping aid.

Kava's active ingredients, called kavalactones, exert their effect by working on the limbic system of the brain, which is the center of our emotions. Research has deemed kava to be effective in the treatment of anxiety. One study found that menopausal women with anxiety disorders obtained significant relief with kava kava, without the negative side effects of traditional drugs like Valium®.

Buy a product that's standardized to contain 30 percent kavalactones. According to the research, this is the most effective extract. The doses of kava extracts used in the studies range from 60 to 120 milligrams of kavalactones. For most products, this translates into one to three tablets or capsules a day. Start with one standardized tablet. If you find this doesn't help your symptoms, increase the dose.

Kava can start working within one week, but it can take up to eight weeks for a maximum effect. Kava has a wide margin of safety. Side effects occur rarely and include mild stomach upset, headaches and dizziness. However, due to recent concerns from Europe that taking kava may cause liver damage, *consult your physician before starting kava.*

Ginkgo Biloba for Memory

This herb is touted to improve memory loss and slow the progression of Alzheimer's disease. Ginkgo's claims are very likely true. The most recent study to make news was a 52-week American trial conducted on 309 patients with mild to moderate dementia as a result of Alzheimer's disease or stroke.[6] Patients were given either 40 milligrams of ginkgo (a special standardized extract called EGb 761) or a placebo pill at each meal. After one year, the placebo group showed a decline in cognitive function whereas the ginkgo group did not show an overall decline. When the researchers looked at Alzheimer's patients only, there were modest but significant changes in memory and other brain functions.

Ginkgo may act in one of two ways to enhance memory. A number of studies suggest that ginkgo increases circulation and oxygen delivery to the brain. The herb's active ingredients make platelet blood cells less sticky, making circulation more efficient. Ginkgo also has a strong antioxidant effect in the brain—free radical damage to brain cells may be a contributing factor in Alzheimer's disease.

Although studies have not been done on perimenopausal women, I do recommend ginkgo to help reduce the effects of aging on brain cells. The active ingredients responsible for ginkgo's beneficial effects are called terpene lactones and ginkgo flavone glycosides. Guidelines for buying a top quality ginkgo supplement are as follows:

- Choose a product that is standardized to contain 24 percent ginkgo flavone glycosides and 6 percent terpene lactones.
- The EGb 761 extract used in the scientific research is sold as Ginkoba® in the United States and Canada.

The recommended daily dose is a 40-milligram tablet taken three times daily. On rare occasions, ginkgo may cause gastrointestinal upset, headache or an allergic skin reaction in susceptible individuals. Safety has not been established during pregnancy and breastfeeding. Ginkgo has a slight blood-thinning effect and the potential to enhance the effects of other blood-thinning medications (e.g., warfarin, aspirin). If you take blood thinners, let your doctor know if you start on ginkgo.

THE BOTTOM LINE....
Leslie's recommendations for managing perimenopause

Hot Flashes

1. Add one serving of soy food to your diet each day. Once you've found a few soy foods you like, ensure you're getting 40 milligrams of isoflavones each day.
2. Try a standardized extract of black cohosh root. Take 40 milligrams of the herb twice daily, morning and evening. If you want maximum effectiveness, take two 40-milligram tablets twice daily. Cut back to one if you experience stomach upset.
3. Consider taking a menopausal formula that contains a combination of herbs that have been shown to ease many symptoms. Kyolic® Estro-Logic™ contains standardized black cohosh, soy isoflavones and other supportive herbs. Other brands include Menopause Multiple and Menopause Formula.

Insomnia

1. To help you sleep soundly, cut back your caffeine intake to less than 200 milligrams per day. Aim for no more than seven alcoholic drinks a week. To lessen alcohol's effect on your brain, have your drink with food or a snack.
2. If you can't fall asleep at night, try a light carbohydrate-rich snack 30 minutes before bed to increase the level of serotonin in your brain.
3. Make sure you get enough B12 in your diet to help promote deep sleep. If you can't get enough B12 through food, or if you don't produce enough stomach acid for its absorption, take a B12 supplement of 500 micrograms or a B complex.
4. Consider taking 400 to 900 milligrams of valerian root extract. Buy a product standardized to contain at least 0.5 percent essential oils or 0.8 percent valerenic acid. Take the herb 30 to 60 minutes before going to bed.
5. Don't forget to investigate other possible causes of sleep disturbances: a lack of exercise, too much stress, or a possible medical problem. If you've tried everything you can and you still have fitful sleep, consult your family physician. Read chapter 6, "Insomnia," for more strategies to help you sleep.

Memory

1. Eat breakfast every day to provide your brain cells with their preferred fuel source—carbohydrate. To sustain your blood-glucose levels, make sure your breakfast has carbohydrates and protein.

2. To help your brain make more of the memory neurotransmitter acetylcholine, increase your intake of foods rich in choline, a fatlike B vitamin. Good sources are eggs, legumes and organ meats. If these foods aren't on your A list, consider taking a choline or lecithin supplement.

3. Even though it might not improve a healthy woman's short-term memory, a standardized extract of ginkgo biloba probably will protect your brain cells from the ravages of aging. Look for an extract that contains 24 percent ginkgo flavone glycosides. Take one 40 milligram tablet with breakfast, lunch and dinner.

Heavy Bleeding

1. If you experience heavy flow during your periods, increase your intake of iron-rich foods.

2. Make sure your multivitamin and mineral supplement has 15 to 18 milligrams of iron. At menopause, when you are no longer menstruating, switch to a regular formula that has no more than 8 milligrams of iron.

3. If heavy flow has plagued you for some time and your energy level is dragging, ask your family doctor to measure your iron level to determine if you have an iron deficiency. If you are diagnosed with iron-deficiency anemia, take a 100-milligram iron supplement two or three times a day after meals.

Once iron supplements are discontinued, return to your multivitamin and mineral supplement.

19

Polycystic Ovary Syndrome (PCOS)

Sometimes referred to as Stein-Leventhal syndrome, polycystic ovary syndrome (PCOS) is the most common cause of menstrual problems in women. The disorder affects as many as 10 percent of all premenopausal women, and many don't even know they have it. In the United States alone, it's estimated that as many as four million women suffer from PCOS. Furthermore, up to 10 percent of women with PCOS are infertile. PCOS also affects other body systems and is linked with a number of serious long-term health problems, including diabetes and heart disease.

For reasons not yet fully understood, women with PCOS produce unusually high levels of estrogen, luteinizing hormone and male hormones called androgens. This disrupts the normal menstrual cycle and encourages the formation of cysts in the ovaries, making PCOS one of the leading causes of infertility. The hormone imbalances observed in PCOS produce symptoms such as severe acne, excessive hair growth and obesity. There is no cure for PCOS and its treatment varies according to the symptoms.

What Causes PCOS?

Hormones are responsible for controlling many of your body's internal processes. These hormones are produced and regulated by an interrelated series of glands that make up your endocrine system. Two tiny glands located in the brain—the hypothalamus and the pituitary gland—are responsible for monitoring and balancing the normal activity of your endocrine system.

The pituitary gland helps control the cycles of the female reproductive system. This gland secretes luteinizing hormone (LH), which stimulates your ovaries to release mature eggs and to produce the female sex hormones estrogen and progesterone. LH is also necessary for the production of androgens, male sex hormones that are present in small quantities in every woman. PCOS is thought to develop when the pituitary gland malfunctions and secretes an overabundance of luteinizing hormone. The abnormally high level of LH triggers an increase in the production of androgens, which results in a corresponding increase in estrogen levels. PCOS causes the production of these three hormones to remain at high levels, disrupting the natural hormonal balance of the menstrual cycle.

PCOS usually develops during puberty at the time when menstruation would normally begin. The elevated level of LH in the bloodstream interferes with the normal functioning of the ovaries. The excess hormones prevent eggs from maturing properly, which often results in failure to ovulate, called anovulation. Anovulation will prevent or delay the onset of menstruation in young girls and may cause mature women to experience irregular periods or to miss a period altogether. PCOS can also cause heavy vaginal bleeding that can lead to iron-deficiency anemia. Because the majority of women with PCOS don't ovulate, this disorder causes infertility in many women.

The hormonal imbalance seen in women with PCOS also causes cysts or fluid-filled sacs to accumulate in the ovaries. These cysts are eggs that have matured but, due to abnormal hormone levels, were never released. Polycystic (meaning "many cysts") ovaries are covered with a tough, thick outer layer and may grow to become as much as two to five times larger than normal. These cysts interfere with the activity of the ovaries and contribute to the infertility problems associated with PCOS.

While the hormonal abnormalities and symptoms resulting from PCOS are well documented, the exact cause of the disorder is still unknown. It is thought that a susceptibility to PCOS may be inherited, but at this time there is not enough evidence to prove a genetic link to the disease.

↯

Symptoms and Associated Medical Conditions

The symptoms of PCOS are physically debilitating and often psychologically damaging. Although the syndrome affects each woman a little differently, the primary symptoms include

- infertility
- abnormal, irregular or absent periods
- mood swings
- weight problems or obesity
- high blood pressure
- increased hair growth (hirsutism)
- male-pattern baldness
- aggravated acne
- heavy, persistent vaginal bleeding
- iron-deficiency anemia

In addition to infertility, women with PCOS face other reproductive concerns. Approximately one-third of all pregnancies in women with the condition end in miscarriage. There's also an increased risk of pregnancy disorders such as preeclampsia, gestational diabetes, premature labor and stillbirth. The reproductive problems that plague women suffering from PCOS make it one of the most heartbreaking and frustrating medical disorders.

PCOS disrupts normal physical development by stimulating the production of higher levels of androgens, or male hormones. This causes some women to acquire secondary male characteristics such as frontal balding, deepening of the voice and increased muscle mass. One of the most common symptoms in women with PCOS is hirsutism, a condition that causes body and facial hair to follow a male growth pattern. Women with hirsutism grow excessive amounts of coarse hair on their face, legs, chest and groin. Studies have shown that hirsutism causes high levels of stress and frequent bouts of depression in women.

Obesity is another serious complication that affects nearly 50 percent of all women with PCOS. Obesity contributes to the already high levels of estrogen associated with this disorder. Androgens are converted to estrogen in body fat, and the greater the amount of body fat a woman has, the higher the level of estrogen. Excess estrogen in the bloodstream can trigger severe acne and has been associated with increased risk of endometrial, ovarian and breast cancer.

PCOS is a disorder that progresses fairly slowly, but unfortunately the symptoms tend to worsen over time. Studies suggest that there may be racial differences in PCOS symptoms. In North America a large percentage of women with PCOS are obese and develop hirsutism. On the other hand, only 10 to 20 percent of Asian women with PCOS develop hirsutism, and obesity is not a commonly seen symptom. Scientists have not been able to determine why symptoms vary in women with PCOS.

Research indicates that women with PCOS have a higher risk of developing insulin resistance, a condition that is further aggravated by obesity. Insulin is a hormone secreted by your pancreas. By attaching to special receptors on your cells, insulin promotes your cells to take in and store glucose and protein, the nutrients your body needs to function and produce energy. Unfortunately, insulin activity can break down as a result of insulin resistance. Insulin resistance is caused by defective insulin receptors to which insulin cannot attach properly. As a result, insulin is not able to do its job properly and glucose sugar is unable to enter the cells, where it is needed for energy.

Insulin resistance causes a high level of insulin to remain in the bloodstream, causing hyperinsulinemia. These high insulin levels can lead to diabetes and heart disease. In fact, studies indicate that women with PCOS have at least seven times the risk of heart attack compared to other women. Many women with PCOS and insulin resistance have high blood pressure, low levels of good HDL cholesterol and high levels of blood triglycerides, a type of blood fat implicated in the development of heart disease. High blood insulin can also cause weight gain, since the body will try protecting itself by turning excess insulin into fat.

Most women with PCOS have some degree of insulin resistance and many go on to develop glucose intolerance or full-blown diabetes. It's been estimated that by the age of 40, as many as 40 percent of women with PCOS will have type 2 diabetes or impaired glucose tolerance. It is becoming more evident that insulin resistance plays a very important role in both the cause and symptoms of PCOS. Treatment directed at reducing insulin resistance can restore ovulation, decrease the levels of male hormones, lower triglycerides and elevated blood pressure and promote weight loss.

❧

Who's at Risk?

Women can develop PCOS as early as their pre-teens, or it may appear at any time throughout their childbearing years. Most women, however, begin to experience symptoms at menarche, the onset of menstruation. PCOS becomes less common as women get older and rarely develops after menopause. But the health consequences of the disorder, such as diabetes resulting from insulin resistance, persist into the menopausal years.

Many women with PCOS have a close female relative with similar symptoms, so there is some indication that it is an inherited condition.

❧

Diagnosis

There is no single test for PCOS. A preliminary diagnosis will usually be made on the basis of symptoms. Identifying PCOS is often very difficult since the symptoms can vary significantly from woman to woman. To diagnose the condition, your physician will normally begin with a full physical exam and a medical history. He or she will be looking for signs such as menstrual irregularities and the presence of male characteristics such as hirsutism, balding and acne.

Blood tests will be performed to check for excessive levels of androgens, estrogen and luteinizing hormone. An ultrasound may be suggested to look for polycystic ovaries. However, it is important to keep in mind that close to one-quarter of women who don't have PCOS show evidence of cysts in their ovaries. Enlarged ovaries may be a symptom of another medical disorder, so ultrasound results are not considered to be true indicators of PCOS. Blood-screening tests for cholesterol, glucose and insulin may also be required to determine the full extent of PCOS-related health risks.

⟳

Conventional Treatment

Since PCOS has no cure, treatment is usually directed at managing the primary symptoms, especially hirsutism, menstrual irregularities and infertility. The choice of treatment will depend on the type and severity of your symptoms, your age and your plans regarding pregnancy.

If you are not planning to become pregnant, taking an oral contraceptive can control menstrual irregularities. Birth control pills inhibit the production and activity of androgens. Oral contraceptives are not recommended for menopausal women or for women with risk factors for certain heart or blood diseases.

By limiting the secretion of androgens, oral contraceptives can help to control other PCOS symptoms. They often reduce acne, lower the risks of ovarian and endometrial cancer and slow hair growth for women with hirsutism. Anti-androgen drugs—e.g., spironolactone, Aldactone®—are also effective in reducing growth of unwanted hair. To further minimize the effects of hirsutism, many women remove excessive hair by shaving, waxing, using depilatories or electrolysis.

If you do plan to have children, the treatment of choice is usually a fertility drug called Clomid® (clomiphene citrate). Clomiphene is effective in stimulating the ovaries to release eggs. Studies indicate that 80 percent of women with PCOS ovulate in response to clomiphene. Unfortunately, only 50 percent of these women become pregnant. If clomiphene does not work well for you, your physician may try to induce ovulation with a variety of hormone supplements, including follicle-stimulating hormone (FSH) and gonadotropin-releasing hormone (GnRH) drugs such as Lupron® (leuprolide) and Synarel® (nafarelin).

Once you have explored all of your treatment options, you may consider undergoing surgery to remove a wedge of your ovary. In the past, this procedure was a standard treatment for infertility caused by PCOS. Today surgery is a last-resort treatment choice, since it can cause scar tissue to form in your pelvis, further reducing your chance of becoming pregnant.

To lower health risks such as diabetes and heart disease, your doctor may prescribe an insulin-sensitizing drug to decrease insulin resistance (e.g., Metformin®, Avandia®). These medications have the added benefit of reducing androgen production and restoring normal menstrual cycles.

While medications such as the ones discussed above do have proven benefits, don't overlook one of the simplest and most effective methods of treating PCOS: weight loss. Obesity aggravates most of the symptoms of PCOS and is an overall health risk all by itself. If you are overweight or obese and you make an effort to lose weight through a program of diet and exercise, you will reduce your insulin resistance, lower the secretion of androgens and lower your estrogen levels. This may help eliminate excessive hair growth, restore regular menstrual periods and improve your chances of becoming pregnant, as well as improving your overall health and well-being.

At present, PCOS is treated on a symptom-by-symptom basis by medication, dietary changes and exercise. Researchers are continuing to investigate both the causes of this syndrome and improved treatment options. If you have PCOS, the changes I list below may help you manage your condition so that you can lead a healthier and more satisfying life.

❧

Managing PCOS

DIETARY STRATEGIES

Weight Loss

Obesity is present in 44 percent of women with PCOS. As I told you earlier in this chapter, being overweight worsens the symptoms of PCOS by increasing insulin resistance and further elevating levels of male hormones. Because of this, weight loss is one of the main goals of treatment for PCOS. In fact, studies find that losing more than 5 percent of body weight can restore fertility in obese women with PCOS.[1] For a woman who weighs 180 pounds, this means losing at least 9 pounds—very do-able!

I strongly recommend that you consult with a registered dietitian to help you lose weight safely and effectively. To find a private practice dietitian in your community check out **www.eatright.org**. Working one-on-one with an expert means you will get an eating plan that is customized to your schedule and food preferences. Regular follow-up visits allow you to monitor your progress, adjust your plan as needed and discuss ways to overcome challenges and potential obstacles to success. I see many women in my private practice with PCOS who successfully lose weight. See my weight-loss tips in chapter 2 to help you get started, and pay special attention to the following:

1. *Reduce your portions of carbohydrate-containing foods.* Low-carbohydrate diets are recommended with PCOS. Eating smaller portions of carbohydrates not only reduces your calorie intake, it also helps to reduce high levels of blood insulin. That's because, once digested into glucose units, carbohydrate foods trigger the release of insulin in the bloodstream. But don't give up all carbohydrate-containing foods. I do not recommend diets like Dr. Atkin's or Protein Power, where followers are told to avoid all starch, fruit and milk products. Over the long run this is not healthy, nor is it sustainable.

2. *Get rid of excess sugar—natural and refined.* Too much sugar in the diet contributes to high blood triglyceride levels, something that a number of women with PCOS show on blood tests.

Low Glycemic Carbohydrates

Unfortunately, insulin resistance makes weight loss more difficult to achieve. To help improve insulin resistance and lower blood insulin levels it is important to eat smaller portions of carbohydrate-rich foods *and* choose the right types of carbohydrate foods. When you eat a carbohydrate-rich food, whether it's pasta, yogurt, an apple or fruit juice, the carbohydrate is broken down into glucose and absorbed into your bloodstream. Your blood sugar rises, and this tells your pancreas to release insulin into the blood. Insulin then clears sugar from your blood, taking it into your cells, where it's used for energy. If you have insulin resistance, insulin cannot perform this task properly. Some sugar remains in the blood, causing more insulin to be released. This can result in a chronically high insulin level.

You're probably wondering what the type of carbohydrate food has to do with it all. Well, it turns out that carbohydrate foods are digested and absorbed at different rates. Some foods are digested slowly and result in a steady, slow rise in blood sugar. That means that less insulin will be secreted into the blood. Slow carbohydrates have what is called a low glycemic index. Foods with a high glycemic index are digested and absorbed more quickly and cause much higher insulin levels.

It's probably obvious by now that your meals and snacks should emphasize foods with a low glycemic index (for a list of foods ranked by their glycemic index value, see page 97 in chapter 5, "Hypoglycemia"). Use the chart below to help you replace higher glycemic carbohydrates with lower glycemic ones.

HIGH GLYCEMIC FOOD	LOW GLYCEMIC FOOD
Bread, white or whole-wheat	Whole-grain pumpernickel, whole-grain rye sourdough
Most processed breakfast cereals (Corn Flakes, Puffed Rice, Special K)	100% bran (All-Bran, Bran Buds), Mueslix, oatmeal
Instant rice	Brown rice, basmati rice
Mashed potato	Pasta or beans or sweet potatoes
Bananas	Apples, oranges, peaches, nectarines
Snack foods: crackers, cookies, chips	Low-fat smoothie, yogurt, milk, latte, dried apricots, fruit (as above), popcorn

VITAMINS AND MINERALS

Calcium and Vitamin D

Women who take gonadotropin-releasing hormone (GnRH) drugs—e.g., Lupron® (leuprolide), Synarel® (nafarelin)—to improve PCOS symptoms should know that these drugs cause accelerated bone loss, which may be partially irreversible. These drugs work by causing a deficiency of estrogen; estrogen prevents bone cells from releasing calcium from the bone into the bloodstream, and causes calcitonin and vitamin D to be released, stimulating new bone growth to occur.

A six-month Italian study of 44 women with PCOS showed that women receiving such a medication experienced a significant decrease in bone density.[2] Women given the drug in combination with the anti-androgen drug spironolactone did not show any change in bone density. It seems that spironolactone offers a bone-sparing effect in this situation. Indeed, your doctor may prescribe another medication along with a GnRH drug to offset the bone loss. The jury is still out on whether some of these drug combinations, called addback regimens, actually prevent bone loss.

If you are taking a GnRH drug, meet your daily recommended intakes for calcium and vitamin D, two nutrients critical for bone health. This is important to help minimize bone loss. See the RDA tables on pages 13 and 16 in chapter 1 to see how much you need every day. Use the tables in chapter 1 to help you boost your intake of these nutrients from foods. Unfortunately, there are only a few good food sources of vitamin D. We meet the majority of our vitamin D requirements by exposing our skin to sunlight during the summer months.

Calcium and Vitamin D Supplements

If you are not meeting your daily targets for calcium and vitamin D through your diet, I strongly recommend that you take a supplement. If you take a multivitamin and mineral supplement it should have 400 IU of vitamin D in it (most brands do). But calcium is a large mineral and manufacturers can't fit very much in a multivitamin and mineral pill. For this reason you have to rely on a separate calcium supplement. Here are a few guidelines to help you choose among a multitude of products:

- If you consume at least three to four servings of dairy products or calcium-fortified beverages each day, you're getting approximately 900 to 1200 milligrams of calcium. For every serving you're missing and not making up with other calcium-rich foods, consider taking a 300 milligram calcium supplement.

- When choosing a supplement look at the source of calcium. Studies show that calcium citrate supplements are better absorbed than those made from calcium carbonate. This is an important consideration if you're over 50 years old or you take medication that blocks the production of stomach acid, as calcium carbonate supplements require more stomach acid for absorption.

- Check the ingredient list to see how much elemental calcium each pill gives you. This is what you base your daily dose on.

- Choose a formula with vitamin D and magnesium, two nutrients that work with calcium to keep bones healthy.

- Spread larger doses throughout the day. If you must take more than 500 milligrams from a supplement, split your dose over two or three meals.

- The daily safe upper limit is 2500 milligrams of calcium from food and supplements combined. Too much calcium may cause constipation, gas and kidney stones in people with a history of the disease.

Chromium

Chromium is needed by the body to make glucose tolerance factor (GTF), which researchers believe increases insulin receptor sensitivity and enhances glucose uptake by cells to maintain normal blood-sugar levels. In a nutshell, chromium, as a critical component of GTF, helps insulin work properly. With adequate amounts of chromium present, your body uses less insulin to do its job. A deficiency of chromium causes impaired glucose tolerance, increased cholesterol and triglyceride levels and decreased good HDL cholesterol levels. And if you work out a lot, you might want to know that heavy exercise causes chromium to be excreted from the body. Studies suggest that, when taken as a supplement, chromium can help reduce high blood cholesterol and triglycerides, and stabilize blood-sugar levels.

Healthy adult women need to consume 25 micrograms of chromium each day. Good food sources include apples with the skin, green peas, chicken breast, refried beans, mushrooms, oysters, wheat germ and brewer's yeast. Processed foods and refined, white starchy foods like bread, rice and pasta, sugar and sweets all contain very little chromium. So if you're a runner who loads up on white bagels, regular pasta and white rice you're probably falling short on chromium.

If you're concerned you're not getting chromium through food, check your multivitamin and mineral supplement to see how much it contains. If it's less than 25 micrograms, you can always consider taking a separate 200-microgram supplement each day. Studies show that chromium picinolate is absorbed more easily than other forms like chromium chloride and chromium nicotinate. At this time, chromium picinolate is available in the United States but not in Canada. Chromium supplements are extremely safe.

HERBAL REMEDIES

Ginseng

In the Orient, this herbal remedy has been used to treat diabetes for centuries, and current research suggests it may help regulate blood sugar even if you don't have full-blown diabetes. Animal studies have shown that the herb enhances the release of insulin from the pancreas and increases the body's sensitivity to insulin. In doing so, ginseng may be able to maintain more stable blood-sugar levels.

A Finnish study investigated the effect of 100 and 200 milligrams of Panax ginseng on blood-sugar control in 36 people with type 2 diabetes—adult onset diabetes that does not require insulin.[3] After eight weeks, both doses of ginseng reduced fasting blood sugar, which is the amount of sugar in the bloodstream after 12 hours of not consuming any foods or beverages. The 200-milligram dose improved glycosylated hemoglobin levels, a measure of long-term blood-sugar control. The researchers concluded that ginseng might indeed be a useful adjunct in the management of type 2 diabetes.

More recently, Toronto researchers at St. Michael's Hospital found that ginseng can help improve blood-sugar control in people with and without diabetes.[4] The researchers gave study participants two 3-gram doses of American ginseng: the first dose was given 40 minutes before consuming 25 grams of sugar (glucose); the second dose was given during this 25-gram sugar challenge. After the sugar challenge, blood-glucose levels were measured every 15 to 30 minutes for up to 2 hours. In people with diabetes, ginseng significantly lowered blood sugar, whether it was given before or during the 25 gram sugar challenge. In non-diabetics, ginseng had no effect on blood sugar when given during the challenge, but did significantly lower blood-sugar levels 45 and 60 minutes after the challenge.

Two types of ginseng are recommended:

1. *Asian (Panax) ginseng* Scientific research has focused mainly on ginseng extracts standardized to contain 4 to 7 percent ginsenosides. Ginsenosides are believed to be the main active ingredients in the ginseng root. When buying a ginseng supplement, look for a statement of standardization and G115 on the label. G115 indicates that the product contains the specific Rg1 and Rb1 extract used in research.

The usual dosage of a standardized extract is 100 or 200 milligrams once daily. I strongly recommend that you buy a standardized extract. It offers you a guarantee that the product is, in fact, ginseng and that it contains a certain amount of the active ingredients. If you take the whole root, which is very expensive, use 1 to 3 grams of the dried root in the form of a tea. People usually take ginseng for periods of from three weeks to three months. Take a two-week break between courses of ginseng.

2. *American (Canadian) ginseng* For healthy young people, the standard dose is 0.25 to 0.5 grams of the root two times daily as a tea. If you are buying a standardized extract, look for a product that contains 4 percent ginsenosides. Follow the manufacturer's directions.

Ginseng is relatively safe at the doses recommended above. In some people, taking the herb may cause mild stomach upset, irritability and insomnia. To avoid overstimulation, start with 100 milligrams a day and avoid taking the herb with caffeine. Ginseng should not be used during pregnancy or breastfeeding, or in individuals with uncontrolled high blood pressure. And there have been a few case reports of spotting in postmenopausal women. If you experience this side effect, stop taking the herb; if spotting continues, consult your physician.

If you are taking a medication to help improve your insulin resistance, be sure to let your physician and pharmacist know before you start on ginseng. Your blood glucose levels should be monitored in order to prevent potential low-blood-sugar reactions (hypoglycemia). Taking ginseng with a meal will also help offset a potential low-blood-sugar reaction.

OTHER NATURAL HEALTH PRODUCTS

Ipriflavone
When it comes to preventing medication-induced bone loss, ipriflavone is a supplement you might consider taking. In a double-blind study ipriflavone taken in combination with calcium prevented loss of bone density in women taking Lupron® (leuprolide).[5] Research suggests that ipriflavone, taken alone or with calcium, is more

effective at maintaining bone density than calcium alone. Studies show that ipriflavone enhances the effects of calcium and vitamin D in preventing osteoporosis.

Ipriflavone is a semi-synthetic isoflavone that is manufactured from daidzein, a natural chemical found in soybeans. (If you read my chapters on menopause or heart disease, you'll learn plenty about soy isoflavones.) Ipriflavone enhances the action of cells that build bone and inhibits the activity of cells that break down bone.

Based on the research showing the effectiveness of ipriflavone on preventing bone loss, you might consider looking for a calcium supplement that has added ipriflavone. Look for a supplement that contains a branded form of ipriflavone called Ostivone™, a high-quality extract of ipriflavone used in clinical research.

The standard dose is 200 milligrams three times daily taken with food. Choose a product that has other nutrients important for bone health, including calcium, vitamin D, magnesium and vitamin C. Such a supplement can replace your standard calcium pill. Brand names of calcium supplements with Ostivone™ include Rx-Bone Ostivone, Bone Renew and Bone Protector. (To learn more about the role these nutrients play in bone health read chapter 10, "Osteoporosis.") Side effects are uncommon but may include stomach upset, diarrhea and dizziness.

Women with hormone-sensitive health conditions, such as breast, uterine and ovarian cancer, endometriosis and uterine fibroids, should seek the advice of a physician, as ipriflavone may potentiate some effects of estrogen. As with many natural health products, women with liver and kidney disease should use the supplement with caution—inform your healthcare practitioner if you start taking ipriflavone.

Inositol

Although not an official vitamin, this natural compound is closely related to the B vitamin family. Inositol is found in foods mainly as phytic acid, a fibrous compound. Good sources include citrus fruits, whole grains, legumes, nuts and seeds. When you eat these foods, bacteria in your intestine liberate inositol from phytic acid.

Once in the body, inositol is an essential component of cell membranes. It promotes the export of fat from cells in the liver and intestine. Supplements of inositol are thought to improve insulin sensitivity and have therefore been used to treat symptoms of PCOS. In one study of 44 obese women, 1200 milligrams of inositol taken once daily for six to eight weeks decreased blood triglycerides and testosterone levels, reduced blood pressure and caused ovulation.[6] Previous studies suggest that people with insulin resistance and type 2 diabetes might be deficient in inositol.

Inositol supplements are hard to find since few companies manufacture them. In the United States, I have found the following products readily available:

- Inositol tablets (Puritan's Pride): 650 milligrams inositol per tablet
- Inositol powder (Puritan's Pride, Source Naturals): 600 milligrams per 1/4 teaspoon (mix into water)
- IP6 Powder (Jarrow Formulas): 1 scoop contains 1.2 grams of inositol

Based on research conducted in women with PCOS, a dose of 1200 milligrams taken once daily is warranted. No adverse effects have been reported. Some brands have added chromium.

THE BOTTOM LINE...
Leslie's recommendations for managing polycystic ovary syndrome (PCOS)

1. If you are overweight, embark on a weight-loss program. Losing weight is a cornerstone in the management of PCOS. Enlist the help of a professional. Contact the American Dietetic Association (**www.eatright.org**) for a referral to a nutritionist in your community.

   - To get you started losing weight, practice my tips in chapter 2. Remember that portion size counts, whether a food is fat-free or not!

   - Follow a diet that is low in carbohydrates, but do not eliminate all carbohydrate foods. This will help women with insulin resistance lose weight more effectively.

2. Choose low glycemic index carbohydrate foods.

3. Increase your intake of calcium and vitamin D, especially if you are taking a gonadotropin-releasing hormone drug such as Lupron® or Synarel®. These medications promote an estrogen deficiency that can cause bone loss.

4. Buy a calcium supplement that contains ipriflavone, a synthetic isoflavone manufactured from a natural compound found in soybeans. Take 150 to 200 milligrams three times daily. Choose a product that contains a high-quality form of ipriflavone called Ostivone™.

5. Consider taking a 200-microgram chromium supplement if you have insulin resistance.

6. Consider supplementing your daily diet with 1200 milligrams of inositol, a relative of the B vitamins.

7. Instead of chromium and inositol, you might consider taking the herbal remedy ginseng to help improve insulin sensitivity and blood-sugar levels. Start by taking 100 milligrams of Asian ginseng once daily. Look for a product that has the G115 statement on the label.

20
Thyroid Disease

There are more than 20 million Americans with thyroid disease and most are unaware they have the disease. Your thyroid gland is a tiny, butterfly-shaped gland that's located in front of your windpipe. While it weighs only an ounce, this gland is the command center for many organs in your body, including your heart, brain and liver. As such, the thyroid gland is responsible for regulating metabolism and cell growth. The symptoms of thyroid disorders are often difficult to read, for both the woman affected and her physician. In fact, many women don't even know they have a thyroid problem. If left untreated, thyroid disease can cause serious health problems.

Thyroid disease affects the production of thyroid hormones. Hypothyroidism results from an underactive gland that produces insufficient thyroid hormones. In hyperthyroidism, the opposite is true. As you will read below, each disorder has unique causes, symptoms and treatments.

ଏ

Hypothyroidism

Hypothyroidism develops when your thyroid gland does not produce enough thyroid hormones to meet your body's needs. An underactive thyroid gland will cause your metabolic rate to slow down, making you feel slow, sluggish and constantly tired. Thyroid deficiencies have also been known to cause infertility or miscarriages in early pregnancy.

Hypothyroidism affects ten times more women than men. It usually strikes after age 40 and is common in elderly women. Hypothyroidism usually develops when your body's immune system malfunctions, causing damage to the thyroid gland. It can also occur after treatment for hyperthyroidism, an overactive thyroid. In most cases, hypothyroidism is a permanent condition that requires lifelong treatment with thyroid hormone drugs.

WHAT CAUSES HYPOTHYROIDISM?

The thyroid gland is a small organ with a big job. Located in your neck, just below your Adam's apple, the thyroid controls and coordinates your body's main body functions, or metabolism. It produces two thyroid hormones, thyroxine (T4) and triiodothyronine (T3), which circulate through your bloodstream and act on almost every organ in your body. These hormones maintain a healthy metabolic rate by controlling the speed at which your body burns calories to use energy.

A well-functioning thyroid gland is essential to normal growth and development. If your thyroid does not produce enough thyroid hormones, all your bodily functions will slow down. You will begin to feel sluggish and tired and may develop a variety of other uncomfortable symptoms. As the condition becomes more advanced, you could experience serious health problems.

The most common type of hypothyroidism is known as Hashimoto's thyroiditis or chronic thyroiditis. It is an auto-immune disease, caused by a malfunction of your immune system. In this case, the immune system begins to produce anti-thyroid antibodies that attack your thyroid gland. The damage caused by these antibodies prevents the thyroid from producing adequate levels of thyroid hormones. People with Hashimoto's thyroiditis often develop a painless thyroid lump or goiter that can be seen at the lower front of their throat.

Hypothyroidism can also be caused by

- surgery to remove the thyroid gland (usually a treatment for thyroid cancer, in some cases for overactive thyroid)
- radioactive iodine therapy (usually used to treat overactive thyroid conditions)

- x-rays, especially of the head and neck
- treatment with certain medications, such as lithium
- obesity
- pregnancy and postpartum conditions
- iodine deficiencies
- absence of a thyroid gland at birth (all babies in the United States are screened for hypothyroidism to detect this condition)
- having a genetic predisposition

Another version of the disorder, known as secondary hypothyroidism, may develop if you have an abnormality in an area of your brain called the hypothalamic-pituitary axis. The pituitary gland helps the thyroid gland regulate the production of T3 and T4 by releasing thyroid-stimulating hormone (TSH). The hypothalamus gland performs a similar function by producing thyrotropin-releasing hormone (TRH). If these two glands do not secrete enough hormones to trigger your thyroid gland to function, you may experience the hormonal deficiencies that lead to hypothyroidism.

SYMPTOMS

The symptoms of hypothyroidism vary in severity, depending on the decrease in thyroid hormone levels and the length of time that a deficiency has been present. Most of the time, the symptoms are fairly mild. In the early stages of the disorder, symptoms may not be noticeable at all and you may still feel quite well. However, research indicates that people with mild hypothyroidism go on to develop more severe thyroid problems in later years.

When you have more severe hypothyroidism, you may begin to feel slow, sluggish, tired and run down. You may also feel depressed and lose interest in your normal activities. Additional hypothyroid symptoms include

- increased sensitivity to cold
- muscle swelling or cramps, especially in your arms and legs
- weight gain
- dry, itchy skin

- constipation

- increased menstrual flow

- tingling or numbness in your hands and feet

- coarseness or loss of hair

- memory loss and mental impairment

- infertility or miscarriages

- a slow heart rate

- dull facial expression, droopy eyelids and hoarse voice

- high blood pressure

Naturally, you won't develop all of these symptoms, but you can certainly expect to experience some of them. Because hypothyroidism progresses gradually, worsening over a period of months or years, you may not even realize how unwell you feel until your thyroid condition is corrected with hormone medication.

WHO'S AT RISK?

Hypothyroidism is a fairly common condition that affects almost 5 percent of the population. More than 5 million Americans have an underactive thyroid gland. Although thyroid disease can affect anyone, statistics indicate that hypothyroidism is 10 times more common in women than in men. This comes as no surprise, since research has shown that 75 percent of all auto-immune diseases occur in women. To underline the high prevalence of this disease in women, consider the fact that Hashimoto's thyroiditis, the most common form of hypothyroidism, strikes women as much as 50 times more often than men.

The risk of hypothyroidism increases considerably as you age. The condition is so common in postmenopausal women that up to 10 percent of women over the age of 65 show evidence of hypothyroidism.

It also seems that auto-immune diseases, such as Hashimoto's thyroiditis, have been associated with a genetic component. Research indicates that this particular type of hypothyroidism clusters in families, so your risk may be greater if you have a close female relative with a related auto-immune disease.

Some women also develop thyroid conditions during or immediately after pregnancy. Some type of thyroid dysfunction complicates approximately 5 to 9 percent of all pregnancies. Thyroiditis is especially common during the period of time following the birth of the baby, when the condition can often be confused with postpartum depression.

For reasons that are still unknown, one out of every 4000 infants is born without a working thyroid gland, a condition known as congenital hypothyroidism. If undetected, this disorder can cause mental retardation and serious growth defects. Fortunately, it has been virtually eliminated in North America, where all babies are tested for the condition at birth.

If you have had surgery or received radioactive iodine therapy to treat thyroid conditions such as hyperthyroidism, Graves' disease or thyroid cancer, then you may be predisposed to hypothyroidism. Irradiation of the head and neck through x-rays or cancer treatment may also predispose you to thyroid problems.

In countries outside of North America, one of the most common causes of hypothyroidism is iodine deficiency. Tiny amounts of this mineral are essential components of the thyroid hormones, and the thyroid gland cannot function properly without them. People who do not have access to natural sources of iodine in their diet, such as fish and other seafood, are at high risk of developing thyroid disorders. In North America, the problem has been virtually eliminated because iodine has been added to our table salt. However, other countries have not yet addressed this issue and iodine deficiency continues to be one of the world's most pressing health problems.

DIAGNOSIS

Current tests for thyroid disorders are quite sensitive and precise, making it possible to get a very accurate diagnosis of hypothyroidism. If your doctor suspects that your symptoms are caused by an underactive thyroid gland, he or she will order blood tests to confirm the diagnosis. One test will measure the level of T4 in your blood; if you have hypothyroidism, the T4 levels will be low. When your condition is mild, however, it's possible that your blood levels of both T4 and T3 could measure in the normal range. In that case, you may be tested for the level of TSH in your blood—a high TSH level will confirm the diagnosis of thyroid failure.

Sometimes, an additional test may be necessary to detect the presence of antithyroid antibodies in your blood. This will help your doctor determine if your hypothyroidism is caused by the immune condition Hashimoto's thyroiditis. Elderly people may also undergo further laboratory testing to find out if the thyroid condition is putting extra stress on the heart or raising blood pressure or cholesterol levels.

CONVENTIONAL TREATMENT

In most cases, hypothyroidism is a permanent condition that requires a lifetime of treatment. The goal of treatment is to provide your body with enough thyroid hormones to maintain an efficient metabolic rate. At present, the prescription of a thyroid supplement is the only effective treatment for this disorder. The supplement is usually a form of synthetic T4 that is taken daily as a small pill. Although the supplements contain only T4, the various organs in your body can convert the hormone into the more powerful T3 as needed.

There are also some thyroid supplements that are made from hormones extracted from animal thyroids. These are not often prescribed today because their potency levels are not consistent. They also contain T3, which can cause heart problems, especially in older people or those with heart conditions.

Your doctor will determine your daily dosage of thyroid replacement hormones, depending on your age, sex, weight, thyroid function and other medications. Usually, you will start with a low dose and increase it gradually until your blood levels of T4 and TSH are within normal range. Hypothyroidism is an on-going process and your dosage may change as your thyroid function continues to deteriorate. Regular blood tests will help your doctor adjust your thyroid hormone medication to suit your needs. If you become pregnant, the dose may need to be increased. Older people need less thyroxine, so your dosage may be lowered as you age. Once your medication levels have been properly adjusted, you should feel energetic, healthy and symptom-free. You should be able to resume a completely normal life.

↶

Graves' Disease (Graves' Hyperthyroidism)

Graves' disease is an auto-immune condition that's caused by an overactive thyroid gland. It occurs approximately five times more often in women than in men and is considered to be the most common cause of hyperthyroidism. Women who suffer from Graves' disease experience symptoms such as rapid weight loss, increased pulse rate, sweating, nervousness, insomnia and a thickening of the skin on the shins. In 50 percent of all cases, Graves' disease causes the eyes to protrude, due to swelling and inflammation of the tissues around the eyes. Fortunately, Graves' disease can be controlled fairly easily. It is treated with anti-thyroid drugs, radioactive iodine or surgical removal of the thyroid gland.

WHAT CAUSES GRAVES' DISEASE?

As you read above, your thyroid gland produces a steady supply of two major thyroid hormones, T4 and T3. When you are healthy, your pituitary gland, located in your brain, releases thyroid stimulating hormone (TSH), which then triggers the release of T3 and T4. These thyroid hormones travel in your bloodstream to various organs in your body and determine the speed of all your internal chemical processes. In a nutshell, thyroid hormones act to control your body's metabolic rate, the speed at which you burn calories. When T3 and T4 are at normal levels, the amount of TSH in your blood will level off.

When your thyroid gland becomes overactive, it secretes too many thyroid hormones, causing your cells to work harder and your metabolism to speed up by 60 to 100 percent. This condition is known as hyperthyroidism and is characterized by a high metabolic rate. Hyperthyroidism causes a range of symptoms, including pounding heartbeats, profuse sweating, increased blood pressure, fatigue, weakness and general feelings of anxiousness, irritability and nervousness. When your levels of T3 and T4 are too high, TSH will be suppressed. Measuring the level of TSH in your blood allows your doctor to check your thyroid function and thyroid hormone levels.

There are several factors that may trigger hyperthyroidism but, in North America at least, Graves' disease causes 90 percent of all cases. This disorder is named after the Irish physician Robert Graves, who first described it in 1835. The condition is also referred to as diffuse toxic goiter, thyrotoxicosis or Basedow's disease.

Graves' disease is an auto-immune condition. Under normal circumstances, the immune system produces antibodies that protect the body from foreign invaders, such as bacteria and viruses. In Graves' disease, the immune system malfunctions and produces a protein called thyroid-stimulating antibody that causes the thyroid gland to overproduce thyroid hormones.

At this point, little is known about the exact causes of Graves' disease. Scientists have determined that Graves' disease tends to run in families, but they don't understand the circumstances that trigger the condition in certain individuals. It's thought that severe emotional stress may be a factor. Stress can increase the blood levels of cortisone and adrenaline, two hormones that help prepare the body for a stressful event. Cortisone and adrenaline may affect the production of antibodies in the immune system. Yet many women with Graves' disease have very little stress in their lives, which suggests that there must be other factors at work. It's possible that environmental conditions may cause immune system malfunctions, triggering the problems of an overactive thyroid.

Graves' disease has a strong association with eye disease. The antibodies that stimulate the overproduction of thyroid hormones also react with the proteins in the eye muscle, as well as the connective tissue and fat around the eyeball. This causes swelling and inflammation of the tissues, resulting in protruding eyes. Again, very little is known about the connection between Graves' hyperthyroidism and eye disease.

Thyroid hormones also have an effect on the reproductive system. Women with Graves' disease may find that their menstrual periods decrease, and younger girls may experience a delay in the onset of menstruation. For many women, an overactive thyroid gland is connected with infertility. Fortunately, once the condition has been treated successfully, fertility is usually quickly restored.

If left untreated, Graves' disease increases the risk of miscarriage or birth defects and may, in rare cases, lead to death. However, if properly diagnosed, the condition can be safely and effectively controlled.

SYMPTOMS

Women with Graves' hyperthyroidism experience many of the following symptoms:

- nervousness and irritability
- fast heartbeat
- sleeplessness
- heat intolerance
- high blood pressure
- increased perspiration
- shakiness and tremors
- muscle weakness, especially in upper arms and thighs
- confusion
- increased appetite
- weight loss
- frequent bowel movements

- eye changes, including puffiness and a constant stare
- sensitivity to light, increased tear formation
- fine, brittle hair and thinning skin
- lighter or less frequent menstrual periods

In addition to the symptoms of hyperthyroidism listed above, Graves' disease is characterized by three other distinctive symptoms:

1. The thyroid gland may become quite enlarged, causing a bulge in the neck. This is called a goiter and develops because the immune antibodies overstimulate the entire gland.

2. Sometimes people with Graves' disease develop a lumpy, reddish thickening of the skin in front of the shins, known as pretibial myxedema. If you develop this symptom, you will find that the thickened skin may be itchy and red and may feel quite hard.

3. Fifty percent of women with Graves' disease will have eyes that protrude out of their sockets, due to a buildup of deposits and fluid in the orbit of the eye. As a result, the muscles that move your eye are not able to function properly, causing double or blurred vision. Your eyelids may not close properly because they are swollen with fluid, exposing your eye to injury from foreign particles. Most of the time, your eyes will be painful, red and watery.

Today, we all lead such busy and demanding lives that it's easy to mistake the symptoms of hyperthyroidism and Graves' disease for the normal signs of stressful living. The onset of hyperthyroidism is very gradual and it may take weeks or months before you realize that you are ill. The skin and eye changes associated with Graves' disease complicate the situation even further, as they may appear long before or many months after the other symptoms of hyperthyroidism are identified. In some cases, the eye symptoms may continue to appear or become worse, even after the excessive thyroid hormone production has been treated and controlled. On the positive side, both the eye and the skin changes have been known to disappear without treatment, after a period of months or sometimes years.

WHO'S AT RISK?

About 75 percent of all auto-immune diseases occur in women, hitting them most often during the ages of 30 to 40. In the United States, hyperthyroidism from all causes affects approximately 2 percent of women, compared to 0.2 percent of men.

Diseases of the immune system also tend to run in families. Graves' disease has been identified as an inherited condition, although not every member of an afflicted family will develop the disorder. Cigarette smoking may also increase your risk for Graves' disease. One study found that, compared to women who smoked the least, those who smoked the most had a five-fold greater risk of developing the disease.[1] The same study revealed that the risk of Graves' disease was almost eight times higher among women with the highest stress scores.

Graves' disease has also been linked with other auto-immune conditions, such as Hashimoto's thyroiditis, diabetes mellitus, rheumatoid arthritis, lupus, pernicious anemia and vitiligo.

You may be at risk of developing this type of hyperthyroidism if you

- are a woman between the ages of 20 and 40
- are a woman who has given birth within the last six months
- have experienced thyroid disease before
- have been overtreated for hypothyroidism
- have other auto-immune conditions

DIAGNOSIS

Usually, your doctor will be able to make an initial diagnosis of hyperthyroidism based on a history and investigation of your symptoms. The appearance of a goiter and protruding eyes are strong indicators of Graves' disease.

To confirm the diagnosis, your physician may suggest a simple blood test to measure the level of thyroid hormone in your bloodstream. If the laboratory results are unclear, a test to measure your blood levels of thyroid stimulating hormone (TSH) may be necessary. The TSH test is a very sensitive diagnostic tool and is often used to identify cases of hyperthyroidism, even before symptoms appear. Once hyperthyroidism has been diagnosed, your doctor may also send you for a CAT scan, an ultrasound or an MRI. These tests are used to obtain a clear picture of your thyroid gland, which will help determine the exact cause of your overactive thyroid problems.

CONVENTIONAL TREATMENT

The treatment for hyperthyroidism varies according to the needs and symptoms of each woman. In developing a treatment plan, your physician will consider your age, the severity of your illness, the symptoms you are experiencing and other medical conditions that you may have.

There are three main approaches to treating the problems associated with hyperthyroidism and Graves' disease.

1. *Medication* Anti-thyroid drugs such as Tapazole® (methimazole) are most commonly used to treat hyperthyroidism. They slow down the activity of the thyroid gland by suppressing the release of thyroid hormones. The doses of these medications are adjusted according to the level of thyroid hormone in your blood. Anti-thyroid medication will usually bring your condition under control if taken for a period of six weeks to three months, but it may be necessary to continue taking the drugs for months or years to ensure that your disease stays in remission. If you stop taking the medication, there's a 50 percent chance that your disease will flare up again. Anti-thyroid drugs are usually prescribed in mild cases of hyperthyroidism and in cases where the disease affects children, young adults or the elderly. Occasionally, these drugs may cause mild allergic reactions, such as rashes, hives and nausea. In very rare instances, anti-thyroid medication may dangerously lower your white blood count, making you susceptible to serious and potentially life-threatening infections.

2. *Radioactive iodine* Since anti-thyroid drugs do not cure hyperthyroidism, you may be treated with radioactive iodine to achieve a long-term solution. A small dose of radioactive iodine is taken by mouth and travels from your stomach to your thyroid gland, where it destroys some of the cells. Only a very small amount of radioactivity is introduced into your body with this treatment, and it disappears from your system without any harmful effects in a matter of hours or days. Treatment is usually designed to destroy only enough thyroid cells to bring thyroid hormone production back to a normal level. In reality, though, treat-

ment with radioactive iodine usually causes your thyroid gland to slow down to the point where it underproduces thyroid hormones, creating hypothyroidism. Hypothyroidism is easily treated by taking a daily thyroid hormone pill called Synthroid® (levothyroxine) to restore normal blood levels.

3. *Surgery* Hyperthyroidism can be permanently cured by surgically removing your thyroid gland in a procedure called a thyroidectomy. This is an option to consider if you have a large goiter, if you have a negative reaction to anti-thyroid medication or if you are in a younger age group. Once your thyroid gland is removed, the cause of your hyperthyroidism is eliminated. In most cases, surgery will control your symptoms, but you may require thyroid replacement pills for the rest of your life.

In addition to these treatment options, your doctor will usually prescribe beta-blocking drugs such as Inderal® (propranolol), Tenormin® (atenolol) and Lopressor® (metoprolol). Beta-blockers do not control your abnormal thyroid function, but they are very useful in managing symptoms, such as increased heart rate and nervousness, until other forms of treatment can be started. These drugs block the action of the thyroid hormone circulating in your bloodstream, slowing your heart rate and reducing feelings of nervousness and irritability. They are not suitable for people who have asthma or heart failure because they may cause these conditions to become worse.

Fertility

Women who have been treated for Graves' hyperthyroid usually have no difficulty becoming pregnant, since normal fertility is restored once the condition is under control. If you've been given radioactive iodine, you should wait six months after treatment before becoming pregnant.

If you are pregnant and require treatment for Graves' disease, you should be aware that radioactive iodine treatment is not recommended during pregnancy and surgery, and should be avoided for fear of causing a miscarriage. Because pregnancy has a suppressive effect on the immune system, you can consider treatment with a low-dose anti-thyroid drug. However, be careful to avoid larger doses, as these medications can cross the placenta and affect your baby's thyroid gland. Radioactive treatments should also be avoided while breastfeeding, but anti-thyroid drugs in lower doses appear to be safe for both nursing mothers and babies.

Eye Symptoms

If you are experiencing the eye changes associated with Graves' disease, the symptoms may improve once your hyperthyroidism is under control. In some cases, however, the condition progresses, despite all thyroid gland treatments. In these situations strong drugs such as oral steroids (prednisone) or immunosuppressants (cyclosporin) can be used to minimize swelling and reduce pressure on the optic nerve.

Cyclosporin drugs have produced good results in controlling eye symptoms in the earlier stages of Graves' disease but they are less effective once the disease reaches an advanced stage. Your specialist may consider radioactive treatments and surgery to remove some bone from the eye orbit to reduce swelling and prevent nerve damage. Simple ways to help you cope with your eye changes include using eye drops and eye lubricants, sleeping with the head of your bed elevated and wearing eyeglasses with prisms to improve double vision. If you are a cigarette smoker, bear in mind that smoking makes eye symptoms worse and reduces your response to treatment.

❧

Managing Thyroid Disease

DIETARY STRATEGIES

Weight Control

Weight gain is a concern for women with both types of thyroid disease—hypothyroidism and hyperthyroidism. In the case of an underactive thyroid gland, a deficiency of thyroid hormones leads to a general decline in the rate at which your body burns carbohydrates, protein and fat for energy. As a result, weight gain is common in hypothyroidism. And it is more difficult (but not impossible) to lose weight if your thyroid hormone levels are not in a correct balance.

If you've been treated for hyperthyroidism, you are also at risk for gaining weight. In fact, some research suggests that up to 50 percent of women with hyperthyroidism report weight problems after therapy. Weight gain can occur for two reasons. When your thyroid hormones return to lower, normal levels your metabolic rate slows down. This means your body will burn fewer calories each day. Secondly, if you do not reduce your food intake to match your lower metabolism, the pounds can creep on. Many women increase their food intake when they are experiencing the disease to prevent weight loss. It can be easy to get used to eating more, even once treatment has ended.

If you are suffering from hypothyroidism and have difficulty controlling your weight, or if you have Graves' disease and you now weigh more than you did before you were afflicted with the condition, examine your eating habits to determine where you are going wrong. Keep a food diary for two weeks. Just writing down what you eat often highlights your dietary discrepancies. I always have my clients keep a food diary before they come to see me. They are often surprised to learn how much and what they eat. There's nothing like seeing it in black and white! For some women, keeping a daily journal is all the motivation you need to make healthy food choices and lose weight.

For some other strategies that will help you lose your excess weight, read the section on weight control in chapter 2.

VITAMINS AND MINERALS

Iodine

This trace mineral is an integral part of T3 and T4, the two thyroid hormones released by the thyroid gland. Our major source of iodine is the ocean—seafood and seawater are excellent sources of the mineral. As you move further inland, the amount of iodine in foods varies and generally reflects the amount in the soil that plants grow in or animals graze on. Land that was once under the ocean contains plenty of iodine. In the United States and Canada, the soil around the Great Lakes is iodine-poor. However, the fortification of table salt with iodine in America has eliminated health problems caused by iodine deficiency.

If your body were short-changed of iodine on an on-going basis, the production of thyroid hormones would slow down. This would eventually lead to hypothyroidism. But if you eat salty processed foods and fast foods, or if you add table salt to your meals, you're certainly not at risk for consuming too little iodine.

It may seem odd, but too much iodine in the diet can also cause hypothyroidism. Excess iodine can result in low thyroid hormone levels by halting the activity of enzymes needed for their production. There have been cases of people who develop hypothyroidism by taking in too much iodine in the form of iodine-rich seaweed and kelp on a daily basis.

Obviously a lack of iodine will not lead to Graves' hyperthyroidism. But if you do have Graves' disease, short-changing your diet of this indispensable mineral might influence your remission rate after treatment with anti-thyroid drugs. An American study of 69 patients who took anti-thyroid medication for Graves' disease suggests that the more iodine in the diet, the longer the rate of remission, or how long the disease remained dormant.[2]

The daily recommended intake for iodine is 150 micrograms per day. During pregnancy and breastfeeding, women need to consume an additional 70 and 140 micrograms each day, respectively. North Americans are estimated to be consuming 200 to 600 micrograms of iodine per day, well above our requirements. Some of this iodine excess may come from our growing dependence on fast and processed foods, since these foods contribute a generous amount of salt to our daily diet. Besides iodized salt, other food sources of iodine include seafood, bread, dairy products, plants grown in iodine-rich soil, and meat and poultry from animals raised on iodine-rich soil.

If you have Graves' disease and anti-thyroid drugs are a part of your treatment regime, make sure you include iodine-rich foods in your diet. This is particularly true if you live in an area with iodine-poor soil, if you avoid fast food and salty foods, and if you don't add table salt to your meals. Consider bringing back the salt shaker—a little is all you need; don't exceed 600 micrograms per day.

≫

Managing Hypothyroidism

DIETARY STRATEGIES

Lowering High Blood Cholesterol

Hypothyroidism is linked with a greater risk of early heart disease as thyroid hormones influence the level of blood cholesterol. Indeed, many studies find that patients suffering from a deficiency of thyroid hormones, whether they have overt symptoms or not, have higher levels of total cholesterol, bad LDL cholesterol and triglyceride levels.[3] And the more severe the hypothyroidism, the higher the cholesterol level was.

Researchers have also learned that people with a sluggish thyroid gland have LDL cholesterol particles that are more readily oxidized by harmful free radical molecules. Free radicals are reactive oxygen molecules that roam the body and damage cells. When free radicals oxidize your LDL cholesterol, this cholesterol has a greater tendency to stick to artery walls. While having a high level of LDL cholesterol is not good, having oxidized LDL cholesterol is worse. Your body does have ways of protecting itself from free radicals though. Special enzymes in the body and certain nutrients in foods act as antioxidants and help to keep free radical activity in check.

If you have high blood cholesterol, there are many dietary changes you can make to help lower your levels to the normal range. I strongly recommend that you read the cholesterol-lowering strategies in chapter 11, "Heart Disease and High Cholesterol." You'll learn what foods and nutrients to add to your diet and what foods to limit. You will also read about the important role that vitamin E plays in protecting your LDL cholesterol from free radical damage. Interestingly, one study found that the vitamin E content of LDL cholesterol particles was significantly lower in hypothyroid patients compared to those with normal thyroid function.

Soy Foods

If you do read chapter 11 on how to lower high blood cholesterol levels, you will notice that I am a big fan of soy foods. Indeed, I encourage all my clients to incorporate a certain amount of soy protein in their daily diet to help bring down their blood cholesterol. And this is a very effective dietary strategy.

You may have heard that eating soy foods can harm your thyroid gland and cause hypothyroidism. This simply isn't true. It is true that raw soybeans contain compounds that interfere with the body's ability to use iodine. But heating soybeans eliminates these effects, and all soy foods, from tofu to soy nuts, are manufactured using heat.

The misinformation may have stemmed from the observation that, back in the 1950s, a small number of goiter cases developed in infants fed soy formula. Since the 1950s, there have been no cases of infant goiter in babies fed soy formulas. What's more, over the past five years a handful of studies have found no effect of soy foods on thyroid function or thyroid hormone levels. So rest assured, you can continue to enjoy your tofu.

VITAMINS AND MINERALS

B Vitamins

Preliminary research suggests that people with hypothyroidism may have higher blood levels of homocysteine, a known risk factor for heart disease. Homocysteine is an amino acid that everyone produces. Under normal circumstances, we convert it to other harmless amino acids with the help of three B vitamins: folate, B6 and B12. When this conversion does not occur rapidly enough, due to a deficiency of B vitamins or a genetic defect, homocysteine can accumulate in the blood. High levels of homocysteine can damage blood vessel walls and promote the build-up of cholesterol deposits.

Getting the right amounts of these B vitamins is an important way to keep your blood homocysteine at a healthy level. See the table on B vitamins on page 4 in chapter 1. The best food sources for each of these B vitamin are as follows:

B VITAMIN	GOOD FOOD SOURCES
Folate	Spinach, orange juice, lentils, wheat germ, broccoli, artichokes, asparagus, leafy greens and whole grains
Vitamin B6	Whole grains, bananas, potatoes, legumes, fish, meat and poultry
Vitamin B12	All animal foods including meat, poultry, fish, dairy products and eggs as well as fortified soy and rice beverages

Taking a multivitamin and mineral pill ensures you are meeting your daily requirements for all B vitamins, not just folate, B6 and B12. A standard multivitamin will provide 100 to 300 percent of the RDA for each nutrient.

"High potency," "mega" or "super" multivitamins have higher amounts of the B vitamins. I often refer to these supplements as a multivitamin/mineral and B complex supplement rolled into one pill. There is certainly no harm in taking a high-potency multi, or a B complex tablet for that matter. Most B complex supplements contain 50 to 100 milligrams or microgram amounts of all eight B vitamins; many brands also add vitamin C.

One word of warning if you are shopping for a super-charged supplement. One B vitamin called niacin can cause flushing when taken in amounts greater than 35 milligrams. This is a harmless reaction that causes your face, chest and arms to feel hot and tingly. Although it can be uncomfortable, it doesn't last long. The reaction is usually gone in 20 to 30 minutes. There are a few ways to avoid the niacin flush:

- take your supplement right after eating a meal
- buy a supplement with less than 35 milligrams of niacin
- buy a multivitamin or B complex that contains niacinamide, the non-flushing form of niacin, instead of niacin

Selenium

This trace mineral is an important component of an enzyme that produces the thyroid hormone T3. Researchers have learned that a selenium deficiency in older adults is strongly associated with lower levels of the T3 hormone. The relationship between impaired selenium status and reduced thyroid hormone levels may be partially responsible for the hypothyroidism that's often diagnosed in elderly women.

To keep your thyroid hormone producing enzymes working efficiently, be sure you get enough selenium each day.

Recommended Dietary Allowance (RDA) of Selenium for Females

AGE	RDA (MICROGRAMS)
9–13 years	40 mcg
14–18 years	55 mcg
19–50 years	55 mcg
51+ years	55 mcg
Pregnancy	60 mcg
Breastfeeding	70 mcg

Reprinted with permission from Dietary Reference Intakes for Vitamin C, Vitamin E, Selenium and Carotenoids, *Copyright © 1999 by the National Academy of Sciences. Courtesy of the National Academy Press, Washington, D.C.*

It's been estimated that American women consume somewhere between 113 and 220 micrograms of selenium each day, an amount above our daily requirements. The best food sources of selenium include seafood and meat. Whole-wheat bread, wheat bran, wheat germ, oats, brown rice, Brazil nuts, Swiss chard and garlic are other good sources. Dietary intake from plant foods will vary according to the selenium content of the soil in which these foods were grown.

Women at greatest risk for a selenium deficiency are those who eat a vegetarian diet that's based on plant foods grown in low-selenium areas. But because we eat supermarket foods that have been transported from areas throughout the United States and Canada (not to mention Mexico and South America), selenium deficiency is uncommon.

If you're considering a supplement, check your multivitamin first. Some high-potency brands contain up to 100 micrograms of selenium. If you are buying single selenium supplements, a 200 microgram dose is plenty. You might want to choose one that contains selenomethionine or selenium-rich yeast, since these organic forms of the mineral appear to be more available to the body.

The daily upper limit for selenium for foods and supplements is 400 micrograms per day. Consuming too much selenium over a period of time has toxic effects, including hair and nail loss, gastrointestinal upset, skin rash, garlic breath odor, fatigue, irritability and nervous system abnormalities.

Iron and Iron Supplements

If you are taking Synthroid® (levothyroxine) and you are also being treated for an iron deficiency, don't take your medication and your iron pill at the same time. It's a good idea to take them two to three hours apart. That's because recent experimental studies have found that iron supplements may reduce the body's absorption of levothyroxine. It is possible that impaired absorption of your medication could make you hypothyroid and increase your medication requirements.

If you are taking iron supplements to correct an iron deficiency, your doctor will monitor your thyroid hormone levels closely. Iron pills should be taken only if your doctor has diagnosed you with iron deficiency. If you are taking them on your own accord, be sure to let your physician know.

Managing Graves' Hyperthyroidism

The nutritional approaches I discuss below are intended to help offset side effects associated with various types of treatment for Graves' disease. In addition to keeping you well during and after your course of therapy for this disease, my strategies will also improve your overall health and feeling of well-being.

VITAMINS AND MINERALS

Antioxidants

Studies suggest that hyperthyroidism is associated with a decrease in antioxidants and an increase in oxidative stress brought on by free radical molecules. Free radicals are highly reactive oxygen molecules that are produced by normal body processes. Dietary antioxidants such as vitamins C and E and beta-carotene quench harmful free radicals and prevent them from causing damage to body cells.

Studies that measure levels of antioxidant nutrients in the blood and thyroid tissue of women with Graves' hyperthyroidism have observed decreased levels of beta-carotene.[4] Another study looked at the effect of a daily vitamin C supplement in 24 women undergoing anti-thyroid drug therapy for Graves' disease.[5] At the beginning of the study, the researchers found that, compared to healthy women who served as controls, those with hyperthyroidism had higher levels of oxidized compounds and lower levels of antioxidant enzymes in their blood. After taking 1000 milligrams of vitamin C for one month, these women had significant increases in antioxidant enzymes.

While the link between antioxidants and hyperthyroidism is preliminary at best, there is no harm in boosting your intake of these nutrients as they have many other potential health benefits. Here's what you need to know about these nutrients.

BETA-CAROTENE

This antioxidant is plentiful in dark green vegetables and orange fruits and vegetables. Currently there is no daily recommended intake for beta-carotene, but many experts believe that 5 to 15 milligrams (9000 to 27,000 international units) per day offer plenty of protection. Here are the best food sources:

FOOD	BETA-CAROTENE (MILLIGRAMS)
Sweet potato, cooked, 1/2 cup (125 ml)	15
Collard greens, cooked, 1 cup (250 ml)	7
Carrot, 1 medium	5

Cantaloupe, 1/2 cup (125 ml)	5
Squash, winter, 1 cup (250 ml)	5
Apricots, fresh, 3 medium	4
Kale, cooked, 1 cup (250 ml)	3
Spinach, cooked, 1 cup (250 ml)	3
Mango, sliced, 1 cup (250 ml)	2

Nutrient Values of Some Common Foods, *Health Canada, Ottawa, 1999.*

The body is not very efficient at absorbing beta-carotene from raw foods. For instance, less than 5 percent of carotenoid compounds have been shown to be available in raw carrots. But the good news is you can enhance absorption by cooking your vegetables—even steaming increases the available beta-carotene in carrots and spinach. And you might want to add a little fat to your meal to optimize beta-carotene absorption. Try a little vegetable dip the next time you snack on those baby carrots. Or add a teaspoon or two of olive oil to your sweet potato purée. And forgo the fat-free salad dressing—I've always been in favor of using a small amount of the real thing.

If you're looking for supplemental beta-carotene, buy a multivitamin and mineral with added beta-carotene. Most brands provide 1000 to 10,000 international units (0.5 to 5.5 milligrams). A word of warning to women who smoke: use of separate beta-carotene supplements (not in a multivitamin format) in doses of 20 milligrams per day for five to eight years has been associated with an increased risk of lung cancer in men who smoke.[6] While these findings may not apply to women, it makes sense to be cautious. If you are a smoker, I recommend that you avoid beta-carotene supplements and stick to getting your daily fix from foods and a multivitamin pill. A higher risk of lung cancer has not been found in smokers who eat a diet plentiful in beta-carotene-rich foods.

If you do take a separate beta-carotene supplement, be advised that when doses of 30 milligrams per day or more are taken for a period of time, a yellow discoloration of the skin can occur. This adverse effect can even occur when people eat plenty of carrots day after day. The condition is called carotenodermia; it's considered harmless and disappears when supplements are discontinued.

Vitamin C

For the amount of vitamin C women should be getting each day, see the RDA table on page 11 in chapter 1. You'll find your best food bets in the Vitamin C in Foods table on page 12.

If you don't eat at least two vitamin-C-rich foods each day, a supplement is a good idea. Keep in mind though that fruits and vegetables contain many other natural chemicals that may work with vitamin C to keep you healthy. So, even if you do take a vitamin C pill, I recommend that you still add foods rich in vitamin C to your daily diet. Here's what you need to know about vitamin C supplements:

- If you're looking for the most C for your money, choose a supplement labeled Ester C. Studies in the lab have found that this form of vitamin C is more available to the body.

- If you don't like to swallow pills and prefer a chewable supplement, make sure it contains calcium ascorbate or sodium ascorbate. These forms of vitamin C are less acidic and therefore less harmful to the enamel of your teeth.

- Take a 500-milligram supplement once or twice a day. There's little point in swallowing much more at once, since your body can use only about 200 milligrams at one time. If you want to take more, split your dose over the day.

- The daily upper limit for vitamin C has been set at 2000 milligrams to avoid diarrhea.

Vitamin E

Like the antioxidants discussed above, vitamin E is a potent scavenger of harmful free radical molecules. Hyperthyroidism is associated with a significantly higher level of LDL cholesterol oxidation. This means that free radical molecules damage your LDL cholesterol particles much more readily. And when your LDL cholesterol particles become oxidized, they adhere to artery walls more easily, increasing the risk for heart disease.

This is where vitamin E enters the story. Once consumed, vitamin E makes its way to the liver, where it is incorporated into cell membranes and lipoproteins, like LDL particles, that transport cholesterol. It is here that vitamin E works to protect these compounds from oxygen damage caused by free radicals.

Until we learn more about the role of vitamin E in hyperthyroidism, strive to meet the daily targets you'll find in the RDA table on page 15 in chapter 1.

Wheat germ, nuts, seeds, soybeans, vegetable oils, corn oil, whole grains and kale are all good sources of vitamin E, so be sure to include a few of these in your daily diet. But it can be a challenge to reach the daily recommended intake of 22 IU when you consider that adding 2 tablespoons of wheat germ to your morning smoothie gives you 4 IU of the vitamin. And wheat germ is one of the best sources. For this reason many women opt for a daily supplement to help them meet their target intakes.

To help you choose the right vitamin E supplement, consider the following suggestions:

- Take 100 to 400 IU per day. There's no evidence to warrant taking more.

- Buy a natural source vitamin E supplement (or look for *d-alpha-tocopherol* on the label; synthetic forms are labeled *dl-alpha tocopherol*). Although the body absorbs both synthetic and natural forms equally well, your liver prefers the natural form, as it incorporates more natural vitamin E into transport molecules. Studies have shown that twice as much vitamin E ends up in the blood of people taking natural E as in those taking the same amount of synthetic E.

- If you're taking a blood-thinning medication like Coumadin® (warfarin), don't take vitamin E without your doctor's approval, since it has slight anti-clotting properties.

- The daily upper limit for vitamin E is 1500 IU of natural vitamin E or 2200 IU of the synthetic form.

Calcium and Vitamin D

It's well documented that hyperthyroidism causes a higher rate of bone breakdown. In fact, the latest research shows that even low-level Graves' disease is associated with bone turnover. A study soon to be published in the *Annals of Internal Medicine* (in press at the time of writing this book) revealed that among 9400 older women, those with low-grade hyperthyroidism had a three-fold greater risk of hip and vertebral fractures.[7]

Some studies have found a harmful effect of anti-thyroid medication on bone density. To explore further the effect of thyroid medication on bone loss, French researchers summarized the results from 41 studies in 1250 patients.[8] Their results showed that medications like Tapazole® (methimazole) and Propyl-Thyracil® (propylthiouracil) that suppress thyroid hormone secretion cause significant bone loss in the lower spine and hip in postmenopausal women.

There is also evidence that women with Graves' disease are more susceptible to calcium and vitamin D deficiency during the winter months. Deficiencies of these two nutrients are linked with a higher risk of tetany following surgery for Graves' disease. Tetany is a condition of mineral imbalance in the body that results in severe muscle spasms. Mild tetany is characterized by tingling in the fingers, toes and lips. More severe forms can lead to death. Tetany occurs when the concentration of calcium in body fluids falls below normal. Low calcium levels can be caused by a lack of vitamin D. Fortunately, most forms of tetany can be successfully treated with adequate calcium and vitamin D.

To protect your bones and lower the risk of postoperative tetany, make sure you meet your daily requirements for each of these essential nutrients—see the RDA tables on pages 14 and 16 in chapter 1. Use the Calcium in Foods and Vitamin D in Foods tables there to help you boost your intake of these nutrients from foods. Unfortunately, there are only a few good food sources of vitamin D. We meet the majority of our vitamin D requirements by exposing our skin to sunlight during the summer months.

CALCIUM AND VITAMIN D SUPPLEMENTS

If you are not meeting your daily targets for calcium and vitamin D through your diet, I strongly recommend that you take a supplement. If you take a multivitamin and mineral supplement, it should have 400 IU of vitamin D in it (most brands do). But calcium is a large mineral and manufacturers can't fit very much in a multivitamin and mineral pill. For this reason, you have to rely on a separate calcium supplement. Here are a few guidelines to help you choose among a multitude of products:

- If you consume at least three to four servings of dairy products or calcium-fortified beverages each day, you're getting approximately 900 to 1200 milligrams of calcium. For every serving you're missing and not making up with other calcium-rich foods, consider taking a 300 milligram calcium supplement.

- When choosing a supplement look at the source of calcium. Studies show that calcium citrate supplements are better absorbed than those made from calcium carbonate. This is an important consideration if you're over 50 years old or you take medication that blocks the production of stomach acid (calcium carbonate requires more stomach acid for its absorption).

- Check the ingredient list to see how much elemental calcium each pill gives you. This is what you base your daily dose on.

- Consider choosing a calcium supplement with ipriflavone, a synthetic isoflavone that's been shown to enhance the bone-building potential of calcium and vitamin D. To learn more about ipriflavone, turn to page 173 in chapter 10, "Osteoporosis."

- Choose a calcium formula with vitamin D and magnesium, two nutrients that work with calcium to keep bones healthy.

- Spread larger doses throughout the day. If you must take more than 500 milligrams from a supplement, split your dose over two or three meals.

- The daily safe upper limit is 2500 milligrams of calcium from food and supplements combined. Too much calcium may cause constipation, gas and kidney stones in people with a history of the disease.

THE BOTTOM LINE...
Leslie's recommendations for managing thyroid disease

1. If you have hypothyroidism and you're concerned about your body weight, or if you've gained excess weight after treatment for Graves' disease, embark on a healthy eating and exercise program. Start by keeping a food diary for two weeks to pinpoint areas that need to be improved upon.

2. Don't skimp on iodine. The best sources of iodine are iodized table salt (all salt in America is fortified with iodine), seafood, plants grown on iodine-rich soil and animal foods from animals that graze on iodine-rich soil. But don't get too much iodine, as intakes greater than 600 micrograms per day may lead to hypothyroidism. To keep your iodine intake within reason, avoid eating large quantities of kelp, dulse or other sea vegetables on a daily basis.

Hypothyroidism

1. If your doctor has determined that you have high blood cholesterol levels, read chapter 11 to get all my nutrition strategies to bring it down.

2. Boost your intake of B vitamins, in particular folate, B6 and B12.

3. Be sure you're getting enough selenium. The best food sources include seafood, meat, whole-wheat products, wheat bran, wheat germ, Brazil nuts, Swiss chard and garlic. If you take a supplement, don't exceed 200 micrograms per day.

4. If you are taking single iron supplements for iron-deficiency anemia, do not take iron pills with your thyroid medication, since iron can reduce your body's absorption of the drug. Take your iron pill two hours before or two hours after taking your medication.

Graves' Disease

1. Boost your intake of dietary antioxidants including vitamins C, E and beta-carotene.

2. Get more calcium and vitamin D in your daily diet. You need 1000 to 1200 milligrams of calcium and 200 to 600 IU of vitamin D each day.

Part 7

Pelvic and Urinary Tract Health

21

Cervical Dysplasia

If you are diagnosed with cervical dysplasia, it means that abnormal changes are beginning to take place in the cells lining the surface of your cervix, the part of your reproductive system that forms the entrance to your uterus. The word *dysplasia* means abnormal cell growth. The cells of your cervix will begin to show microscopic changes and will start to divide at a faster rate than normal.

If left untreated, cervical dysplasia could progress to become cervical cancer. Despite improvements in diagnosis and treatment over the past 50 years, cancer of the cervix continues to threaten the health of American women. It is the second most common cancer in women, most often striking those between the ages of 35 and 55. It is a cancer that progresses very slowly and may take up to ten years to develop. If detected in the early stages, it can be treated effectively and the long-term prognosis is very good.

There are no warning signs or symptoms for cervical dysplasia. The only reliable way to detect this pre-cancerous condition is to have an annual Pap smear, a laboratory test of a small sample of your cervical tissue.

What Causes Cervical Dysplasia?

Scientists don't know what causes the cell changes of cervical dysplasia, but they suspect that it is something spread through sexual contact. Current research indicates that the human papillomavirus (HPV), a virus that causes sexually transmitted genital infections, may be the trigger that begins the sequence of abnormal cell growth.[1]

There are three stages of cervical dysplasia. If abnormal cells are found only on the surface of the cervix, the condition is considered mild. Unfortunately, these precancerous cells often spread deeper into the tissue of the cervix lining. When this happens, cervical dysplasia is labeled as moderate or severe, depending on the extent of the tissue penetration. Up to 60 percent of women with mild cervical dysplasia find that these cell changes are only temporary. Within 6 to 12 months, the cells of the cervix return to normal and health is no longer at risk. However, once cervical dysplasia reaches the moderate or severe stage, there is a much greater chance that the condition will progress to cervical cancer within the next ten years.

Symptoms

As I mentioned earlier, there are no warning signs of cervical dysplasia. Without the appropriate medical testing, you probably won't realize that anything is wrong until the disease is well advanced. If you have regular medical check-ups, your doctor may notice a growth or a sore or suspicious area on your cervix during a routine pelvic examination.

But usually cell changes take place long before they can be seen by the naked eye. In most cases, identifiable symptoms don't appear until the cervical dysplasia has progressed to cervical cancer. At that time, a woman may experience some pain or some intermittent bleeding or spotting between menstrual cycles. To prevent cervical cancer, it is critical that you test for cervical dysplasia by having a Pap smear on a regular basis.

Who's at Risk?

Women who begin having sexual intercourse at an early age (16 years or younger) and those who have multiple sexual partners are at higher risk for developing cervical dysplasia. So are women who have a history of sexually transmitted disease, especially human papillomavirus (HPV) infection. Other conditions that may predispose you to cervical dysplasia include

- smoking cigarettes or exposure to second-hand smoke
- using oral contraceptives for more than five years
- having a history of a gynecological cancer
- following a diet that's low in vitamin A, beta-carotene and folate

Studies indicate that many women, including women over the age of 60, recent immigrants and Native American women, do not go to their doctor for annual Pap smears. If you're sexually active and you don't get tested regularly for cervical dysplasia, you have a greater chance of developing cervical cancer.

Diagnosis

Ever since the Pap test was introduced in North America after World War II, we've seen a dramatic decline in the number of deaths caused by cervical cancer. To perform a Pap test, your doctor will conduct a regular pelvic examination. Using a small spatula and a brush, he or she will scrape some cells from the surface of your cervix and smear these cells on a slide. This tiny tissue sample will then be sent to a laboratory and examined under a microscope for abnormal cells.

The Pap smear identifies pre-cancerous changes in cervical cells and it also indicates the presence of invasive cancer cells. But an abnormal result does not always mean your health is at risk. Sometimes a virus may cause temporary cell changes that will disappear after a short period of time.

A normal Pap smear result is reassuring because it indicates that you have a very low risk of cervical cancer. However, it is not a guarantee that your cervix is cancer-free. It is possible that cancer cells or abnormal cells can be missed if they are not part of the tissue sample collected for the test. For that reason doctors recommend that women who are sexually active or who are over 18 years old have a Pap smear once every year.

ॐ

Conventional Treatment

Approximately 8 percent of all Pap smears show abnormal results. The treatment for cervical dysplasia varies, depending on the extent and severity of the dysplasia. Treatment may involve removal of the abnormal cervical tissue.

If you are diagnosed with mild dysplasia and have no other risk factors for cervical cancer, your doctor will probably just monitor your condition and wait to see if the affected cells return to normal. Your doctor will perform a second Pap smear in four to six months and, if cell growth is normal at that time, no treatment will be necessary. With mild dysplasia, it is recommended that you continue to monitor the health of your cervix by returning for a pelvic examination and Pap smear twice a year for at least two years.

A diagnosis of moderate or severe dysplasia is treated a little differently. Your doctor will check the surface of your cervix for abnormalities by performing a colposcopy: using a viewing tube with a magnifying lens, he or she will inspect your cervix and will take a *biopsy* of tissue from the abnormal area. There are two types of biopsy used in this procedure: a *punch biopsy* samples a tiny piece of your cervix; *endocervical curettage* is used to scrape tissue from the cervical canal. These samples are sent to a laboratory to determine the extent of changes in cervical cells.

Once the severity of the cervical dysplasia is known, the treatment involves removing all the abnormal growth that can turn into cervical cancer. Your doctor may perform a surgical procedure called a *cervical conization*, which removes a cone-shaped area of tissue. Other ways of removing the abnormal area include cauterizing the tissue with heat, freezing it with cryosurgery, vaporizing it with lasers or removing it with an electrified wire loop procedure known as LEEP. These treatments usually do not affect your ability to become pregnant. But because cervical dysplasia can return, it is important to monitor yourself carefully and have Pap smears every three months for the first year after surgery and every six months after that.

In more severe cases, a hysterectomy to remove your uterus may be necessary. This decision will prevent you from having children in the future.

The sooner you detect and treat cervical dysplasia, the lower your risk for developing cervical cancer. In the meantime, there are dietary and nutritional strategies that can help prevent cervical dysplasia from developing in the first place. If your recent Pap test has revealed abnormal cervical cells, some of the strategies I discuss below might even reverse the dysplasia.

⅜

Preventing and Treating Cervical Dysplasia

VITAMINS AND MINERALS

Antioxidants

Many studies have found a link between cervical dysplasia and low blood levels of antioxidant nutrients, especially beta-carotene and vitamin C. Women with cervical dysplasia are also more likely to have poor dietary intakes of these and other antioxidants. Antioxidants are vitamins, minerals or natural plant chemicals that protect cells in the body from damage caused by free radicals—highly reactive oxygen molecules that are produced by normal body processes. Excess free radicals can also be formed by pollution, cigarette smoke and heavy exercise. These compounds can damage the genetic material of cells, which, in turn, may lead to cancer development. Antioxidants neutralize free radicals, preventing them from causing damage to cells.

Our body has built-in antioxidant enzymes for keeping free radical activity in check, but levels decline as we age. Scientists are learning every day that a daily supply of dietary antioxidants is important for reducing the risk of certain cancers (not to mention heart disease, cataracts and possibly Alzheimer's disease).

When it comes to cervical dysplasia (a precursor to cervical cancer), a handful of dietary antioxidants have been identified that may prevent free radical damage to cervical cells. These include beta-carotene, lycopene, vitamin C and vitamin E. Below I discuss the antioxidants that have been studied the most with respect to cervical dysplasia. To boost your intake of all these antioxidants, try to eat at least five to ten servings of fruits and vegetables each day. One serving equals a piece of fruit, 1/2 cup (125 milliliters) of vegetables, 1 cup (250 milliliters) of green salad, or 3/4 cup (175 milliliters) of unsweetened juice.

BETA-CAROTENE

When you think of beta-carotene, no doubt you think of carrots. In fact, this antioxidant is also plentiful in dark green vegetables and orange fruits and vegetables. It's been hypothesized that beta-carotene may protect from cervical dysplasia and cervical cancer in a few ways. First of all, we know that beta-carotene is a potent antioxidant and therefore may protect cervical cells from free radical damage.

In addition to its antioxidant powers, beta-carotene is used to make vitamin A in the body. Vitamin A is essential for normal cellular growth and development. A number of laboratory studies have shown the ability of vitamin A to prevent abnormal cell growth. What's more, women with cervical dysplasia have been shown to have lower blood levels of vitamin A. One study of 134 Japanese women diagnosed with cervical dysplasia found that the rate of progression of cervical cancer was 4.5 times higher in women with low blood vitamin A levels than in those with higher blood levels.[2]

Beta-carotene has been the focus of many studies of women with cervical dysplasia. Researchers have found that, compared to women free of cervical dysplasia, those with the condition have significantly lower blood levels of this antioxidant nutrient. Furthermore, some studies have revealed that women with dysplasia consume a smaller amount of dietary antioxidants, including beta-carotene.

This does not necessarily mean that beta-carotene can reverse the course of dysplasia once you are diagnosed with the condition. To date, two randomized control trials (the gold standard of scientific studies) have compared women taking a 30-milligram beta-carotene supplement to women taking a placebo.[3] The researchers found no difference in regression of dysplasia in either group of women. It is possible that these studies were too short to notice an effect—one was three months, the other nine months.

A recent randomized control trial from Australia investigated the effects of supplemental 30 milligrams of beta-carotene, alone or in combination with 500 milligrams of vitamin C, and did notice better regression rates in the women who took beta-carotene alone and with vitamin C.[4] However, these findings were not statistically significant.

At the time of writing this book, there is a two-year trial nearing completion in the United States. The study involves 120 women with moderate to severe dysplasia who were randomized to receive either 30 milligrams of beta-carotene or an inactive placebo each day. Hopefully, this trial will be long enough to find if there is a protective effect of beta-carotene supplements.

In the meantime it makes good sense to get more beta-carotene in your diet, especially if you are a smoker. You may recall that cigarette smoking increases the risk of cervical dysplasia. Well, cigarette smoking also leaches antioxidants from your body, especially beta-carotene and vitamin C. Currently there is no daily recommended intake for beta-carotene, but many experts believe that 5 to 15 milligrams (9000 to 27,000 IU) per day offers plenty of protection. If you have cervical dysplasia you might up your intake to 30 milligrams from food and a supplement. Here are the best food sources.

Beta-carotene in Foods

FOOD	BETA-CAROTENE (MILLIGRAMS)
Sweet potato, cooked 1/2 cup (125 ml)	15 mg
Collard greens, cooked, 1 cup (250 ml)	7 mg
Carrot, 1 medium	5 mg
Cantaloupe, 1/2 cup (125 ml)	5 mg
Squash, winter, 1 cup (250 ml)	5 mg
Apricots, fresh, 3 medium	4 mg
Kale, cooked, 1 cup (250 ml)	3 mg
Spinach, cooked, 1 cup (250 ml)	3 mg
Mango, sliced, 1 cup (250 ml)	2 mg

Beta-carotene in raw foods is not absorbed that well by the body. For instance, less than 5 percent of carotenoid compounds have been shown to be available in raw carrots. But the good news is you can enhance absorption by cooking your vegetables—even steaming increases the available beta-carotene in carrots and spinach. And you might want to add a little fat to your meal to optimize beta-carotene absorption. Try a little vegetable dip the next time you snack on those baby carrots.

Or add a teaspoon or two of olive oil to your sweet potato purée. And forgo the fat-free salad dressing—I've always been in favor of using a small amount of the real thing.

Beta-carotene Supplements You can see from the list above that you would need to eat many large servings of fruits and vegetables each day to achieve an intake of 30 milligrams of beta-carotene. While this is a very good habit, as it ensures you are getting many other protective nutrients and antioxidants, it may not be practical for some women on a daily basis.

To boost your intake, buy a multivitamin and mineral supplement with added beta-carotene. Most brands provide 1000 to 10,000 international units (0.5 to 5.5 milligrams). If you opt for a separate beta-carotene supplement, I recommend you choose a product that offers a mix of carotenoids including beta-carotene and lycopene.

One word of warning to women who smoke: use of beta-carotene supplements in doses of 20 milligrams per day for five to eight years has been associated with an increased risk of lung cancer in men who smoke. While these findings may not apply to women, it makes sense to be cautious. If you are a smoker, I recommend that you avoid beta-carotene supplements and stick to getting your daily fix from foods. This potential health risk has not been found in smokers who eat a diet with beta-carotene-rich foods.

If you take a beta-carotene supplement, be advised that, when taken in doses of 30 milligrams per day or more for a long period of time, supplements can cause a yellow discoloration of the skin. In fact, this adverse effect has been known to occur when people eat many carrots day after day. This condition is called carotenodermia; it's considered harmless and disappears when supplements are discontinued.

LYCOPENE

This antioxidant belongs to the same family of carotenoid compounds that beta-carotene comes from. But compared to beta-carotene, lycopene is twice as potent an antioxidant. As such, lycopene is yet another dietary defense mechanism against free radical damage to the genetic material of cells.

A few studies have suggested that lycopene protects women from cervical dysplasia. One study from the University of Pennsylvania School of Medicine found that women with the highest intake of lycopene were one-third as likely to have dysplasia compared to those who consumed the least.[5]

Lycopene is found in red-colored fruits and vegetables. It's the natural chemical that gives these foods their bright color. Tomatoes are the richest source of lycopene, but you'll also find some in pink grapefruit, watermelon, guava and apricots.

While more work needs to be done to unravel the precise role lycopene plays in cervical health, there's no reason why you shouldn't be getting a good supply in your daily diet. Based on the research that has been conducted in the area of heart disease, it appears that an intake of 5 to 7 milligrams offers protection. And that's easy to get if you eat heat-processed tomato products.

Lycopene in Foods

FOOD	LYCOPENE (MILLIGRAMS)
Tomato, raw, 1 small	0.8–3.8 mg
Tomatoes, cooked, 1 cup (250 ml)	9.25 mg
Tomato sauce, 1/2 cup (125 ml)	3.1 mg
Tomato paste, 2 tbsp (30 ml)	8.0 mg
Tomato juice, 1 cup (250 ml)	23.0 mg
Ketchup, 2 tbsp (30 ml)	3.1–4.2 mg
Apricots, dried, 10 halves	0.3 mg
Grapefruit, pink, 1/2	4.2 mg
Papaya, 1 whole	6.2–16.5 mg
Watermelon, 1 slice (25 cm × 2 cm)	8.5–26.4 mg

Heat-processed tomato products provide a source of lycopene that is much more available to the body. Even though one fresh tomato packs 4 milligrams of lycopene, your body doesn't absorb all of it. And here's another tip to increase the amount of lycopene you absorb—add a little olive oil to your pasta sauce. Lycopene is a fat-soluble compound and is better absorbed in the presence of a little fat.

If you're looking for a boost of lycopene, all you really have to do is add a glass of low-sodium tomato juice to your lunch. However, lycopene supplements are available in health food and drug stores. If you opt for supplements, I recommend that you choose a brand that's made with the Lyc-O-Mato™ or LycoRed™ extract. This source of lycopene comes from Israel and is derived from whole tomatoes. It is also the extract that has been used in clinical studies. Most supplements offer 5 milligrams of lycopene per tablet, so one a day is all you need.

VITAMIN C

Much less research has been done on this antioxidant vitamin and its potential role in protection from cervical dysplasia. A few studies have determined that women with low blood levels of vitamin C have a greater risk of cervical dysplasia compared to women with higher levels. Furthermore, cigarette smoke decreases the level of vitamin C in the body. One American study found a strong association between a woman's history of smoking and her level of vitamin C, whether or not she had cervical dysplasia.[6]

In the section above on beta-carotene, I mentioned the results of a randomized controlled trial from Australia that did suggest vitamin C supplements in combination with beta-carotene increase the rate of regression of cervical dysplasia.

To see how much vitamin C women should be getting each day see the RDA table on page 11 in chapter 1. Also check out the Vitamin C in Foods table to find the best bets for food containing this antioxidant. You'll notice that some foods with beneficial amounts of vitamin C—cantaloupe, grapefruit, mango, tomato juice—are also good sources of beta-carotene and/or lycopene.

Vitamin C Supplements If you don't eat at least two vitamin-C-rich foods each day, a supplement is a good idea. Keep in mind, though, that fruits and vegetables contain many other natural chemicals that may work with vitamin C to keep you healthy. So even if you do take a vitamin C pill, I recommend that you still add foods rich in vitamin C to your daily diet. Here's what you need to know about vitamin C supplements.

- If you're looking for the most C for your money, choose a supplement labeled Ester C. Studies in the lab have found that this form of vitamin C is more available to the body.

- If you don't like to swallow pills and prefer a chewable supplement, make sure it contains calcium ascorbate or sodium ascorbate. These forms of vitamin C are less acidic and therefore less harmful to the enamel of your teeth.

- Take a 500-milligram supplement once or twice a day. There's little point in swallowing much more than that at once, since your body can use only about 200 milligrams at one time. If you want to take more, split your dose over the day.

- The daily upper limit for vitamin C has been set at 2000 milligrams to avoid diarrhea.

VITAMIN E

A discussion of dietary antioxidants cannot exclude vitamin E. Chances are you've already heard about this heart-healthy nutrient (read chapter 11 for all the facts on vitamin E and heart disease). As with vitamin C, less research has been done in the area of vitamin E and cervical dysplasia. Nevertheless, observational studies have found a link between the risk of dysplasia and blood levels of the vitamin. For instance, one study from the Cancer Research Center of Hawaii revealed that women with the highest blood vitamin E levels had a 70 percent lower risk of cervical dysplasia than those with the lowest blood levels.[7] The researchers also noticed what's called a dose-response effect. That means the higher the level of vitamin E, the lower the risk of dysplasia.

Like the antioxidants discussed above, vitamin E is a potent scavenger of harmful free radical molecules and may keep cervical cells healthy in this way. Until we learn more about the role of vitamin E in cervical health, strive to meet your daily targets—see the RDA table on page 15 in chapter 1.

Vitamin E Food Sources and Supplements Wheat germ, nuts, seeds, soybeans, vegetable oils, corn oil, whole grains and kale are all good sources of vitamin E, so be sure to include a few of these in your daily diet. But it can be a challenge to reach the daily recommended intake of 22 IU (international units), when you consider that adding 2 tablespoons of wheat germ to your morning smoothie gives you only 4 IU of the vitamin—and wheat germ is one of the best sources. For this reason, many women opt for a daily supplement to help them meet their target intakes. To help you choose the right vitamin E supplement, consider the following suggestions:

- Start taking 100 to 400 IU per day. There's no evidence to warrant taking more.
- Buy a natural source vitamin E supplement (or look for *d-alpha-tocopherol* on the label; synthetic forms are labeled *dl-alpha tocopherol*). Although the body absorbs both synthetic and natural forms equally well, your liver prefers the natural form, as it incorporates more natural vitamin E into transport mole-

cules. Studies have shown that twice as much vitamin E ends up in the blood of people taking natural E as in those taking the same amount of synthetic E.

- Consider choosing a vitamin E supplement that is labeled "mixed tocopherols." Preliminary research shows that one form of vitamin E called gamma-tocopherol has potent anti-inflammatory effects in addition to its antioxidant properties. This may play a role in cancer prevention.

- If you're taking a blood-thinning medication like Coumadin® (warfarin), don't take vitamin E without your doctor's approval, since it has slight anti-clotting properties.

- The daily upper limit for vitamin E is 1500 IU of natural vitamin E or 2200 IU of the synthetic form.

Folate

Moving away from the antioxidant connection, let's turn our attention to a vitamin that appears to have a very important role in preventing the development of dysplasia. Research shows that, as one's intake of folate-rich foods decreases, the risk of cervical dysplasia increases. An American study found that women consuming less than 400 micrograms of folate each day were 2.6 times more likely to develop dysplasia than women who consumed more than 400 micrograms.[8]

A lack of this B vitamin may promote the development of dysplasia in a number of ways. Folate may act in some way to protect cervical cells. Studies have found that many women with dysplasia have normal blood levels of folate but low levels of the vitamin in cervical tissue. A deficiency of folate may also enhance the harmful effect of human papillomavirus (HPV) infection on cervical cells.

Folate is critical for the synthesis of DNA (deoxyribonucleic acid), the genetic material of cells. Low levels of folate in cervical tissue can make cellular DNA more susceptible to damage. Even a marginal folate deficiency can cause damage to DNA in cells, damage that resembles cervical dysplasia. It is possible that this alteration to DNA is an early step in the progression of cervical dysplasia and cervical cancer. Furthermore, this damage to a cell's genetic material may be stopped or reversed if you are given supplements of the B vitamin. In fact, two trials have found that folic acid supplements improved dysplasia in women taking birth control pills.[9] However, trials conducted in women not taking oral contraceptives did not find folic acid supplements to alter the course of dysplasia. The researchers concluded that a deficiency of the B vitamin may be involved in the initiation of dysplasia but, once you have the disease, supplements do not appear to reverse it.

What these studies suggest is that getting enough folate every day is an important strategy in the prevention of cervical dysplasia. See how much folate women should be striving for every day in the RDA table on page 6 in chapter 1. Be sure to choose whole-grain breads, cereals and pasta more often than refined grain foods. While refined grain products are enriched with folic acid in the United States and Canada, whole grains provide more. For more folate-rich foods, see the Folate in Foods table on page 7 of chapter 1.

FOLIC ACID SUPPLEMENTS

For some women, consuming 400 micrograms of folate every day can be challenging. As you can see from the list in chapter 1, you pretty much have to make sure your daily diet includes beans, spinach and orange juice. Some of you might want to take a multivitamin and mineral supplement to ensure you're reaching your target. Look for a supplement that gives 0.4 to 1.0 milligrams of folic acid (check the ingredient list for this information).

By the way, you may have noticed that I have been using the terms folate and folic acid throughout this section. Folate refers to the B vitamin as it is found naturally in foods. Folic acid refers to the synthetic form—whether it's in a supplement or added back to foods like enriched breakfast cereals.

If you take a separate folic acid supplement, be sure to buy one that has vitamin B12 added. High doses of folic acid taken over a period of time can hide a B12 deficiency and result in progressive nerve damage. The upper limit for folic acid intake from a supplement is 1000 micrograms (1 milligram) per day.

THE BOTTOM LINE...

Leslie's recommendations for preventing and managing cervical dysplasia

1. First things first. If you are sexually active, make sure you get an annual Pap test.

2. Whether you are sexually active or not, don't smoke cigarettes.

3. Boost your antioxidant intake by eating a diet that's loaded with fruits and vegetables. Strive for at least five to ten servings of fruits and vegetables each day.

4. To get more beta-carotene, reach for bright orange and dark green produce. The best choices are sweet potato, carrots, winter squash, mango, cantaloupe, kale and collard greens.

5. If you are a non-smoker and want to increase your daily intake of beta-carotene, buy a multivitamin and mineral supplement with added beta-carotene. Most brands will offer 5000 to 10,000 international units (IU). If your multivitamin does not include this antioxidant, consider taking a separate beta-carotene supplement.

6. If you are a smoker, avoid taking a beta-carotene supplement. Increase your daily intake of beta-carotene from foods only.

7. Boost your intake of lycopene, found in red-colored fruits and vegetables. The best sources are heat-processed tomato products such as tomato sauce, stewed tomatoes, tomato juice and ketchup. Other foods to add to your diet include pink grapefruit, guava juice, apricots and papaya.

8. If you opt for a lycopene supplement, choose one that has Lyc-O-Mato™ or LycoRed™ on the label.

9. Try to get more vitamin C into your diet. If you take a daily vitamin C pill, consider buying a supplement made from Ester C, a high-quality form of the supplement that's more available in your body.

10. Be sure vitamin E is included in your daily antioxidant regime. Vegetable oils, corn oil, nuts, seeds, wheat germ and kale are good sources. Consider taking a separate vitamin E supplement that's natural source and offers "mixed tocopherols."

11. Eat more foods rich in folate. Foods that offer the most folate and should be eaten on a regular basis include asparagus, spinach, lentils, kidney beans, unsweetened orange juice and whole-grain enriched breakfast cereals.

12. To ensure you meet the RDA for folate, make sure your multivitamin and mineral supplement contains 0.4 to 1.0 milligram (400 to 1000 micrograms) of the vitamin (look for folic acid on the ingredient list). If you decide to take a separate folic acid supplement, make sure you buy one with vitamin B12 added, since high doses of folic acid can hide a B12 deficiency.

22

Endometriosis

Endometriosis is a poorly understood disease that afflicts as many as one in ten women. The condition develops when uterine-type cells grow outside of the uterus. These cells may travel throughout the body and attach to a number of different areas. The misplaced cells develop into nodules, lesions, implants or growths that are affected by the hormonal fluctuations of the menstrual cycle. These growths cause pelvic pain, pain during intercourse, infertility and other problems. There's no question that endometriosis can influence every aspect of a woman's life—her ability to have children, to work and to relate with loved ones.

❧

What Causes Endometriosis?

The uterus, a reproductive organ located within the abdominal cavity, is lined with a type of tissue called *endometrium*. When you have endometriosis, tissue that looks and acts like endometrium is found living outside of your uterus. In most cases, the misplaced tissue is discovered growing somewhere within the abdominal cavity. It may be found attached your ovaries, bowel, bladder, fallopian tubes or cervix. Although rare, the appearance of endometrial tissue in other sites around the body including the lung, arm and thigh, is possible. Endometrial growths can vary in size and penetration of the surrounding tissue. Rest assured that endometrial growths are generally not cancerous—they are normal types of tissue found growing outside the normal location.

During the course of a normal menstrual cycle, the endometrial lining of your uterus gradually builds up in preparation for pregnancy. If you don't become pregnant, the lining breaks down, bleeds and is discharged from your body during your period. Unfortunately, the endometrial tissue living outside of your uterus responds to the hormonal cycles of menstruation in exactly the same way. But, unlike the menstrual flow from the uterus, the blood from the misplaced tissue has no place to go. This causes episodes of internal bleeding and inflammation that can result in internal scarring, severe pain and infertility.

Scientists still don't know what causes endometriosis. The most commonly held view is the *retrograde menstruation theory*. This theory suggests that menstrual tissue occasionally flows backwards through the fallopian tubes during menstruation. The tissue is discharged from the fallopian tubes into the abdomen, where it becomes implanted and develops into endometrial growths. Another theory proposes that endometrial tissue may be distributed from the uterus to other parts of the body through the lymph glands or blood vessels. In some cases, endometrial tissue may be accidentally transplanted into distant sites through surgical procedures. It's possible that hereditary factors are involved making some families more susceptible to the disease. Eventually, scientists may discover that endometriosis is caused by a combination of factors.

⁊

Symptoms

The most common symptom of endometriosis is pain before and during menstruation. Symptoms include

- severe menstrual cramps
- irregular vaginal bleeding
- pelvic pain
- painful sexual intercourse

- painful bowel movements
- pain during exercise
- painful and frequent urination
- backache
- constipation or diarrhea
- fatigue

The symptoms of endometriosis have little to do with the extent of the endometrial growths. Some women with mild endometriosis and small growths may experience excruciating pain, while other women with large growths and severe endometriosis may have no painful symptoms at all. Each case of endometriosis is unique. Symptoms usually start after the onset of menstruation and subside after menopause, when the growths tend to shrink or disappear.

Infertility affects 30 to 40 percent of women with endometriosis. Severe endometriosis, which causes extensive scarring and organ damage, is considered one of the three major causes of infertility. While many women with endometriosis fear cancer, the condition is rarely associated with endometrial cancer—fewer than 1 percent of women with endometriosis go on to develop endometrial cancer.[1]

THE BOWEL

Many women with endometriosis experience on-going gastrointestinal discomfort, including diarrhea, painful bowel movements and general intestinal distress. In fact, the data registry of the Endometriosis Association (a U.S.-based nonprofit organization) reported that 79 percent of women with endometriosis experience these symptoms.[2] Gastrointestinal symptoms were the most commonly reported symptoms, along with painful periods and fatigue.

Indeed, many of my clients with endometriosis complain of pain, nausea, feeling full, bloating and altered bowel habits. Occasionally women report vomiting. Studies have revealed that endometriosis is associated with changes to the intestinal tract, such as altered motility and bacterial overgrowth. There are four possible reasons why women with endometriosis experience bowel problems:

1. Endometrial growths develop directly on the bowel, usually the latter part of the large intestine. This usually causes painful bowel movements, a sense of rectal pressure, urgency to defecate or bloody stools. Most specialists carefully check the

bowel for the presence of endometriosis but, because the intestine is so long, it is possible for growths to be missed. For the most effective treatment, many endometriosis experts recommend surgically removing the portion of bowel affected.

2. Adhesions can result from the endometriosis itself, or from past surgeries. Adhesions are fibrous bands or structures by which parts abnormally adhere. These adhesions pull on the bowel and cause pain.

3. Prostaglandins may cause intestinal symptoms—such as diarrhea, nausea and vomiting—in women who do not have any evidence of endometriosis on their bowels. During a woman's period, these symptoms can be caused by prostaglandins, compounds produced by the body that control the smooth muscle of the uterus, bowel and blood vessels.

4. Symptoms may be caused by an overgrowth of *Candida albicans (candidiasis)*, a fungus responsible for causing yeast infections in women. In this case, intestinal symptoms often include constipation and/or diarrhea, stomach pain, gas, bloating and rectal itching. Women with this yeast infection often develop food sensitivities, which can contribute to gastrointestinal upset. Usually treatment of the candidiasis provides women relief of these symptoms. Unfortunately, diagnosis of yeast overgrowth is not easy to obtain, as this condition is new and controversial among the medical community.

Women with endometriosis are often told by their doctor that they have irritable bowel syndrome (IBS). Unfortunately this diagnosis is not very helpful because it does not indicate what the underlying problem is. IBS is really just an umbrella term used to describe gastrointestinal distress when no other diagnosis can be made. During IBS, the muscular contractions of the bowel become uncoordinated, resulting in alternating constipation and diarrhea, gas, bloating and nausea. These symptoms can be caused by any of the four reasons listed above. Having your doctor thoroughly investigate the cause of your bowel problems is important for effective treatment.

Who's at Risk?

More than 5.5 million North American women and girls have endometriosis. The disease occurs most often in women of childbearing age, affecting 10 to 15 percent of women between the ages of 25 and 44, but teenagers can also suffer from endometriosis.

The disease is believed to run in families, so you are more at risk if you have a first-degree relative (e.g., mother, sister) with endometriosis. Other risk factors include being of Caucasian descent, having your first child after the age of 30 and having an abnormal uterus.

Diagnosis

If you are suffering from the symptoms listed above, or you are having difficulty becoming pregnant, your doctor may suspect that you have endometriosis. He or she will evaluate your medical history and conduct a complete physical examination, including a pelvic exam. It is sometimes possible to actually feel an endometrial growth during the pelvic exam.

Most often, an accurate diagnosis can be made only if patches of endometrial tissue can be seen. To determine the presence of misplaced tissue, your doctor will conduct a minor surgical procedure called a laparoscopy. A small surgical tube with a light attached is inserted through a small incision in your abdomen. This allows your doctor to examine your abdominal organs and to evaluate the size and extent of any endometrial growths. In some cases, tissue samples may be removed and sent to a laboratory for microscopic examination.

Conventional Treatment

The management of endometriosis is tailored to each individual woman. The choice of treatment is guided by the extent of your symptoms, your age and your plans to have a family. If your condition is mild and you want to become pregnant, your doctor may choose to simply wait and see how the disease will progress. The only treatment may be pain-relief medication such as aspirin or ibuprofen. Exercise, heat from a bath or heating pad, massage and relaxation may also help to ease painful symptoms.

If you are not planning to have children, your doctor may suggest hormone suppression treatment. This involves taking a combination of drugs to prevent ovulation and limit the amount of estrogen that stimulates the endometrial growths. It is hoped that this will slow the growth of the misplaced tissue and minimize injury to surrounding organs. Drugs commonly prescribed include

- *Birth control pills* to control irregular vaginal bleeding and improve pain with a regulated, low-dose combination of estrogen and progesterone

- *Progestins* to prevent ovulation and reduce estrogen levels

- *Gonadotropin releasing hormone (GnRH) agonists* (to enhance the secretion of these hormones) such as Lupron® (leuprolide) or Synarel® (nafarelin), to create a temporary and reversible menopause by stopping estrogen production by the ovaries. Endometriosis shrinks and symptoms improve during treatment in 90 percent of women with this treatment. Side effects include hot flashes, mood swings, headache, vaginal dryness and some bone loss.

- *Danazol*, a synthetic testosterone, to reduce the production of estrogen from the ovaries and stop menstruation. Possible side effects include water retention, weight gain, oily skin, muscle cramps, mood changes and hot flashes. Occasionally a rash, facial hair or deepening of the voice may occur, in which case treatment with danazol should be stopped.

Medication does not cure endometriosis. Once you stop taking the drugs, the disease will usually return.

Pregnancy is another way of relieving the symptoms of endometriosis. During pregnancy, ovulation and menstruation stop and hormone levels change. Many women find that their endometriosis is much less active during the months of their pregnancy. Unfortunately, the disease will return once pregnancy and nursing have ended.

If you have moderate or severe endometriosis, surgery may be necessary. Your doctor will remove as much misplaced tissue as possible, while preserving your ability to have children by retaining your ovaries and uterus. This type of surgery usually provides only temporary relief of symptoms, since endometriosis recurs in most women.

A more radical approach involves preventing ovulation by removing all your reproductive organs in a surgical procedure called a *hysterectomy*. A complete hysterectomy will be considered only if you are not planning to become pregnant and have severe pelvic pain that is not relieved by medication. Once your reproductive organs are removed, the endometriosis will not recur.

It may not be possible to remove all endometrial growths during the hysterectomy. But because they will be deprived of hormonal stimulation, the growths will eventually shrink and disappear. Until that time, women may continue to feel some of the symptoms of endometriosis. After surgery, estrogen replacement therapy may be prescribed to counteract the menopausal symptoms that will develop.

৵

Managing Endometriosis

The nutritional approaches I list below are aimed at easing endometriosis-associated pain, improving fertility and minimizing the side effects of certain medications. While these are not cures for endometriosis, and are not intended to be stand-alone treatments for the condition, they can help women feel better.

DIETARY STRATEGIES

Essential Fatty Acids and Omega-3 Fats

Dietary fat is composed of building blocks called fatty acids. These fatty acids are incorporated into cell membranes, where they affect the integrity and fluidity of the membrane. The body is able to make all but two fatty acids: linoleic acid and alpha-linolenic acid. Because these two fatty acids are indispensable to our health, they must be obtained from the diet and are therefore referred to as *essential fatty acids*.

Linoleic acid is the main member of the omega-6 family of fats. Major food sources include vegetable oils and margarines made from corn, safflower, sunflower, sesame and soybeans, as well as nuts, seeds and meat. Alpha-linolenic acid is the primary member of the omega-3 family. Oils such as canola, flaxseed and walnut are rich in alpha-linolenic acid. Other sources of this omega-3 fat include Omega-3 eggs, wheat germ, soybeans, soy nuts and tofu.

The body uses these two essential fatty acids to produce hormonelike compounds called *prostaglandins* (PGs), sometimes referred to as eicosanoids. Prostaglandins regulate our blood pressure, blood clot formation, blood fats, immune compounds and hormones. They are produced by the lining of the uterus, by endometrial lesions and by immune compounds called macrophages. Researchers have learned that prostaglandin formation is altered in women with endometriosis.[3] Studies have revealed that these women have significantly higher levels of prostaglandins than women who are free of endometriosis.[4] What's more, there appears to be a direct relationship between the degree of pain experienced by these women and the amount of prostaglandins produced.[5] A high level of prostaglandins can alter the contractility of the uterus and fallopian tubes, resulting in painful menstrual periods and infertility. Some of these PGs can enter the bloodstream and affect smooth muscle in other parts of the body. PGs can stimulate the gastrointestinal tract, causing it to contract in an uncontrolled manner.

The body makes different types of prostaglandins. Prostaglandins can either increase inflammation or they can decrease it. In the case of endometriosis, two inflammatory prostaglandins called PGE and PGF appear to be involved. A diet that's high in fatty acids from animal foods and processed fat favors the production of prostaglandins that cause inflammation. On the other hand, if the fat in your diet consists of mainly omega-3 fatty acids found in flaxseed oil, canola oil, walnuts, soybeans and fish, more non-inflammatory prostaglandins will be formed.

The omega-6 oils containing linoleic acid can be used by your body to produce either series-1 PGs (non-inflammatory) or series-2 PGs (inflammatory). Arachadonic acid is a fatty acid found in animal foods; it is used to form inflammatory compounds in the body. Omega-3 oils, whether from foods that contain alpha-linolenic acid or fatty fish, are transformed into non-inflammatory series-3 PGs. So the balance of omega-6 to omega-3 oils in your diet is very important for proper prostaglandin formation. The optimal ratio is thought to be 4:1, or four times the amount of omega-6 oils to omega-3 oils. It's estimated that most women are currently consuming more than 20 times more omega-6 than omega-3 oils. A diet with such an imbalance will lead to a greater production of inflammatory PGs.

To achieve a better balance of omega-6 oils to omega-3 oils, practice the following tips:

1. *Reduce the amount of animal fat in your diet.* Remember that these foods contain arachadonic acid that is used to produce unfavorable PGs. Choose lean cuts of meat and poultry (e.g., flank steak, inside round, sirloin, eye of round, extra-lean ground beef, venison, center-cut pork chops, pork tenderloin, baked ham, deli ham, skinless chicken breast, turkey breast, lean ground turkey). Choose 1 percent or skim milk, cheeses made with less than 20 percent milk fat, and yogurt with less than 2 percent milk fat.

2. *Avoid foods with trans fat*, an unhealthy fat formed when manufacturers hydrogenate vegetable oils for commercial foods such as margarines and baked goods. To help you achieve this goal, look for the words "partially hydrogenated vegetable oil" on the list of ingredients, and eat foods that contain them less often. Up to 40 percent of the fat in foods like french fries, fast food, doughnuts, pastries, snack foods and commercial cookies is trans fat. If you eat margarine, choose one that's made with non-hydrogenated fat. At the time of writing, the U.S. Food and Drug Administration is moving quickly to require trans fat on nutrition labels after a report from the Institute of Medicine found there is no safe level in people's diets. The FDA says it will publish a final rule requiring the mandatory listing of trans fat content within the Nutrition Facts panel early in 2003. Until the new labeling becomes law, read ingredient lists carefully.

3. *Add 1 to 2 tablespoons of flaxseed oil to your daily diet.* This oil is one of the richest sources of omega-3 fat. Flaxseed oil is easily broken down by heat, so you can't cook with it. If you want to add it to a hot dish like pasta sauce, add it at the end of cooking. Use the oil in salad dressing and dip recipes. And be sure to store it

in the fridge. You'll find bottles of flaxseed oil sold in the refrigerator section of your local health food store. Check out **www.omegaflow.com** for recipe ideas. If you don't want to add the oil to your diet, supplements of flaxseed oil are available. Keep in mind that it takes four capsules (4 grams) to give you a teaspoon of oil. It's much easier to use the oil, not to mention less expensive.

4. *Eat fish at least three times a week.* Not only will eating more fish improve the ratio of omega-6 to omega-3 fats in your diet and improve endometriosis pain caused by inflammation, but it also might protect your heart (read chapter 11, "Heart Disease and High Cholesterol" for more on this). The oilier the fish, the higher the omega-3 content. Salmon, trout, sardines, herring, mackerel, and albacore tuna are good choices. If you plan to rely on tuna fish sandwiches to get your omega-3, you're going to be out of luck—canned tuna has very little omega-3 fat.

Dietary Fiber

I mentioned earlier that many women with endometriosis experience painful gastrointestinal symptoms such as bloating, distention, stomach cramps and altered bowel habits. There's no question that getting enough fiber is an important way to help regulate bowel habits and ease symptoms.

Dietary fiber is actually made up of two types of fiber, *soluble* and *insoluble*. Both types are present in varying proportions in different plant foods, but some foods may be rich in one or the other. And both types of fiber function differently in your body to promote health.

Soluble fibers, as their name suggests, dissolve in water. Dried peas, beans and lentils, oats, barley, psyllium husks, apples and citrus fruits are good sources of soluble fiber. When you consume these foods, the soluble fibers form a gel in your stomach and slow the rate of digestion and absorption.

Foods like wheat bran, whole grains and some vegetables contain mainly insoluble fibers. Although these fibers do not dissolve in water, they do have a significant capacity for retaining water. In this way they act to increase stool bulk and promote regularity.

A high-fiber diet with adequate fluids is the best way to prevent and treat constipation. The sponge-like action of insoluble fiber enables it to absorb plenty of water, producing larger, softer stools that your body can eliminate easily and quickly.

It's estimated that Americans are getting 11 to 14 grams of fiber each day, only half of what is recommended. Experts agree that a daily intake of 25 grams of total dietary fiber is needed to reap its health benefits. It's important to gradually build up to 25 grams of fiber. Too much too soon can cause bloating, gas and diarrhea. When adding fiber to your diet, spread it out over the course of the day, since getting all your fiber at once may reduce the benefits and increase the discomfort. And don't forget that fiber needs water to work—aim for a minimum of 8 ounces of fluid with every high-fiber meal and snack.

To help you sneak more fiber into your diet, try the following:

- Eat a variety of foods every day to get the benefits of both soluble and insoluble fiber.

- Strive for five or more servings of fruits and vegetables each day.

- Eat at least five servings of whole-grain foods each day.

- Buy high-fiber breakfast cereals. Aim for at least 4 grams of fiber per serving (check the nutrition information panel).

- Top your breakfast cereal with banana, berries or raisins.

- Add 2 tablespoons of natural wheat bran, oat bran or ground flaxseed to cereals, yogurt, casseroles and soup.

- Eat legumes more often—add white kidney beans to pasta sauce, black beans to tacos, chickpeas to salads, lentils to soup. Start with small portions to minimize gas.

- Add a few tablespoons of walnuts, soynuts, sunflower seeds or raisins to salads.

- Reach for high-fiber snacks like popcorn, dried apricots or dates.

Probiotics

Research suggests that women with endometriosis may have bacterial or yeast overgrowth in their gastrointestinal tract, which may aggravate bloating, stomach pain, early satiety diarrhea and/or constipation. In one study conducted at the Women's Hospital of Texas in Houston, 40 out of 50 women studied had excessive levels of bacteria.[6]

The term *probiotic* literally means "to promote life" and refers to living organisms that, upon ingestion in certain numbers, improve microbial balance in the intestine and exert health benefits. Such friendly bacteria are known collectively as lactic acid bacteria and include *L. acidophilus, L. bulgaricus, L. casei, S. thermophilus* and bifidobacteria.

The human digestive tract contains hundreds of strains of bacteria, making up what is called the normal intestinal flora. Among the intestinal flora are lactic acid bacteria that inhibit the growth of unfriendly, or disease-causing, bacteria by preventing their attachment to the intestine and by producing lactic acid and other antibacterial substances to suppress harmful bacteria. Plenty of studies have shown that consuming probiotic foods or supplements increases the number of lactic acid bacteria in the intestinal tract.

Today scientists are learning that these friendly bacteria may do a whole lot more than keep our intestinal tract healthy. Several well-controlled clinical studies have shown that lactic acid bacteria, when taken as a supplement or as yogurt, speed recovery from diarrhea in children and adults.

Lactose intolerance is caused by a deficiency of lactase, the enzyme in the small intestine that digests the milk sugar. If lactose remains undigested in the gut it draws water into the intestine, which can lead to diarrhea. Bacteria then ferment the lactose, causing bloating, gas and pain. Most people with a mild to moderate lactose intolerance can consume probiotic foods like yogurt and kefir without any gastrointestinal complaints. The fact that lactose is better digested in these foods is attributed, in part, to their live bacteria content. Not only do lactic acid bacteria digest some of the lactose present in the food, but they also contain enzymes that have been shown to increase the level of the lactase enzyme in the small intestine.

Lactic acid bacteria can also inhibit the growth of *Candida albicans,* a yeast responsible for vaginal yeast infections. One American study found that women who consumed 8 ounces of *L. acidophilus* yogurt each day for six months had a three-fold decrease in candida infections compared to women who did not eat yogurt. Another study found that taking the probiotic supplement Kyo-Dophilus™ once or twice daily resulted in 89 percent of women having lower candida symptom scores.

Lactic acid bacteria in fermented milk products and supplements will exert their health effects only if they reach the intestine in sufficient numbers. That means you must consume an adequate "dose" of live bacteria. Counts of 1 to 10 billion viable cells of bacteria have been shown to be clinically effective. The amount of live bacteria in a 175-milliliter serving of yogurt ranges from 175 to 17,500 million and can decrease by a factor of 10 to 100 during storage. In the United States, all commercial yogurts are made using *L. bulgaricus* and *S. thermophilus*. Some manufacturers have added other strains, such as bifidobacteria, *L. acidophilus* and *L. casei*. To begin reaping the health benefits of probiotics, include one serving of yogurt in your daily diet. If you're a little more adventurous you might try kefir or sweet acidophilus milk, fermented milk beverages available in most supermarkets.

Probiotic Supplements

If you don't eat dairy products, probiotic capsules or tablets are a good alternative. In fact, many health experts believe that taking a high-quality supplement is the only way to ensure you're getting a sufficient number of friendly bacteria. So even if you enjoy yogurt, you might consider adding a supplement to your daily nutrition regime. Here are a few considerations when choosing a product:

- *Buy a product that offers 1 billion to 10 billion live cells* per dose. Taking more than this may result in gastrointestinal discomfort.

- For greater convenience, *choose a product that is stable at room temperature* and does not require refrigeration. This allows you to continue taking your supplement while traveling. Good manufacturers will test their products to ensure that they maintain their viability over a long period of time. For example, Wakunaga's probiotic supplement Kyo-Dophilus™ has been tested and found to retain high bacteria counts for up to six years at room temperature.

- *Know the type and source of bacteria in the supplement.* Many experts believe that supplements made from human strains of bacteria are better adapted for growth in the human intestinal tract. When choosing a product, you might ask the pharmacist or retailer if the formula contains human or non-human strains.

- *Always take your supplement with food.* When eating a meal, the stomach contents become less acidic due to the presence of food. This allows live bacteria to withstand stomach acids and reach their final destination in the intestinal tract.

PREBIOTICS

Believe it or not, you can actually eat foods that promote the growth of these friendly, protective bacteria in your intestinal tract. These foods are called prebiotics and they contain components called fructo-oligosaccharides (FOSs). The human intestine does not digest FOSs; FOSs stay in the intestinal tract and feed the lactic acid bacteria. Good food sources include Jerusalem artichokes, asparagus, onions and garlic. The amount we consume in our daily diet is considered too low to have any significant effect on the growth of friendly bacteria. Jerusalem artichokes, also called sunchokes, are available in most supermarkets. Chop them and add to salads and stir-fries. I suspect we will see purified FOSs added to commercial food products one day in the not too distant future, as is already the case in Japan.

Caffeine

A study from the Harvard School of Public Health found that women with endometriosis who consumed 5 to 7 grams of caffeine per month had almost double the risk of not conceiving compared to women who didn't drink any caffeinated beverages.[7] This study would suggest that, among women with endometriosis, caffeine can delay conception and therefore further aggravate infertility. You're probably wondering how much coffee you have to drink to consume 5 to 7 grams of caffeine. Well, it works out to one to two cups of coffee per day. If you are trying to conceive (whether you have endometriosis or not), I recommend giving up caffeine.

There are two other reasons why you should cut back your caffeine intake if you have endometriosis. Gonadotropin-releasing hormone drugs like Lupron® (leuprolide) or Synarel® (nafarelin) cause bone loss—if you take one of these medications, read the section on calcium and vitamin D on page 421. Caffeine causes bone loss, too. It's been estimated that every 6-ounce cup of coffee leaches 48 milligrams of calcium from your bones. If you can't give up your morning brew, make sure you're getting 1000 to 1500 milligrams of calcium each day.

Caffeine can also wreak havoc on your gastrointestinal tract. If you are one of the many women with endometriosis who suffers intestinal upset, caffeine can stimulate your bowel and cause more frequent bowel movements and diarrhea.

See the Caffeine in Common Beverages, Foods and Medications table on page 38 in chapter 1 to see where your caffeine may be coming from. Most experts agree that a daily upper limit for caffeine of 450 milligrams per day does not pose a health risk for most healthy people; however, it certainly can cause problems for women with endometriosis.

If you have assessed your daily caffeine intake and determined that you're overdoing it, gradually cut back over a period of two to three weeks to minimize withdrawal symptoms such as headaches, tiredness or muscle pain. Start by eliminating caffeine from the latter part of your day. Stick to a "no caffeine" rule after noon. Switch to low-caffeine beverages like tea or hot chocolate, or caffeine-free alternatives such as decaf coffee, herbal tea, cereal coffee, juice, milk or water. If you're still hooked on coffee, order a latte or cappuccino to get extra calcium. And if your gut is sensitive to lactose in milk, try a soy latte (make sure the soy beverage is calcium-fortified).

Alcohol

When it comes to fertility, alcohol is something else you should consider giving up. The same researchers from the Harvard School of Public Health that investigated caffeine and conception in women with endometriosis looked at the effect of alcohol.[8] They determined that women who drank a moderate amount of alcohol—i.e., one or two drinks a day—had a 60 percent higher risk of infertility compared to non-drinkers. Instead of having a glass of wine, pour yourself a glass of sparkling mineral water with a slice of lime. Or try some of the non-alcoholic wines or beers available in supermarkets and liquor stores. If you're looking for a cocktail, I suggest a virgin Caesar, tomato juice or a glass of soda water with a splash of cranberry juice.

Like caffeine, alcohol can also increase your bowel discomfort. If you are not trying to get pregnant and just want to minimize the effect of alcohol on your gut, try the following: drink alcohol with a meal or snack; drink no more than one drink every hour; try alternating one alcoholic drink with a non-alcoholic drink.

Food Sensitivities

If your endometriosis is causing bowel discomfort, there are a handful of foods and spices that may aggravate your symptoms. You might already know what these are. If you are unsure, I recommend you keep a food and symptom diary for a two-week period. Record everything you eat, how much of the food you eat and any symptoms you feel. If you are working with a consulting dietitian, she or he will use this tool to identify culprits.

It can be difficult to detect foods that are causing you grief because a particular food may not bother you all of the time. Sometimes it isn't what you ate, but how much of the food you ate, how quickly you ate, how many trigger foods you ate in one day or how much stress you were under at the time. Use your food diary to look for patterns, not just specific foods.

To help you pinpoint potential trigger foods, here is a list of foods that often cause intestinal problems in my clients with endometriosis:

- *Caffeine and alcohol* (as discussed above)

- *Artificial sweeteners*

- *High-fat and/or high-calorie meals* Both dietary fat and large meals have a greater stimulating effect on colon contractions.

- *Excessive sugar* from soft drinks, candy and sweets. Often soft drinks cause problems due to the sugar, caffeine and carbonation.

- *Dairy products* Some women don't produce enough of an enzyme called lactase in their intestinal tract. Lactase breaks down the natural milk sugar, lactose. In this case, lactose remains undigested in the intestinal tract, causing bloating, gas and diarrhea. If you have moderate lactose intolerance, chances are you can still handle yogurt, as it has much less lactose than milk. And hard cheeses have even less lactose. If you are symptomatic, try lactose-reduced milk and yogurt (e.g., Lactaid®). Or buy Lactaid® pills at the pharmacy; take a pill before a meal with dairy. Alternatives to dairy include calcium-fortified soy and rice beverages.

- *Wheat* In some women with endometriosis, bloating, distention and gas is caused by an intolerance to wheat-based foods. This can be a problem since wheat is such a staple in our diet. Just think of all the wheat we eat each and every day—bread, bagels, muffins, pasta, ready-to-eat breakfast cereals, crackers and baked goods are all made from wheat flour. If you are unsure if wheat is causing your gas and bloating, try eliminating it from your diet for two weeks. Do your symptoms improve? Then, slowly add it back to your diet. Every two days, add a new wheat food. Do your symptoms return? Alternatives to wheat include rice, rice pasta, rice crackers, quinoa, quinoa pasta, millet, potato, sweet potato, corn, rye and oats. A good health food store will have many products—breakfast cereals, pasta, crackers, cookies and breads—that are made from grains other than wheat. Some of these foods, like rice pasta and rice crackers, are available in large grocery stores.

- *Raw vegetables* Be sure to cook your veggies to reduce potential gas formation. Gassy vegetables include bok choy, broccoli, brussels sprouts, cabbage, cauliflower, kale, radishes, rutabaga, onions and fresh garlic.
- *Legumes* such as kidney beans, chickpeas and black beans. A natural sugar in dried peas, beans and lentils often causes gas and bloating. To reduce potential symptoms, rinse your beans before you add them to recipes and eat a smaller portion. Try Beano™, a natural enzyme available at pharmacies and health food stores that breaks down the sugar—just a few drops on your food is all it takes.
- *Certain fruits*, including berries, apple with the peel, melon and prunes.
- *Nuts and seeds*
- *Spices* such as chili powder, curry, ginger, garlic, hot sauce

VITAMINS AND MINERALS

Vitamin E

Some researchers theorize that oxygen damage caused by free radical molecules contributes to endometriosis by promoting the growth of endometrial tissue. Free radicals are highly reactive oxygen molecules that are produced by normal body processes, including the body's own immune response. It is thought that damaged red blood cells and misplaced endometrial tissue signal the recruitment and activity of immune compounds in the abdominal cavity. In the process of engulfing foreign particles and protecting the body, these activated immune compounds generate harmful free radicals, which cause oxidation.

Research has shown that compounds called lipoproteins in the fluid of the abdominal cavity do indeed have lower levels of vitamin E, an important antioxidant. Antioxidants are vitamins, minerals or natural plant chemicals that protect cells in the body from damage caused by free radicals. Other dietary antioxidants include vitamin C and beta-carotene.

To boost your intake of vitamin E reach for vegetable oils, nuts, seeds, soybeans, olives, wheat germ, whole grains and leafy green vegetables like kale. See the RDA table on page 15 in chapter 1 for the recommended daily intake of vitamin E for women.

It can be challenging to get ample amounts of vitamin E in your daily diet, particularly if you use vegetable oils sparingly. If this is the case, you might want to take a daily vitamin E supplement. When buying vitamin E, consider the following:

- Take 100 to 400 IU per day. There's no evidence to warrant taking more than this.

- Buy a natural source vitamin E supplement (or look for *d-alpha-tocopherol* on the label; synthetic forms are labeled *dl-alpha tocopherol*). Although the body absorbs both synthetic and natural vitamin E supplements equally well, your liver prefers the natural form, as it incorporates more natural vitamin E into transport molecules. Studies have shown that twice as much vitamin E ends up in the blood of people taking natural E as in those taking the same amount of synthetic E.

- If you're taking a blood-thinning medication like Coumadin® (warfarin), don't take vitamin E without your doctor's approval, since vitamin E has slight anti-clotting properties.

- The daily upper limit for vitamin E is 1500 IU of natural vitamin E or 2200 IU of the synthetic form.

Calcium and Vitamin D

If you are taking a GnRH drug such as Lupron® (leuprolide) or Synarel® (nafarelin), your bone health is a concern. That's because these drugs suppress estrogen production, resulting in accelerated bone loss. A review of studies in women taking GnRH drugs determined the average bone loss to be 1 percent per month or 6 percent in total.[9] If you compare that to an average bone loss of 3 percent in the first year of menopause, it seems considerable. And while that may not be important at age 25, it may be very relevant at 65. Because of their negative effect on bone density, the U.S. Food and Drug Administration has limited the use of GnRH drugs to six months.

Scientists have tried to determine whether this bone loss is reversible. Once women stop taking this medication, do they regain their lost bone? In some women it seems so. But other studies have not found this to be true, leading some experts to believe that bone loss brought on by GnRH drugs is partially irreversible.

All this being said, you can now see that it is more important than ever to meet your calcium and vitamin D requirements while taking these drugs. Here's how much you need every day.

Recommended Dietary Allowances (RDAs) of Calcium and Vitamin D for Females

AGE	RDA (MILLIGRAMS/INTERNATIONAL UNITS)
13–18 years	
Calcium	1300 mg
Vitamin D	200 IU
19–50 years	
Calcium	1000 mg
Vitamin D	200 IU
51–70 years	
Calcium	1200 mg
Vitamin D	400 IU
71+ years	
Calcium	1200 mg
Vitamin D	600 IU
Pregnancy and Lactation	
Calcium	1000 mg
Vitamin D	200 IU

Reprinted with permission from Dietary Reference Intakes for Calcium, Phosphorus, Magnesium, Vitamin D and Fluoride, *Copyright © 1999 by the National Academy of Sciences. Courtesy of the National Academy Press, Washington, D.C.*

Use the Calcium in Foods and Vitamin D in Foods tables in chapter 1 to help you boost your intake of these nutrients from foods. Unfortunately, there are only a few good food sources of vitamin D. We meet the majority of our vitamin D requirements by exposing our skin to sunlight during the summer months.

If you are not meeting your daily targets for calcium and vitamin D through your diet, I strongly recommend that you take a supplement. If you take a multivitamin and mineral supplement it should have 400 IU of vitamin D in it (most brands do). But calcium is a large mineral and manufacturers can't fit very much in a multivitamin and mineral pill. For this reason you have to rely on a separate calcium supplement. Here are a few guidelines to help you choose from among a multitude of products:

- If you consume at least three to four servings of dairy products or calcium-fortified beverages each day, you're getting approximately 900 to 1200 milligrams of calcium. For every 300 milligram serving you're missing and not making up with other calcium-rich foods, consider taking a 300 milligram calcium supplement.

- When choosing a supplement, look at the source of calcium. Studies show that calcium citrate supplements are better absorbed than those made from calcium carbonate. This is an important consideration if you're over 50 years old or you take medication that blocks the production of stomach acid—calcium carbonate supplements require more stomach acid for their absorption.

- Check the ingredient list to see how much elemental calcium each pill gives you. This is what you base your daily dose on.

- Choose a calcium formula with vitamin D and magnesium, two nutrients that work with calcium to keep bones healthy.

- Spread larger doses of calcium throughout the day. If you must take more than 500 milligrams from a supplement, split your dose over two or three meals.

- The daily safe upper limit is 2500 milligrams of calcium from food and supplements combined. Too much calcium may cause constipation, gas and kidney stones in people with a history of the disease.

THE BOTTOM LINE...
Leslie's recommendations for managing endometriosis

1. To help your body produce friendly, non-inflammatory prostaglandins choose the right fats and oils in your diet. Reduce the amount of animal fat in your diet by selecting lean cuts of beef, poultry breast and lower-fat dairy products. As much as possible avoid foods with partially hydrogenated vegetable oils. To boost your intake of omega-3 oils, supplement your diet with 1 or 2 tablespoons of flaxseed oil. For even more omega-3, eat fish three times a week.

2. To help ease bowel discomfort, gradually increase your intake of dietary fiber. Aim for a daily intake of 25 grams. Be sure to increase your water intake, too, since fiber needs fluid to work properly.

3. Eat 1 cup (250 milliliters) of yogurt each day for a dose of friendly lactic acid bacteria. If you don't eat fermented dairy products, consider taking a probiotic supplement each day. Look for a product that is stable at room temperature and provides 1 billion to 10 billion live cells per dose.

4. If you are trying to get pregnant, avoid caffeine-containing beverages, foods and medications. Cutting back on your caffeine intake may also reduce bowel discomfort.

5. Eliminate alcoholic beverages, as alcohol may reduce your chances of conceiving and aggravate diarrhea.

6. Keep a food and symptom diary to pinpoint trigger foods that you might be sensitive to.

7. Increase your intake of vitamin E, an antioxidant vitamin. Food sources include vegetable oils, nuts, seeds, soybeans, wheat germ, whole grains and leafy green vegetables. Consider supplementing your diet with 100 to 400 IU of a natural-source vitamin E.

8. If you take a GnRH drug, make an extra effort to boost your intake of calcium and vitamin D. Aim for 1000 to 1500 milligrams of calcium and 200 to 400 IU of vitamin D.

23

Interstitial Cystitis (IC)

This chronic inflammatory condition of the bladder is very much a woman's disease. Of the estimated half million people who suffer with interstitial cystitis (IC), 90 percent of them are women. Interstitial cystitis causes recurring discomfort or pain in the bladder and pelvic area, and a frequent or urgent need to urinate. Some women with the disease feel only mild discomfort, while others suffer intense pain.

Although the symptoms are often very similar, interstitial cystitis is not a true urinary tract infection. What makes this condition different from common urinary tract infections is the fact that it is resistant to conventional antibiotic therapy.

The cause of interstitial cystitis is unknown but, at this point, it does not seem to be the result of a bacterial infection. Treatment usually involves medication to ease pain and reduce inflammation. Unfortunately, long-term therapy has had limited success in achieving a cure.

❧

What Causes Interstitial Cystitis?

Before I describe what's happening in the body to cause the symptoms of interstitial cystitis, it's important to understand how your urinary tract system works. The bladder is an important part of your urinary tract that's connected to your kidneys by two small tubes called ureters. Your kidneys produce urine and, as urine accumulates, it flows through the ureters into your bladder, which acts as a reservoir or storage tank for the fluid waste. Gradually, your bladder expands to hold a larger quantity of urine. When your maximum bladder capacity is reached, urine is released into another tube, called the urethra, where it flows out of your body in a process called urination.

IC is a chronic inflammation of the bladder wall. When you have this condition, small areas on the walls of your bladder become irritated. This causes the bladder wall to become scarred and stiff, impairing its normal function. The inflammation can also cause your bladder to spasm, which can reduce its capacity to store urine. The consequence of this is an increased, and often urgent, need to urinate—one of the main symptoms of IC. As the irritation becomes more pronounced, small spots of pinpoint bleeding, called glomerulatins, develop on the bladder walls. In rare cases, ulcers appear behind the bladder lining. Almost without exception, IC causes recurring, severe pain in the bladder and surrounding pelvic areas.

While the symptoms of interstitial cystitis are somewhat similar to those of the common urinary tract infection, IC is quite a different disorder. Most urinary tract infections are caused by bacteria and can usually be cleared up with antibiotics. However, people with IC have no bacteria in their urine and their symptoms do not improve with antibiotic therapy.

The exact cause of this disabling disorder remains a mystery. One theory suggests that IC is the result of a defective defense barrier in the bladder lining. This would allow toxins or infective agents in the urine to leak through the lining and irritate the bladder wall. It's also possible that some type of infectious bacteria may be living in the bladder cells. However, urine tests have failed to identify any bacteria in the urine of patients with IC, so it is difficult to prove this theory.

Some researchers believe that IC is an auto-immune disorder and that the chronic inflammation is the body's response to an earlier bladder infection. American scientists have identified auto-antibodies in 50 percent of patients with IC. It's also possible that hereditary factors are involved, but studies have not found any one gene responsible for the disorder. When scientists eventually do identify the cause of IC, it will open the doors to more effective treatments and possibly a cure.

⤳

Symptoms

The most common symptoms of IC include

- *Frequent urination* Women with IC feel the urge to urinate more often, both during the day and at night. In mild cases, this may the only symptom of the disorder. In severe cases, people with IC have been known to urinate up to 60 times a day.
- *Urgent urination* Another symptom is the pressure to urinate immediately; this sensation may be accompanied by pain and bladder spasms.
- *Pain* Women with IC feel mild to severe discomfort in the lower abdomen or vaginal area. IC makes sexual intercourse quite painful and sex drive may be reduced as a result.
- *Other disorders* Muscle and joint pain, gastrointestinal discomfort, allergies and migraine headaches may also occur in some people with IC. There appears to be some unknown connection between IC and other chronic disease and pain disorders, such as fibromyalgia, lupus, endometriosis and irritable bowel syndrome.

⤳

Who's at Risk?

Although very little is known about the risk factors of IC, research now indicates that it is much more prevalent than was previously reported. While the condition affects postmenopausal women most frequently, it is becoming evident that IC can attack people at any age. It can affect men and children, as well as women.

ༀ

Diagnosis

The earlier a diagnosis is made, the better one's chances are of responding to medical treatment. Fortunately, IC is not a progressive disease and symptoms do not usually become worse over time. But symptoms may go into remission for extended periods, only to recur months or years later.

There is no definitive test that will identify IC. Because symptoms such as frequent, urgent urination and pelvic pain are similar to other urinary tract disorders, your doctor will rely on a process of elimination to arrive at a diagnosis of IC. He or she must first rule out the possibility that your symptoms are caused by another disorder, such as a urinary tract infection, bladder cancer, kidney disease, vaginal infection, sexually transmitted disease or endometriosis, to name just a few.

After taking a medical history and discussing your symptoms, your doctor will take a urine culture to determine if a bacterial infection exists. If your urine tests positive for bacteria, then you probably don't have IC. The chances are good that you are simply suffering from a urinary tract infection that can be treated with an antibiotic.

If no bacteria are found in your urine and you don't have any other disorder that could be causing your symptoms, your doctor will perform more tests to confirm a diagnosis of IC. The most reliable test for IC is a *cystoscopy*. Because this procedure can be quite uncomfortable, it is normally conducted under general anesthesia. Your doctor will use a cytoscope, a hollow tube with a light and several lenses, to look inside your bladder and urethra. Your bladder will also be stretched or distended with gas or some type of liquid. A cystoscopy will detect bladder inflammation, a stiff, thick bladder wall and pinpoint bleeding.

In some cases, a biopsy of your bladder may be necessary. If this is the case, a sample of bladder tissue is removed during the cystoscopy and examined under a microscope. A biopsy will help your doctor confirm that you have IC and rule out the possibility of bladder cancer.

The very process of diagnosing IC can be therapeutic for some people. Distending the bladder to perform a cytoscopy occasionally improves symptoms, possibly because the process increases bladder capacity and interferes with pain signals.

~~

Conventional Treatment

At this time there is no cure for IC. Nor is there a single treatment that works effectively in all people who have the disease. Symptoms vary from individual to individual and may appear or disappear at random. Because scientists do not yet know what causes the disorder, treatment is aimed mainly at relieving symptoms.

One of the more recent and effective treatments for IC is an oral drug known as Elmiron® (pentosan polysulfate sodium). This medication seems to repair damage to the bladder wall's defense barrier. The drug is effective at relieving symptoms in 30 percent of people who take it. Side effects of Elmiron® may include upset stomach, diarrhea and hair loss, which disappear when the medication is discontinued.

Pain medications such as aspirin and ibuprofen are helpful in treating the discomfort of IC. Sometimes antidepressants and antihistamines are prescribed to ease the chronic pain and psychological stress associated with IC. If pain is quite severe, narcotic drugs may be necessary to control symptoms.

Another treatment that can be effective is a bladder installation, or bladder wash. A solution of dimethyl sulfoxide (DMSO) is passed into the bladder, where it is held for 15 minutes before being expelled. The DMSO washes are given regularly every one or two weeks for six to eight weeks. They are thought to be effective because they reach the bladder tissue more directly, reducing inflammation and pain.

If all treatment methods have failed and your pain is severe, surgery may be considered. Various procedures, including removing bladder ulcers with a laser, enlarging the bladder with a piece of bowel or removing the bladder altogether, may help improve symptoms. Unfortunately, the results of these types of surgery can be unpredictable and many people continue to have symptoms even after the surgery.

Several alternative treatments have proven to ease the chronic pain of IC. Transcutaneous Electrical Nerve Stimulators (TENS) use mild electrical pulses to relieve daily discomfort and have produced good results for a small percentage of IC sufferers. The electrical pulses generated by TENS may work by increasing blood flow to the bladder, strengthening the pelvic muscles that control the bladder or triggering substances that block pain. Self-help techniques such as exercise, bladder retraining, biofeedback and stress reduction may reduce the severity and frequency of symptom flare-ups. Many people with IC have achieved success in controlling their symptoms with a program of diet modification.

؋

Managing Interstitial Cystitis

DIETARY STRATEGIES

Food Triggers

Many women with IC develop painful symptoms after eating certain foods. Once you know your trigger foods, eliminating them from the diet can help control symptoms and flare-ups. If you have IC, you have probably read through many lists of problematic foods that can cause you grief. The problem is that no two IC sufferers are alike when it comes to food sensitivities. Some of these foods may pose no problem at all for you, while others not on the list may be irritating your bladder wall. Food avoidance lists are compiled by doctors based on patient case histories. They should be used as a general guideline to help you pinpoint your triggers.

Below is a list of foods that have been reported to trigger pain in women with IC. Many of these foods are acidic and can irritate the bladder.

Food List for Women with Interstitial Cystitis

PRESERVATIVES AND ADDITIVES

Avoid: benzol alcohol, citric acid, monosodium glutamate (MSG), aspartame (NutraSweet™), saccharin, artificial colors

FRUIT

Avoid: apples, citrus fruit, figs, cranberries, cantaloupe, strawberries, pineapple, peaches, nectarines, plums, prunes, rhubarb

Okay: melons (not cantaloupe), pears

VEGETABLES

Avoid: asparagus, beets, eggplant, mushrooms, pickles, tomatoes, tomato-based sauces, raw onion, spinach, parsley, beet greens, peppers, corn, sauerkraut, sweet potatoes, dandelion greens, artichokes, turnip greens, Swiss chard, purselane

Okay: other vegetables, home-grown tomatoes (tend to be less acidic)

MEATS AND FISH

Avoid: aged, canned, cured, processed or smoked meats and fish, anchovies, caviar, chicken livers, corned beef and meats that contain nitrates or nitrites

Okay: other meats, fish and poultry

DAIRY PRODUCTS

Avoid: aged and natural cheeses, sour cream, yogurt, goat's milk

Okay: cottage cheese, frozen yogurt, milk

GRAIN FOODS

Avoid: yeast-based products such as leavened bread, wheat, corn, rye, oats and barley. Grain products are usually not well tolerated; try them in small quantities.

Okay: rice, potatoes, rice pasta, pasta

LEGUMES

Avoid: lentils, lima beans, fava beans, soybeans, tofu

Okay: all other beans

NUTS AND SEEDS

Avoid: most nuts

Okay: almonds, cashews, pine nuts

Eggs

may aggravate symptoms

Herbs, Spices and Condiments

Avoid: BBQ sauce, cocktail sauce, mayonnaise, miso, spicy foods, ketchup, salsa, hot sauce, relish, soy sauce, salad dressing, vinegar, Worcestershire sauce

Okay: garlic and other seasonings

Beverages

Avoid: alcohol (especially beer and wine), carbonated drinks, tea, coffee, cranberry juice

Okay: bottled water, decaffeinated coffee or tea, some herbal teas

Other

Avoid: caffeine (chocolate, especially dark chocolate, certain medications), junk foods, tobacco, diet pills, certain vitamins that contain starch fillers

Some of these foods may strike a chord with you. Many others may not, either because you aren't sensitive to them or you don't realize that you are. While painful symptoms often occur up to four hours after eating, making it relatively easy to pinpoint a problem food, sometimes symptoms won't appear until the following day. Identifying foods that aggravate your condition can be challenging and frustrating.

Elimination/Challenge Diet

Here's how you can make detecting your individual food sensitivities a little easier. The steps below outline an elimination diet, followed by a period of gradual reintroduction of potential food triggers. It may pose a short-term hassle but you'll find it's worth the effort. This process should help you decide what foods to avoid and what foods you can continue to enjoy.

1. *Elimination phase* For a period of two weeks, eat only foods identified above as *Okay* unless you already know that one of these foods causes you bladder or pelvic pain.

2. At the same time, keep a *food and symptom diary*. Record everything you eat, amounts eaten and what time you ate the food or meal. Document any symptoms, the time of day you started to feel the symptom, and the duration of time you felt the symptom. You might want to grade your symptoms: 1 = mild, 2 = moderate, 3 = severe.

3. *Challenge phase* After two weeks, start introducing foods from the *Avoid* section. Do this gradually, introducing them one at a time. I recommend the following procedure for testing foods:

   Day 1: Introduce the food in the morning, at or after breakfast. If you do not experience symptoms, try it again in the afternoon or with dinner.

   Day 2: Do not eat any of the test food. Follow your elimination diet, eating only foods considered okay. If you do not experience a reaction on this day, the food is considered safe and can be included in your diet.

   Day 3: If no symptoms occurred, try the next food on your list, according to the above schedule.

You may find that you can tolerate some foods if you eat them once every few days, but not if they are consumed every day. You may also learn that some troublesome foods are better tolerated if eaten in small portions. The good news is you don't have to completely eliminate all problematic foods from your diet, especially if you enjoy them.

Some women with IC have food allergies that contribute to their symptoms. Allergies to wheat, corn, rye, oats and barley are common. If you suspect you have a food allergy, speak to your family doctor about allergy testing. Of course, the elimination diet outlined above will also help you determine allergenic foods.

Determining what foods you need to stay away from can take time. I recommend you consult a registered dietitian in your community. Visit **www.eatright.org** to find a nutritionist in private practice who can work with you to plan a healthy diet for your condition.

LOW-ACID FOODS

Many of the foods in the *Avoid* section of the food list above are acidic and can cause bladder pain and urinary urgency in women with IC. If you find your list of troublesome foods leaves you little left to eat, you may want to try a dietary supplement called Prelief®. This supplement reduces the acid in many foods and beverages so that you don't have to exclude them from your diet. Two studies of more than 200 IC sufferers have revealed that Prelief® does indeed reduce the pain and discomfort associated with consuming foods such as pizza, tomatoes, spicy foods, coffee, fruit juices, alcohol and chocolate.[1] The supplement is made of calcium glycerophosphate and it's available in tablet form to be taken upon eating, or as granules that can be mixed right into foods.

The supplement can be ordered directly from the manufacturer by calling 1-800-994-4711. Visit the company's website at **www.akpharms.com** to learn more. It's important to use the correct amount of Prelief® to reduce the amount of acid in certain foods. The company offers a pocket guide, free of charge, to help you do this.

If eating a certain food brings on bladder symptoms, you can neutralize the acid in your urine by drinking a glass of water mixed with 1 teaspoon of baking soda. Practicing this as a precautionary measure when you're dining out may also help prevent bladder irritation. If you do experience a flare-up after eating, be sure to drink plenty of water to help dilute your urine.

L-arginine

Supplementing your diet with an amino acid called L-arginine may help lessen your symptoms. This amino acid is used to make an enzyme necessary for the formation of nitric oxide, a compound that relaxes the smooth muscle of the bladder. Studies have shown that patients with IC have reduced levels of these compounds in their urine. Evidence suggests that women with a larger bladder capacity and/or a history of recurrent urinary infections may respond more favorably to this amino acid.

Researchers from the Yale University School of Medicine have found that 1500 milligrams of L-arginine taken orally for six months significantly reduced voiding discomfort, urinary frequency, lower abdominal pain and pelvic pain.[2] In another study of 53 patients with IC, the same dose of L-arginine improved symptoms after five weeks of treatment.[3]

Amino acids are the building blocks of protein. Twenty amino acids exist in high-protein foods like meat, poultry, fish, eggs and dairy products. L-arginine is considered a non-essential amino acid; that means we don't have to consume it from food because usually the body is able to make enough on its own. Despite the fact that we get this amino acid from our diet, you need to take a supplement to achieve an intake of 1500 milligrams per day.

L-arginine is available in health food and supplement stores. Pregnant and breastfeeding women are advised to not use L-arginine, as we lack information about its use during these times.

HERBAL REMEDIES

Uva Ursi

This herbal remedy also goes by the name of bear's grape, hogberry and redberry—to name only a few. Studies suggest that when taken on a short-term basis, this herb may be effective for inflammatory conditions of the urinary tract, including IC. The leaf of the plant contains arbutin, tannins and hydroquinone, three components that may be responsible for its effect. When taken orally, uva ursi has antiseptic and astringent effects in the urinary tract and it may reduce inflammation. It is thought that products that reduce the acidity of the urine (like Prelief® or baking soda) may actually enhance the antibacterial properties of uva ursi.

If you experience a flare-up and you want to give this herb a try, there are some things you must know:

- Do not use the herb longer than one week without medical supervision. Tannins can irritate the stomach and limit the herb's duration of use. Hydroquinone can have toxic effects if taken in larger amounts for an extended period of time.
- Your doctor should evaluate urinary tract symptoms that persist for more than 48 hours.
- Limit your use of the herb to five times a year.
- Do not take uva ursi if you are pregnant or breastfeeding. The herb can increase the speed of labor in pregnant women and there is very little information available about its use during lactation.
- Do not use uva ursi if you have a kidney disorder.

You can take the herb as a standardized extract or as a tea. If you are buying the herb in pill or tablet form, buy a product that is standardized to contain 20 percent arbutin; this statement can be found on the front label or the ingredient list. Buying an herb that is standardized means you are purchasing a product that has a guaranteed amount of the active ingredient. If you are using a tea, steep 3 grams of the dried leaf in 150 milliliters of cold water for 12 to 24 hours and then strain; take one cup of tea four times a day. It's recommended that you prepare the tea with cold water to minimize the tannin content (tannins can cause stomach upset). Uva ursi leaves are available from a certified herbalist.

THE BOTTOM LINE...
Leslie's recommendations for managing interstitial cystitis

1. Determine what foods trigger symptoms and/or what foods you may be allergic to. Start by following an elimination diet for two weeks. Next, try potential trigger foods one at a time. Keep a detailed food and symptom diary during the elimination and challenge phases of your diet.

2. If you find your list of comfortable foods is limited, or you really crave a food that brings on symptoms, try using Prelief®, a dietary supplement that neutralizes the acid content of foods.

3. If you're dining out and are not sure about ingredients used, take along Prelief® or a little baking soda. Dissolve 1 teaspoon of baking soda in a glass of water and drink right before you eat.

4. If you eat a food that triggers bladder pain and/or urinary frequency, drink plenty of water to dilute your urine.

5. Try L-arginine, an amino acid supplement. Take 1500 milligrams per day.

6. If you are experiencing painful symptoms, consider trying the herbal remedy uva ursi. Do not take this herb for longer than one week and limit its use to five times a year. Using the product for extended periods of time can have harmful side effects. Buy a product standardized to 20 percent arbutin or drink the herbal tea.

24

Urinary Tract Infections (UTIs)

Urinary tract infections (UTIs) are ten times more common in women than in men. In fact, one in every four adult women will have a urinary tract infection at some time in her life. UTIs are particularly prevalent in elderly women, although they can affect females in any age group, even young girls. Women tend to be more prone to these infections than men because of the differences in the structure of the male and female urinary tract.

The most common symptom of a UTI is pain or a burning sensation during urination. While UTIs are distressing and uncomfortable, they are easily cured and rarely have lasting complications in healthy women. However, if they are left untreated, UTIs can lead to potentially life-threatening problems. Early detection and treatment are essential to prevent a serious health risk.

❧

What Causes a Urinary Tract Infection?

The role of the urinary system is to help your body eliminate waste products in the form of urine. Your urinary tract comprises the kidneys, ureters, bladder and urethra. All of these elements work in harmony to produce, store and eliminate urine. The urinary process begins with the kidneys, which filter and remove waste products from your bloodstream. These waste products become urine, which flows from the kidneys through small tubes called the ureters into the bladder. Your bladder serves as a storage tank, collecting the urine until it can be eliminated. During urination, muscles in your bladder push the urine out through the urethra, which has an opening on the outside of your body to discharge this fluid waste.

Normally, the urine that flows through the urinary tract system is sterile, which means that it does not contain bacteria. Most UTIs begin when bacteria enter the urethra and travel upward through the urinary tract, producing inflammation and irritation. Over 80 percent of all UTIs are caused by *Escherichia coli* (*E. coli*) bacteria, which migrate into the urinary tract from the rectum or the vagina. On rare occasions, bacteria may enter the urinary tract through the bloodstream. When this happens, the infection begins in the kidneys and travels downward to the other organisms.

The differences between the urinary tract of men and women are primarily associated with the urethra. In women, the opening of the urethra is very close to the opening of the rectum or anus. The rectum contains fecal matter, a waste product of the digestive tract. Because of the close proximity of these two openings, bacteria can be easily transferred from the rectum into the urinary tract, causing infection. The female urethra is also considerably shorter than the male urethra, and this allows the bacteria to reach the bladder much more easily. The final difference lies in the fact that the female urethra is purely a urinary duct, whereas the male urethra also carries semen, giving it both a urinary and a reproductive function. It's thought that the male prostate gland secretes a bacteria-killing fluid into the urethra, to protect the semen as it travels through this multi-functional passageway. This fluid may help prevent men from contracting UTIs.

The most common type of UTI is cystitis, which is an infection of the bladder. When cystitis occurs, it may be accompanied by an inflammation of the urethra. Sexually transmitted diseases, such as herpes, chlamydia and gonorrhea, often cause urethritis in both men and women. If the infection is left untreated, bacteria will travel further into the urinary tract, resulting in an inflammation of the ureters. In some cases, the infection may even attack the kidneys, a condition that can cause permanent kidney damage if not treated promptly.

Symptoms

Any woman who has suffered through a UTI will tell you that it is a very uncomfortable condition and can make you feel quite miserable. One of the most recognizable symptoms of a UTI is a burning sensation when you urinate. You will feel the burning either when you begin to urinate or when you are in the middle of urination. As your condition progresses, your urge to urinate may become stronger and more frequent. You may also notice that your urine has a strange odor and is cloudy, dark and even a little blood-tinged.

Sometimes a UTI may produce fever, chills and vomiting, or may cause pain in your back or in your lower abdominal area. It is very important that you do not ignore these symptoms because they may indicate the beginning of a kidney infection, a serious complication of a UTI. Young children and elderly women are particularly prone to developing kidney infections. Fortunately, most UTIs are uncomplicated and, if treated promptly, they are easily cured in just a few days.

Who's at Risk?

Sexually active girls and women are most often at risk for developing a UTI. During intercourse, friction can push bacteria from the anus into the urethra, initiating the cycle of infection. Studies have shown that women who use a diaphragm plus a spermicide, or spermicide-coated condoms, are also quite prone to UTIs.

Pregnant women are at high risk for developing a UTI. Approximately 4 to 7 percent of pregnant women contract a urinary tract infection, often in the first trimester. Pregnancy produces hormonal changes that affect the urinary system, increasing the likelihood of infection. The urinary tract is often dislodged from its normal position by pressure from the growing fetus, which further increases susceptibility. If you are pregnant and develop a UTI, especially during your third trimester, you should be treated promptly to prevent premature delivery, high blood pressure and other serious complications.

Urinary tract infections are also a common concern for elderly women. As women approach menopause, estrogen levels begin to fall, leaving them prone to infections and irritations of the vagina and urinary tract. In rare cases, UTIs may be the result of anatomical problems, causing obstructions within the urinary tract.

❧

Diagnosis

Because the symptoms are so well defined, most doctors are able to identify a UTI fairly easily. To confirm the diagnosis, a urine test will usually be required. An uncontaminated sample of your urine is collected and tested for bacteria. Persistent UTIs may require further testing with ultrasound, x-ray, bladder examination or dye testing to identify any underlying conditions that may prevent a full recovery from the infection.

❧

Conventional Treatment

In some cases urinary tract infections will clear up spontaneously, without any treatment; however, most UTIs are treated with antibiotics. The drugs may be given in a single large dose or may be spread over a course of three to seven days. A repeat infection is treated with a second course of antibiotics. Treatment is normally continued until your symptoms disappear and a urine test shows no bacteria.

It is not unusual for women to experience recurrent urinary tract infections. Some women have as many as three or four a year; others have them even more frequently. Nearly 80 percent of these cases are actually re-infections, caused by the same circumstances that produced the original infection. If you have recurrent UTIs, you should discuss treatment options with your doctor. Low daily doses of antibiotics for a 6-month period or a single dose of antibiotic after sexual activity may prevent long-term problems. Postmenopausal women with recurrent UTIs may find some relief through estrogen replacement therapy, particularly estrogen creams that are applied to the vagina.

~

Preventing and Managing Urinary Tract Infections

DIETARY STRATEGIES

Cranberry Juice

The juice of this native North American fruit has been used for years to treat and prevent urinary tract infection. It was once thought that the juice cleared up infection by acidifying the urine, killing bacteria in the process. It is now known that natural chemicals in the berry, known as proanthocyanins, treat UTIs by preventing the adherence of *E. coli* bacteria to the wall of the urinary tract. Instead of hanging around to multiply, bacteria are flushed out in the urine.

But will cranberry juice help you? Studies show that a daily glass of the juice may not only prevent a UTI, but may be effective at treating one. In a 1994 landmark study, researchers from the Brigham and Women's Hospital/Harvard Medical School in Boston studied 153 women for six months.[1] The women were given either 300 milliliters (10 fluid ounces) of cranberry juice or a placebo to drink once daily. At the end of the study, women drinking the cranberry juice were only about one-quarter as likely as the placebo group to continue to have UTIs. This improvement in UTIs was seen after two months of treatment.

How much do you need? There are no clear recommendations, but a dose of 300 milliliters (10 fluid ounces) per day was used in the 1994 study. The participants drank a cranberry cocktail that was 27 percent juice. Be sure to check labels—most cranberry cocktails contain 10 to 33 percent cranberry juice. To treat and prevent a UTI, 300 milliliters to 1 liter per day is often suggested.

Cranberry juice may not be for everyone, though. Drinking large quantities (1 liter or more) of the juice may aggravate kidney stones in some people. Stones made from oxalate and uric acid are more likely to form in acidic urine. Women with irritable bowel syndrome may experience diarrhea if they drink too much cranberry juice. If you are at risk for such problems, limit your intake to 300 milliliters (10 fluid ounces) per day.

Blueberries

Proanthocyanins, the same phytochemicals in cranberries that prevent bacteria from sticking to the urinary tract wall, are present in blueberries. If you don't like cranberry juice, or you want a little variety, add 1/2 to 1 cup of blueberries to your daily diet. And you don't have to wait until blueberry season to take advantage of their health-enhancing effects. Blueberries are available frozen, canned or dried year round. Be creative . . .

- Add frozen blueberries to a breakfast smoothie.
- Toss dried blueberries into your morning bowl of cold cereal, or mix them into oatmeal.
- Add dried blueberries to a green salad, then toss with a raspberry vinaigrette.
- Thaw frozen berries and mix into yogurt, or use them to top a scoop of low-fat ice cream.
- Use dried or frozen blueberries in baked goods like muffins and loaves.

Water

Every single day, drink plenty of water to help flush the bacteria out of your system. Women who don't exercise need to drink at least 2 to 3 liters (8 to 12 cups) of water each day. If you work out, add another liter (4 cups). Aim to drink 500 milliliters (2 cups) with each meal and with your mid-day snack. Take water with you when you're on the go—have a bottle in the car, in your purse and on your desk at work. There's no question that, if you are not used to it, drinking water is one of the more difficult habits to form. It's all a matter of training yourself. And if you don't have a water bottle around to remind you to drink, you're apt to forget.

Aggravating Foods

During your recovery period, it is wise to avoid coffee, alcohol and spicy foods, which may aggravate your irritable urinary tract. You may find that there are other foods that make your situation worse. Make a mental note of these. You may also want to look at the list of condiments and spices in chapter 23, "Interstitial Cystitis"—some of these irritating foods may also apply to you.

HERBAL REMEDIES

Cranberry Extract

You might not want to take in the extra sugar and calories from a daily glass or two of cranberry juice, and you may want to avoid the artificial sweeteners in the "light" brands of juice. Capsules of dried cranberry contain between 300 and 800 milligrams of dried cranberry powder, and are available in health food stores and pharmacies. Take two 500-milligram capsules to get the equivalent of 300 milliliters of cranberry juice.

Garlic

There is good evidence to support this herbal remedy's immune-boosting power. Studies have shown that garlic, in particular the allyl sulfur compounds plentiful in aged garlic extract, stimulate the body's immune system. Animal studies have found that the amount of garlic equivalent to three aged garlic extract capsules dramatically increases the activity of white blood cells that fight infection—the killer cells, macrophages and leukocytes. You might want to take garlic daily to help maintain a healthy immune system. Or, if you are experiencing a UTI, consider adding this herb to your treatment plan.

Most scientists agree that one-half to one clove of fresh garlic consumed each day will offer health benefits. And most people can take one or two cloves a day without any problems. Use more raw garlic in cooking: add it to salad dressings, pasta sauces and stir-fries.

It's the oil-soluble compounds in fresh garlic that account for its odor and its potential to cause stomach upset. If you decide to take garlic pills, buy a supplement made with aged garlic extract. This form of garlic has the highest concentration of the special sulfur compounds that boost the immune system. Aged garlic extract has two other benefits—it's odorless, and the irritating components present in raw garlic are removed. Take between two to six capsules a day—that's one or two with each meal. Because aged garlic extract can thin the blood, check with your physician first if you are taking blood-thinning medication such as Coumadin® (warfarin).

Uva Ursi

Studies suggest that, when taken on a short-term basis, this herb may be effective for urinary tract problems, including UTIs. (In chapter 23, I discuss its use for interstitial cystitis.) The leaf of the plant is where the three active ingredients are found: arbutin, tannins and hydroquinone. When taken orally, uva ursi has antiseptic and astringent effects in the urinary tract and it may reduce inflammation. Although not proven, it is believed that foods that increase the acidity of the urine, like cranberry juice, may actually diminish the antibacterial properties of uva ursi.

If you experience a UTI and want to give this herb a try, be sure to use it safely.

- *Do not use the herb longer than one week* without medical supervision. Tannins can irritate the stomach and limit the herb's duration of use. Hydroquinone can have toxic effects if taken in larger amounts for an extended period of time.

- Your doctor should evaluate urinary tract symptoms that persist for more than 48 hours.

- Limit your use of the herb to five times a year.

- *Do not take uva ursi if you are pregnant or breastfeeding.* The herb can increase the speed of labor in pregnant women, and there is very little information available about its use during lactation.

- *Do not use uva ursi if you have a kidney disorder.*

You can take the herb as a standardized extract or as a tea. If you are buying the herb in pill or tablet form, buy a product that is standardized to contain 20 percent arbutin; this is the extract used in clinical studies. A statement of standardization can be found on the front label or the ingredient list. Buying an herb that is standardized means you are purchasing a product that has a guaranteed amount of the active ingredient. If you are using a tea, steep 3 grams of the dried leaf in 150 milliliters of cold water for 12 to 24 hours and then strain; take one cup of tea four times a day. It's recommended that you prepare the tea with cold water to minimize the tannin content, as tannins can cause stomach upset. Uva ursi leaves are available from a certified herbalist.

OTHER NATURAL HEALTH PRODUCTS

Lactobacillus acidophilus and **Bifidobacteria**

In addition to garlic, you might want to get a daily dose of *Lactobacillus acidophilus* to help ward off infections caused by *E. coli* bacteria. This friendly bacteria lives in your intestinal tract where it forms a protective barrier, blocking the ability of infection-causing bacteria to grow. *Lactobacillus acidophilus,* like other friendly bacteria called bifidobacteria, produces lactic acid and hydrogen peroxide, compounds that suppress the growth of *E. coli* in the intestinal tract. A number of laboratory studies have shown that these bacteria prevent *E. coli* from attaching to the lining of the intestine and the vagina. One study even found that lactobacillus treatment reduced the recurrence of UTIs in women. These bacteria are often referred to as probiotic agents.

Probiotics may also enhance your body's immune system. Two human studies found an increased number of immune compounds in people who drank fermented milk.[2] In one study, bifidobacteria added to fermented milk led to an increase in white blood cell activity against *E. coli*.

If you are taking an antibiotic medication for your UTI, you should consider adding a probiotic supplement to your treatment regime. Antibiotics kill all bacteria—friendly and disease-causing. Taking a probiotic while you are on antibiotic therapy may lessen the chances of re-infection and decrease gastrointestinal upset caused by the drug.

The recommended dose of a probiotic agent varies. The strength of a supplement is expressed in the number of live bacteria cells per capsule. If you have a UTI, take 1 billion to 10 billion live cells divided into three doses daily. If you are taking a supplement to keep your immune system healthy, one capsule a day is all you need. Take your supplement with a meal when your stomach contents are less acidic due to the presence of food. This allows a greater number of bacteria to withstand stomach acids and reach their final destination in the intestinal tract.

The potency of these supplements can be reduced by storage conditions and the duration of storage; that's why you'll find these products sold in the refrigerator section of your local health food store. Some brands, however, are manufactured to maintain their potency at room temperature. For example, Wakunaga's Kyo-Dophilus™ has been tested and found to retain high bacteria counts for up to six years at room temperature.

Since research has shown that both *Lactobacillus acidophilus* and bifidobacteria offer health benefits, a product that contains both types is recommended. Many experts believe that supplements made from human strains of bacteria are better adapted for growth in the human intestinal tract. When choosing a product, you might ask the pharmacist or retailer if the formula contains human or non-human strains.

Don't forget to add probiotic foods to your diet. Fermented milk products like yogurt, kefir and sweet acidophilus milk all contain live bacterial cultures.

❧

Lifestyle Factors

One of the most important methods of preventing a UTI is to practice good personal hygiene. When you urinate or have a bowel movement, make it a habit to wipe gently from front to back; this will avoid spreading bacteria from the rectum into the urethra. When you feel the urge to urinate, try not to resist. A regular release of fresh, sterile urine will often wash harmful bacterial out of the urethra before it has a chance to travel into the urinary tract.

It is also a wise idea to clean your genital area before having intercourse, as this will remove harmful bacteria that may be accidentally transferred into the urethra. Urinating before and after intercourse will help to wash out any bacteria that has migrated into the urinary tract. If you are experiencing UTIs and are using a diaphragm or spermicide-coated condoms, you may want to consider another method of birth control. Always check the fit of your diaphragm and only leave it in for short periods of time.

Bacteria grow best in a warm, moist environment. Cotton is a fiber that provides good ventilation, so whenever possible you should wear cotton underwear or pantyhose with cotton liners. Avoid tight-fitting pants or other types of clothing that may trap heat, irritate tissues and promote bacterial growth. Washing your underclothes in strong soaps or bleach may cause irritations that could lead to a UTI. If you are susceptible to UTIs, avoid the chemical irritants in bubble bath, perfumed soaps, douches, feminine hygiene deodorants and deodorant tampons and pads.

Many women find that a heating pad, a hot water bottle or a warm bath will go a long way to relieve the pain and discomfort caused by a UTI.

THE BOTTOM LINE...

Leslie's recommendations for managing urinary tract infections

1. To prevent or treat an existing UTI, drink at least 300 milliliters (10 fluid ounces) of cranberry juice each day.

2. If you want a change from cranberry juice, add 1/2 to 1 cup (125–250 ml) of blueberries to your diet.

3. If you are leery about the sugar, excess calories or artificial sweeteners in cranberry juice, try capsules of dried cranberry powder. Two capsules are roughly equivalent to a 300-milliliter (10 fluid ounce) serving of the juice.

4. To help flush bacteria from your urinary tract, drink at least 2 liters (8 cups) of water each day. If you exercise regularly add an extra liter of fluid to your daily intake.

5. If you are experiencing a UTI, avoid foods that can irritate your urinary tract—coffee, alcoholic beverages and spicy foods are a few examples.

6. To give your immune system a hand in fighting off a UTI, add garlic to your nutrition regime. If you decide to supplement, take one or two aged garlic extract capsules with meals.

7. If you are looking for added protection from infection-causing *E. coli* bacteria, take a probiotic supplement with your meals. Use a supplement of *Lactobacillus acidophilus* and bifidobacteria that contains 1 billion to 10 billion live cells per day. You can also add foods to your diet that contain lesser amounts of these friendly bacteria—yogurt, kefir and sweet acidophilus milk are examples.

9. During a UTI, consider trying the herbal remedy called uva ursi. Buy a product that's standardized to 20 percent arbutin, one of the herb's active ingredients. Do not take the herb for longer than one week and limit your use to five times a year. The herb is not safe to take during pregnancy and lactation.

Endnotes

やん

Introduction

1. The American Dietetic Association, *2002 Nutrition Trends Study.* Chicago, IL, October 2002.

Chapter 1

1. Burton, G.W. et al. "Human plasma and tissue alpha-tocopherol concentrations in response to supplementation with deuterated natural and synthetic vitamin E" *Am J Clin Nutr* Apr 1998; 67(4):669–684.
2. Wester, P.O. "Magnesium" *Am J Clin Nutr* 1987; 45(Suppl 5):1305–1312.
3. "Joint Position Statement: Nutrition and athletic performance" American College of Sports Medicine, American Dietetic Association and Dietitians of Canada, *Med Sci Sports Exerc* Dec 2000; 32(12):2130–2145.

Chapter 3

1. Gray-MacDonald, K. et al. "Food habits of Canadians: Reduction of fat intake over a generation" *Can J Public Health* Sept–Oct 2000; 91(5):381–385.
   Kuhnlein, H.V. et al. "Dietary nutrient profiles of Canadian Baffin Island Inuit differ by food source, season, and age" *J Am Diet Assoc* Feb 1996; 96(2):155–162.
   Godel, J.C. et al. "Iron status and pregnancy in a northern Canadian population: Relationship to diet and iron supplementation" *Can J Public Health* Sept–Oct 1992; 83(5):339–343.

2. Kuzminski, A.M. et al. "Effective treatment of cobalamin deficiency with oral cobalamin" *Blood* Aug 15, 1998; 92(4):1191–1198.

Chapter 4

1. Schluederberg, A. et al. "NIH conference. Chronic fatigue syndrome research. Definition and medical outcome assessment" *Ann Intern Med* Aug 15, 1992; 117(4):325–331.
2. Sibbald, B. "Chronic Fatigue Syndrome comes out of the closet" *CMAJ* 1998; 159:537–541.
3. *The Facts about Chronic Fatigue Syndrome,* U.S. Department of Health and Human Services, Atlanta, 1995.
4. Scaglione, F. et al. "Immunodulatory effects of two extracts of Panax ginseng C.A. Meyer." *Drugs Exp Clin Res* 1990; 16(10):537–542.
5. Behan, P.O. et al. "Effect of high doses of essential fatty acids on the postviral fatigue syndrome." *Acta Neurol Scand* 1990; 82:209–216.
6. Plioplys, A.V. et al. "Amantadine and L-carnitine treatment of chronic fatigue syndrome." *Neuropsychology* 1997; 35:16–23.

Chapter 5

1. Kerr, D. et al. "Effect of caffeine on the recognition of and response to hypoglycemia in humans" *Ann Intern Med* 1993; 119(8):799–804.
2. Anderson, R.A. et al. "Effects of supplemental chromium on patients with symptoms of reac-

tive hypoglycemia" *Metabolism* 1987; 36(4):351–355.

3. Clausen, J. "Chromium induced clinical improvement in symptomatic hypoglycemia" *Biol Trace Elem Res* 1988; 17:229–236.

Chapter 6

1. Landolt, H.P. et al. "Caffeine intake (200 mg) in the morning affects human sleep and EEG power spectra at night" *Brain Research* 1995; 675(1–2):67–74.
   Landolt, H.P. et al. "Caffeine reduces low-frequency delta activity in the human sleep EEG" *Neuropsychopharmacology* 1995; 12(3):229–238.

2. Okawa, M. et al. "Vitamin B12 treatment for sleep-wake rhythm disorders" *Sleep* 1990; 13(1):15–23.

3. Mayer, G. et al. "Effects of vitamin B12 on performance and circadian rhythm in normal subjects" *Neuropsychopharmacology* 1996; 15(5):456–464.

4. Lindahl, O. et al. "Double blind study of a valerian preparation" *Pharmacology Biochemistry and Behaviour* 1989; 32:1065–1066.

5. Leathwood, P.D. et al. "Aqueous extract of valerian root improves sleep quality in man" *Pharmacology Biochemistry and Behaviour* 1982; 17:65–71.

6. Leathwood, P.D. et al. "Aqueous extract of valerian root reduces latency to fall asleep in man" *Planta Medica* 1985; 51:144–148.

Chapter 7

1. Schoenen, J. et al. "Effectiveness of high-dose riboflavin in migraine prophylaxis. A randomized controlled trial" *Neurology* 1998; 50(2):466–470.

2. Peikert, A. et al. "Prophylaxis of migraine with oral magnesium: Results from a prospective, multi-center, placebo-controlled and double-blind randomized study" *Cephalalgia* 1996; 16(4):257–263.

3. Murphy, J.J. et al. "Randomised double-blind placebo-controlled trial of feverfew in migraine prevention" *Lancet* 1988; 2(8604):189–192.

Chapter 8

1. Miller, A.B. et al. "The Canadian National Breast Screening Study: Update on breast cancer mortality" *J Natl Cancer Inst Monograms* 1997; (22):37–41.

2. Boyd, N.F. et al. "Effects at two years of a low fat, high carbohydrate diet on radiologic features of the breast: results from a randomized trial" Canadian Diet and Breast Cancer Prevention Study Group, *J Natl Cancer Inst* 1997; 89(7):488–496.

3. Zheng, W. et al. "Well-done meat intake and the risk of breast cancer" *J Natl Cancer Inst* 1998; 90(22):1724–1729.

4. Knept, P. et al. "Intake of dairy products and the risk of breast cancer" *Br J Cancer* 1996; 73(5):687–691.

5. Rose, D.P. et al. "Effect of omega-3 fatty acids on the progression of metastases after surgical excision of human breast cancer cell solid tumors growing in nude mice" *Clin Cancer Research* 1996; 2(10):1751–1756.

6. Thompson, L.U. et al. "Flaxseed and its lignan and oil components reduce mammary tumor growth at a late stage of carcinogenisis" *Carcinogenesis* 1996; Vol. 17(6):1373–1376;
   Thompson, L.U. et al. "Antitumorigenic effect of a mammalian lignan precurser from flaxseed" *Nutrition and Cancer* 1996; Vol. 26(2): 159–165.

7. Thompson, L.U., T. Li, J. Chen, P.E. Goss "Biological effects of dietary flaxseed in patients with breast cancer" *Breast Cancer Research and Treatment* November 2000; 64(1):50.

8. Hunter, D.J. et al. "A prospective study of intake of vitamin C, E and A and the risk of breast cancer" *New England Journal of Medicine* 1993; 329:234–240.

9. Freudenheim, J.L. et al. "Premenopausal breast cancer risk and intake of vegetables, fruits and related nutrients" *J Natl Cancer Inst* 1996; 88(6):340–348.

10. Howe, G.R. et al. "Dietary factors and risk of breast cancer: Combined analysis of 12 case-control studies" *J Natl Cancer Inst* 1990; 82:561–569.

11. Van't Veer, P. et al. "Combination of dietary factors in relation to breast-cancer occurrence" *Int J Cancer* 1991; 47(5):649–653.

12. Biffi, A. et al. "Antiproliferative effect of fermented milk on the growth of a human breast cancer cell line" *Nutr Cancer* 1997; 28(1):93–99.

13. Hunter, D.J. et al. "A prospective study of caffeine, coffee, tea and breast cancer" *Am J Epidemiol* 1992; 136:1000–1001. [Abstract]

14. Longnecker, M.P. et al. "Alcoholic beverage consumption in relation to risk of breast cancer: Meta analysis and review" *Cancer Causes and Control* 1994; 5:73–82.

15. Hankinson, S.E. et al. "Alcohol, height, and adiposity in relation to estrogen and prolactin levels in postmenopausal women" *J Natl Cancer Inst* 1995; 87(17):1297–1302.
Hirose, K. et al. "Effect of body size on breast cancer risk among Japanese women" *Int J Cancer* 1999; 80(3):349–355.
Huang, Z. et al. "Dual effects of weight and weight gain on breast cancer risk" *JAMA* 1997; 278(17):1407–1411.
La Vecchia, C. et al. "Body mass index and post-menopausal breast cancer: An age-specific analysis" *Br J Cancer* 1997; 75(3):441–444.

16. Rohan, T.E. et al. "Dietary fibre, vitamins A, C, and E and the risk of breast cancer: A cohort study" *Cancer Causes and Control* 1993; 4:29–37.

17. Zhang, S. et al. "Dietary carotenoids and vitamins A, C, and E and risk of breast cancer" *J Natl Cancer Inst* 1999; 91(6):547–556.

18. Wu, K. et al. "A prospective study on folate, B12, and pyridoxal-5'-phophate (B6) and breast cancer" *Cancer Epidemiology Biomarkers and Prevention* 1999; 8(3):209–217.

19. Zhang, S. et al. "A prospective study of folate intake and the risk of breast cancer" *JAMA* 1999; 281(17):1632–1637.

Chapter 9

1. Rose, D.P. "Effect of a low-fat diet on hormone levels in women with cystic breast disease I: Serum steroids and gonodotropins" *J Natl Cancer Inst* 1987; 78(4):623–626.
Rose, D.P. et al. "Effect of a low fat diet on hormone levels in women with cystic breast disease II: Serum radioimmunoassayable prolactin and growth hormone and bioactive lactogenic hormones" *J Natl Cancer Inst* 1987; 78(4):627–631.

2. Rose, D.P. et al. "Effects of diet supplementation with wheat bran on serum estrogen levels in the follicular and luteal phases of the menstrual cycle" *Nutrition* 1997; 13:535–539.

3. Russell, L.C. "Caffeine restriction as initial treatment of breast pain" *Nurse Pract* 1989; 14(2):36–37.

4. Meyer, E.C. et al. "Vitamin E and benign breast disease" *Surgery* 1990; 107(5):549–551.
Ernster, V.L. et al. "Vitamin E and benign breast disease: A double-blind, randomized clinical trial" *Surgery* 1985; 97(4):490–494.

5. Pye, J.K. et al. "Clinical experience of drug treatments for mastalgia" *Lancet* 1985; 2(8451):373–377.

6. Tamborini, A. and R. Taurelle "Value of standardized Ginkgo biloba extract (EGb 761) in the management of congestive symptoms of premenstrual syndrome" *Rev Fr Gynecol Obstet* Jul–Sep 1993; 88(7–9):447–457. [French]

Chapter 10

1. Alekel, D. et al. "Isoflavone-rich soy protein isolate exerts significant bone sparing effect in the lumbar spine of perimenopausal women" Third International Symposium on the Role of Soy in Preventing and Treating Chronic Disease, October 1999. [Abstract]

2. Schieber, M.D. et al. "Dietary soy isoflavones favorably influence lipids and bone turnover in healthy postmenopausal women" Third International Symposium on the Role of Soy in Preventing and Treating Chronic Disease, October 1999. [Abstract]

3. Munger, R.G. et al. "Prospective study of dietary protein intake and risk of hip fracture in postmenopausal women" *Am J Clin Nutr* 1999; Vol. 69(1):147–152.

4. Schurch, M.A. et al. "Protein supplements increase serum insulin-like growth factor-I levels and attenuate proximal femur bone loss in patients with recent hip fracture. A randomized, double-blind, placebo-controlled trial" *Annals of Internal Medicine* 1998; Vol. 128(10):801–809.

5. Lloyd, T. et al. "Dietary caffeine intake and bone status of postmenopausal women" *Am J Clin Nutr* 1997; 65(6):1826–1830.

6. Harris, S.S. and B. Dawson-Hughes "Caffeine and bone loss in healthy menopausal women" *Am J Clin Nutr* 1994; 60(4):573–578.

7. Devine, A. et al. "A longitudinal study of the effect of sodium and calcium intakes on regional bone density in postmenopausal women" *Am J Clin Nutr* 1995; 62(4):740–745.

8. Sakhaee, K. et al. "The effect of calcium citrate on bone density in the early and mid-postmenopausal period: a randomized, placebo-controlled study" The Second Joint Meeting of the American Society for Bone and Mineral Research and the International Bone and Mineral Society, 1998. Mission Pharmacal Company. [Abstract]

9. Baran, D.T. et al. "A placebo-controlled study of pre-menopausal women: Calcium supplementation and bone density" Annual Meeting of the American Society for Bone and Mineral Research, 1999. [Abstract]

10. Harris, S.S. and B. Dawson-Hughes "Seasonal changes in plasma 25-hydroxyvitamin D concentrations of young American black and white women" *Am J Clin Nutr* 1998; 67(6):1232–1236.

11. Leveille, S.G. et al. "Dietary vitamin C and bone mineral density: Results from the PEPI study" *Calcif Tissue Int* 1998; (63)3:183–189.

12. Feskanich, D. et al. "Vitamin K intake and hip fractures in women: A prospective study" *Am J Clin Nutr* 1999; 69(1):74–79.

13. Strause, L. et al. "Spinal bone loss in postmenopausal women supplemented with calcium and trace minerals" *J Nutr* 1994; 124(7):1060–1064.

14. Dalsky, G.P. et al. "Weight-bearing exercise training and lumbar bone mineral content in postmenopausal women" *Ann Intern Med* Jun 1988; 108(6):824–828.

Chapter 11

1. Ridker, P.M. et al. "Homocysteine and risk of cardiovascular disease among postmenopausal women" *JAMA* 1999; 281(19):1817–1821.

2. Willett, W.C. et al. "Intake of trans fatty acids and risk of coronary heart disease among women" *Lancet* 1993; 341(8845):581–585.

3. Hu, F.B. et al. "A prospective study of egg consumption and risk of cardiovascular disease in men and women" *JAMA* 1999; 281(15):1387–1394.

4. Anderson, J.W. et al. "Meta-analysis of the effects of soy protein intake or serum lipids" *New England Journal of Medicine* 1995; 333(5):276–282.

5. MacKay, S. and M.J. Ball "Do beans and oat bran add to the effectiveness of a low fat diet?" *European J Clin Nutr* 1992; 46(9):641–648. Olson, B.H. et al. "Psyllium-enriched cereals lower blood total cholesterol and LDL cholesterol, but not HDL cholesterol, in hypercholesterolemic adults: Results of a meta-analysis" *J Nutr* 1997; 127(10):1973–1980.

6. Liu, S. et al. "Whole-grain consumption and risk of coronary heart disease: results from the Nurses' Health Study" *Am J Clin Nutr* 1999; 70(3):412–419.

7. Jacobs, D.R., Jr. et al. "Whole-grain intake may reduce the risk of ischemic heart disease death in postmenopausal women: The Iowa Women's Health Study" *Am J Clin Nutr* 1998; 68(2):248–257.

8. Hu, F.B. et al. "Frequent nut consumption and risk of coronary heart disease in women: Prospective cohort study" *Br Med J* Nov 14, 1998; 317(7169):1341–1345.

9. Sesso, H.D. et al. "Coffee and tea intake and the risk of myocardial infarction" *Am J Epidemiol* 1999; 149(2):162–167.

10. Hankinson, S.E. et al. "Alcohol consumption and mortality among women" *New England Journal of Medicine* 1995; 332(19):1245–1250.

11. Rimm, E.B. et al. "Folate and vitamin B6 from diet and supplements in relation to risk of coronary heart disease among women" *JAMA* 1998; 279(5):359–364.

12. Simon, J.A. et al. "Serum ascorbic acid and cardiovascular disease prevalence" *Epidemiol* 1998; 9(3):316–321.

13. Lopes, C. et al. "Diet and risk of myocardial infarction. A case-control community-based study" *Acta Med Port* 11(4):311–317.

14. Stampfer, M.J. et al. "Vitamin E consumption and the risk of coronary heart disease in women" *New England Journal of Medicine* 1993; 328(20):1444–1449.

15. Agawal, S. and A.V. Rao. "Tomato lycopene and low density lipoprotein oxidation: A human dietary intervention study" *Lipids* 1998; 33(10):981–984.

16. Steiner, M. et al. "A double-blind crossover study in moderately hypercholesterolemic men that compared the effect of aged garlic extract and placebo administration on blood lipids" *Am J Clin Nutr* 1996; 64(6):866–870.

17. Song, K. and J. Milner "The influence of heating on the anticancer properties of garlic." *J Nutr* 2001; 131:10545–10575.

Chapter 12

1. *Depression.* National Depressive and Manic-Depressive Association, 2001. Available www.ndmda.org/depression.html

2. Wyatt, K.M. et al. "Efficacy of vitamin B6 in the treatment of premenstrual syndrome: systematic review" *Br J Med* 1999; 318(7195):1375–1381.

3. Linde, K. et al. "St. John's wort for depression—an overview and meta-analysis of randomized clinical trials" *Br Med J* 1996; 313:253–258.

4. Balon, R. "Ginkgo biloba for antidepressant-induced sexual dysfunction?" *Journal of Sex and Marital Therapy* 1999; 25(1):1–2.

Chapter 14

1. Stoppard, Miriam, MD and Catherine Younger-Lewis, MD, eds. *Woman's Body* The Reader's Digest Association (Canada) Ltd., Quebec, 1995:162.

2. Stanton, C.K. and R.H. Gray "Effects of caffeine consumption on delayed conception" *Am J Epidemiol* 1995; 142(12):1322–1329.

3. Wilcox, A. et al. "Caffeinated beverages and decreased fertility" *Lancet* 1988; 2(8626–8627):1453–1456.

4. Bolumar, F. et al. "Caffeine and delayed conception: A European multicenter study on infertility and subfecundity" European Study Group on Infertility Subfecundity *Am J Epidemiol* 1997; 145(4):324–334.

5. Grodstein, F. et al. "Infertility in women and moderate alcohol use" *Am J Epidemiol* 1994; 84(9):1429–1432.

6. Gulden, K.D. "Pernicious anemia, vitiligo and infertility" *J Am Board Fam Pract* 1990; 3(3):217–220.
Sanfilippo, J.S. and Y.K. Liu "Vitamin B12 deficiency and infertility: A case report" *Int J Fertil* 1991; 36(1):36–38.

7. Gerhard, I. et al. "Mastodynon® bei weiblicher Sterilitat" *Forsch Komplemetarmed* 1998; 5:272–278. [in German; English abstract]

8. El-Nemr, A. et al. "Effect of smoking on ovarian reserve and ovarian stimulation in-vitro fertilization and embryo transfer" *Hum Reprod* 1998; 13(8):2192–2198.

9. Joesoef, M.R. et al. "Fertility and use of cigarettes, alcohol, marijuana, and cocaine" *Ann Epidemiol* 1993; 3(6):592–594.

10. Geva, E. at al. "The effect of antioxidant treatment on human spermatozoa and fertilization

rate in an in vitro fertilization program" *Fertil Steril* 1996; 66(3):430–434.

Suleiman, S.A. et al. "Lipid peroxidation and human sperm motility: Protective role of vitamin E" *J Androl* 1996; 17(5):530–537.

11. Hansen, J.C. and Y. Deguchi "Selenium and fertility in animals and man—a review" *Acta Vet Scand* 1996; 37(1):19–30.

12. Scott, R. et al. "The effect of oral selenium supplementation on human sperm motility" *Br J Urol* 1998; 82(1):76–80.

13. Kumamoto, Y. et al. "Clinical efficacy of mecobalamin in treatment of oligozoospermia: Results of a double-blind comparative clinical study" *Acta Urol Jpn* 1998; 34:1109–1132.

14. Netter, A. et al. "Effect of zinc administration on plasma testosterone, dihydrotestosterone, and sperm count" *Arch Androl* 1981; 7:69–73.

15. Matalliotakis, I. et al. "L-carnitine levels in the seminal fluid of fertile and infertile men: Correlation with sperm quality" *Int J Fertil Womens Med* 2000; 45(3):236–240.

16. Vitali, G. et al. "Carnitine supplementation in human idiopathic asthenospermia: Clinical results" *Drugs Exp Clin Res* 1995; 21(4):157–159.

17. Parazzini, F. et al. "Risk factors for unexplained dyspermia in infertile men: A case-control study" *Arch Androl* 1993; 31(2):105–113.

Chapter 16

1. *Breastfeeding. HHS Blueprint for Action on Breastfeeding.* Department of Health and Human Services, Office of Women's Health, 2000. Available at www.4woman.gov/Breastfeeding/bluprntbk.2.pdf.

2. Ibid.

Chapter 17

1. *Premenstrual Syndrome* Health Oasis Mayo Clinic, August 2000. Available at www.mayohealth.org/home?id=5.1.1.16.11

2. Blum, I. et al. "The influence of meal composition on plasma serotonin and norepinephrine concentrations" *Metabolism* 1992; 41(2):137–140.

3. Sayegh, R. et al. "The effect of a carbohydrate-rich beverage on mood, appetite, and cognitive function in women with premenstrual syndrome" *Obstet Gynecol* 1995; 86(4 pt 1):520–528.

4. Jones, D.Y. "Influence of dietary fat on self-reported menstrual symptoms" *Physiol Behav* 1987; 40(4):483–487.

Boyd, N.F. et al. "Effect of a low-fat high-carbohydrate diet on symptoms of cyclical mastopathy" *Lancet* 1988; 2(8603):128–132.

5. Barnard, N.D. et al. "Diet and sex-horomone globulin, dysmenorrhea, and premenstrual symptoms" *Obstet Gynecol* 2000; 95(2):245–250.

6. Gateley, C.A. et al. "Drug treatments for mastalgia: 17 years experience in the Cardiff Mastalgia Clinic" *J R Soc Med* 1992; 85(1):12–15.

7. Wyatt, K.M. et al. "Efficacy of vitamin B6 in the treatment of premenstrual syndrome: Systematic review" *Br J Med* 1999; 318(7195):1375–1381.

8. De Souza, M.C. et al. "A synergistic effect of a daily supplement for 1 month of 200 mg magnesium plus 50 mg vitamin B6 for the relief of anxiety-related premenstrual symptoms: A randomized, double-blind, crossover study" *J Womens Health Gend Based Med* 2000; 9(2):131–139.

9. London, R.S. et al. "Efficacy of alpha-tocopherol on premenstrual symptomology: A double-blind study II Endocrine correlates" *J Am Coll Nutr* 1984; 3:351–356.

London, R.S. et al. "Efficacy of alpha-tocopherol on premenstrual symptomology: A double-blind study" *J Reprod Med* 1987; 32(6):400–404.

London, R.S. et al. "Efficacy of alpha-tocopherol on premenstrual symptomology:

A double-blind study" *J Am Coll Nutr* 1983; 2:115–122.

10. Thys-Jacobs, S. et al. "Calcium carbonate and the premenstrual syndrome: Effects on premenstrual and menstrual symptoms" Premenstrual Syndrome Study Group, *Am J Obstet Gynecol* 1998; 179(2):444–452.

11. Walker, A.F. et al. "Magnesium supplementation alleviates premenstrual symptoms of fluid retention" *J Womens Health* 1998; 7(9):1157–1165.

12. Wester, P.O. "Magnesium" *Am J Clin Nutr* 1987; 45(Suppl 5):1305–1312.

13. Loch, E.G. et al. "Treatment of premenstrual syndrome with a phytopharmaceutical formulation containing Vitex angus castus" *J Womens Health Gend Based Med* 2000; 9(3):315–320.

14. Tamborini, A. and R. Taurelle "Value of standardized Ginkgo biloba extract (EGb 761) in the management of congestive symptoms of premenstrual syndrome" *Rev Fr Gynecol Obstet* Jul–Sep 1993; 88(7–9):447–457. [French]

15. Linde, K. et al. "St. John's Wort for depression—an overview and meta-analysis of randomized clinical trials" *Br Med J* 1996; 313:253–258.

16. Stevison, C. and E. Ernst "A pilot study of Hypericum perforatum for the treatment of premenstrual syndrome" *BJOG* 2000; 107(7):870–876.

17. Schellenberg, R. et al. "Pharmacodynamic effects of two different hypericum extracts in healthy volunteers measured by quantitative EEG" *Pharmacopsychiatry* 1998; 31 (suppl):44–53.

18. Kinzler, et al. "Arzneim Forsch" *Drug Research* 1991; 41:584–588. [German]

19. Warnecke, G. et al. *Phytotherapy* 1990; 11:81–86. [German]

Chapter 18

1. Albertazzi, P. et al. "The effect of dietary soy supplementation on hot flashes" *Obstet Gynecol* 1998; 91(1):6–11.

2. Okawa, M. et al. "Vitamin B12 treatment for sleep-wake rhythm disorders" *Sleep* 1990; 13(1):15–23.

3. Foster, S. "Black cohosh: A literature review" *Herbalgram* 1999; 45:35–49.

4. Lindahl, O. et al. "Double blind study of a valerian preparation" *Pharmacology Biochemistry and Behaviour* 1989; 32:1065–1066.

5. Leathwood, P.D. et al. "Aqueous extract of valerian root improves sleep quality in man" *Pharmacology Biochemistry and Behaviour* 1982; 17:65–71.
   Leathwood, P.D. et al. "Aqueous extract of valerian root reduces latency to fall asleep in man" *Planta Medica* 1985; 51:144–148.

6. Le Bars, P.L. et al. "A placebo-controlled, double-blind, randomized trial of an extract of Ginkgo biloba for dementia" North American EGb Study Group, *JAMA* 1997; 278(16): 1327–1332.

Chapter 19

1. Franks, S. et al. "Obesity and polycystic ovary syndrome" *Ann N Y Acad Sci* 1991; 626:201–206.
   Kiddy, D.S. et al. "Improvement in endocrine and ovarian function during dietary treatment of obese women with polycystic ovary syndrome" *Clin Endocrinol* (Oxf) 1992; 36(10):105–111.

2. Moghetti, P. et al. "Spironolactone, but not flutamide, administration prevents bone loss in hyperandrogenic women treated with gonadotropin-releasing hormone agonist" *J Clin Endocrinol Metab* 1999; 84(4):1250–1254.

3. Sotaniemi, E.A. et al. "Ginseng therapy in non-insulin-dependent diabetic patients" *Diabetes Care* Oct 1995; 18(10):1373–1375.

4. Vuksan, V. et al. "Similar postprandial glycemic reductions with escalation of dose and administration time of American ginseng in type 2 diabetes" *Diabetes Care* Sep 2000; 23(9):1221–1226.

Vuksan, V. et al. "American ginseng (Panax quinquefolius L) reduces postprandial glycemia in nondiabetic subjects and subjects with type 2 diabetes mellitus" *Arch Intern Med* Apr 10, 2000; 160(7):1009–1013.

5. Gambacciani, M. et al. "Ipriflavone prevents the loss of bone mass in pharmacological menopause induced by GnRH-agonists" *Calcif Tissue Int* 1997; 61 (Suppl 1):S15–18.

6. Nestler, J.E. et al. "Ovulatory and metabolic effects of D-chiro-inositol in the polycystic ovary syndrome" *New England Journal of Medicine* 1999; 340(17):1314–1320.

Chapter 20

1. Yoshiuchi, K. et al. "Stressful life events and smoking were associated with Graves' disease in women, but not in men" *Psychosom Med* 1998; 60(2):182–185.

2. Solomon, B.L. et al. "Remission rates with antithyroid drug therapy: Continuing influence of iodine intake?" *Ann Intern Med* 1987; 107(4):510–512.

3. Vierhapper, H. et al." Low-density lipoprotein cholesterol in subclinical hypothyroidism" *Thyroid* 2000; 10(11):981–984.
Pucci, E. et al."Thyroid and lipid metabolism" *Int J Obes Relat Metab Disord* 2000; (Suppl 2):S109–112.

4. Goswami, U.C. and S. Choudhury "The status of retinoids in women suffering hyper and hypothyroidism: Interrelationship between vitamin A, beta-carotene and thyroid hormones" *Int J Vitam Nutr Res* 1999; 69(2):132–135.

5. Seven, A. et al. "Biochemical evaluation of oxidative stress in propylthiouracil treated hyperthyroid patients" *Clin Chem Lab Med* 1998; 36(10):767–770.

6. Albanes, D. et al. "Effects of alpha-tocopherol and beta-carotene supplements on cancer incidence in the Alpha-Tocopherol Beta-Carotene Cancer Prevention Study" *Am J Clin Nutr* 1995; 62(6 Suppl): 1427S–1430S.

7. Bauer, Douglas, MD "Clinical Dilemmas in Thyroid Disease" *Controversies in Women's Health: December 2000*. Department of Medicine, University of California, San Francisco, School of Medicine. [presentation]

8. Uzzan, B. et al. "Effects on bone mass of long term treatment with thyroid hormones: A meta-analysis" *J Clin Endocrinol Metab* 1996; 81(12):4278–4289.

Chapter 21

1. Schiffman, M.H. "New epidemiology of human papillomavirus infection and cervical neoplasia" *J Natl Cancer Inst* 1995; 87:1345–1347.
Palefsky, J.M. and E.A. Holly "Molecular virology and epidemiology of human papillomavirus and cervical cancer" *Cancer Epidemiol Biomarkers Prev* 1995; 4:415–428.

2. Nagata, C. et al. "Serum retinal level and risk of cervical cancer in cases with cervical dysplasia" *Cancer Invest* 1999; 17(4):253–258.

3. Giuliano, A.R. and S. Gapstur "Can cervical dysplasia be prevented with nutrients?" *Nutr Rev* 1998; 56(1 Pt 1):9–16.
Romney, S.L. et al. "Effects of beta-carotene and other factors on outcome of cervical dysplasia and human papillomavirus infection" *Gynecol Oncol* 1997; 65(3):483–492.

4. Mackerras, D. et al. "Randomized double-blind trial of beta-carotene and vitamin C in women with minor cervical abnormalities" *Br J Cancer* 1999; 79(9–10):1448–1453.

5. Kantesky, P.A. et al. "Dietary intake and blood levels of lycopene: Association with cervical dysplasia among non-Hispanic, black women" *Nutr Cancer* 1998; 31(1):31–40.

6. Basu, J. et al. "Plasma ascorbic acid and beta-carotene levels in women evaluated for HPV infection, smoking, and cervix dysplasia" *Cancer Detec Prev* 1991; 15(3):165–170.

7. Goodman, M.T. et al. "The association of plasma micronutrients with the risk of cervical dysplasia in Hawaii" *Cancer Epidemiol Biomarkers Prev* 1998; 7(6):537–544.

8. McPherson, R.S. "Nutritional factors and the risk of cervical dysplasia" [abstract], in Proceedings and abstracts of papers presented at the 22nd annual meeting of the Society for Epidemiological Research; 1989 June 14–16; Birmingham (Alabama). *Am J Epidemiol* 1989; 130(4):830.

9. Whitehead, N. et al. "Megaloblastic changes in the cervical epithelium: association with oral contraceptive therapy" *JAMA* 1973; 226:1421–1424.
Butterworth, C. et al." Improvement in cervical dysplasia associated with folic acid therapy in users of oral contraceptives" *Am J Clin Nutr* 1982; 35:73–82.

Chapter 22

1. *Facts About Endometriosis* The National Institute of Child Health and Human Development Publications On-line, National Institutes of Health, U.S. Department of Health and Human Services. Available at http://156.40.88.3/publications/pubs/endomet.htm

2. Endometriosis Association ENDOnline. Available at www.endometriosis.org/endo.html

3. Benedetto, C. "Eicosanoids in primary dysmenorrhea, endometriosis and menstrual migraine" *Gynecol Endocrinol* 1989; 3(1):71–94.

4. Koike, H. et al. "Eicosanoids production in endometriosis" *Prostaglandins Leukot Essent Fatty Acids* 1992; 45(4):331–371.

5. Koike, H. et al. "Correlation between dysmenorrheic severity and prostaglandin production in women with endometriosis" *Prostaglandins Leukot Essent Fatty Acids* 1992; 46(2):133–137.

6. Mathias, J.R. et al. "Relation of endometriosis and neuromuscular disease of the gastrointestinal tract: New insights" *Fertil Steril* 1998; 70(1):81–88.

7. Grodstein, F. et al. "Relation of female infertility to consumption of caffeinated beverages" *Am J Epidemiol* 1993; 137(12):1353–1360.

8. Grodstein, F. et al. "Infertility in women and moderate alcohol use" *Am J Public Health* 1994; 84(9):1429–1432.

9. Dawood, M.Y. "Hormonal therapies for endometriosis: Implications for bone metabolism" *Acta Obstet Gynecol Scand Suppl* 1994; 159:22–34.

Chapter 23

1. Whitmore, K. et al. "Survey of the effect of Prelief on food-related exacerbation of interstitial cystitis symptoms" Philadelphia 1998–99, unpublished.
Intersitital Cystitis Support Group "The Therapeutic effects of Prelief in Interstitial Cystitis" January 2000, unpublished.

2. Smith, S.D. et al. "Improvement in interstitial cystitis symptom scores during treatment with oral L-arginine" *J Urol* 1997; 158(3 Pt 1): 703–708

3. Korting, G.E. et al. "A randomized double-blind trial of oral L-arginine for treatment of interstitial cystitis" *J Urol* 1999; 161(2):558–565.

Chapter 24

1. Avron, J. et al. "Reduction of bacteruria and pyuria after ingestion of cranberry juice" *JAMA* 1994; 271:751–754.

2. Nago, F. et al. "Effects of a fermented milk drink containing Lactobacillus casei strain Shirota on the immune system in healthy human objects." *Biosci Biotechnol Biochem* 2000; 64(12):2706–2708; and Schiftrin, E.J. et al. "Immodulation of human blood cells following ingestion of lactic acid bacteria." *J Dairy Sci* 1995; 78(3):491–497.

Index

෨

A

acetylcholine, 339, 345

acid blockers, 10, 74

acupuncture, 123

additives, chemical, 3, 81, 120, 430

adenosine, 315

adenosine triphosphate (ADP), 20, 83

adrenaline, 368

aging: breast cancer risk and, 132; depression and, 215; heart disease risk and, 189; hypothyroidism and, 365

alcohol, 442; breast cancer and, 144–45, 149; while breast-feeding, 296–97; cancer and, 113; dependency, 109, 183; depression and, 216, 225; endometriosis and, 418, 424; fertility and, 250, 255, 418, 424; folate absorption and, 72, 148, 150; heart disease and, 203, 209; hypoglycemia and, 92, 102, 105; insomnia and, 107, 110, 112–13, 116; limiting intake of, 3, 50, 81; migraines and, 120; perimenopause symptoms and, 335, 344; PMS and, 304, 314, 326

Aldactone®, 351

allergies, food. *See* food allergies

allopregnanolone, 304

alpha-fetoprotein test (AFP), 266, 410–11

alpha-linolenic acid (ALA), 86, 139, 202, 208, 283, 312

Alzheimer's disease, 11, 14, 107, 343

American Academy of Pediatrics, 286, 290

American Cancer Society, 153

American College of Obstetrics and Gynecologists, 332

American Dietetic Association, 360

American Headache Society, 119

American Heart Association, 196, 197

American Medical Association, 110

amino acids, 32, 434

amniocentesis, 266

analgesics, 122, 307

anaphylaxis, 56–57

Anaprox®, 307

androgens, 346, 347, 349, 350, 351

anemia, 62–75; causes of, 63–64; defined, 62; diagnosis of, 67, 267; folate deficiency and (megaloblastic anemia), 6, 62, 64, 67, 71–73, 75; iron-deficiency, 62–71, 74–75, 274–75, 288, 298, 332, 339, 345; prevention and treatment of, 63, 67, 68–75; recommendations, 75; risk factors, 66; symptoms of, 62, 65; vitamin B12 deficiency and (pernicious anemia), 62, 64, 67, 73–74, 75, 250

Annals of Internal Medicine, 384

anorexia nervosa, 226–31; causes of, 227–28; conventional treatment of, 230–31; diagnosis of, 230; risk factors, 229–30; symptoms of, 228–29

antacids, 72, 114, 338

antibiotics, 445

anticonvulsants, 72

antidepressants, 217–18, 222, 307, 322; for eating disorders, 231, 235; for migraines, 122; SSRIs, 80, 217–18, 221, 223, 225, 307; tricyclic, 80, 218

antihistamines, 80

antioxidants, 3, 11, 30, 139, 140, 144, 145, 149, 203; cervical dysplasia and, 394–401, 402–403; Graves' hyperthyroidism and, 381–84; male fertility and, 252–53, 255. *See also* free radicals; *specific antioxidants*

anti-thyroid drugs, 372, 373, 376, 384–85

anxiety, 107, 109, 304, 324, 327, 342–43

arachadonic acid, 411, 412

Asian ginseng. *See* Panax ginseng

aspartame, 120

aspirin, 72

assisted reproductive technologies (ART), 240, 248

atherosclerosis, 189

auto-immune diseases, 365, 366, 368, 371, 426

Avandia®, 352

Azulfidine® (sulfasalazine), 72

B

balding, frontal, 348

barbiturates, 72

basal temperature records, 247, 248

Basedow's disease. *See* Graves' disease (Graves' hyperthyroidism)

beet greens, 31, 140

behavioral therapy, 111

beta-blockers, 122, 373

beta-carotene, 11, 30, 139, 140, 145, 181, 381–82, 387; cervical dysplasia and, 394–97, 403; food sources of, 146, 381–82, 396–97, 403; smoking and taking supplements of, 382, 397, 403; supplements, 382, 397, 403

bifidobacteria, 445–46, 447

binge eating disorder (BED), 226, 234–35

bingeing and purging (bulimia nervosa), 226, 231–34

biofeedback, 111, 123, 325, 429

biopsy, 154, 393

biotin, 4

bipolar disorder, 213, 214. *See also* depression

birth control pills. *See* oral contraceptives

birth defects, 6, 277–80, 369

bisphosphonates, 170–71

black cohosh root *(Cimifuga racemosa),* 340–41, 344

black tea, 144, 149, 202

bladder problems. *See* interstitial cystitis (IC); urinary tract infections (UTIs)

bleeding: heavy menstrual bleeding, 331–32, 339–40, 345; iron-deficiency anemia caused by, 63–64, 67

blood clots, 189

blood pressure: diastolic, 192; garlic and, 208; high (*see* high blood pressure); measuring, 193; systolic, 192

blood sugar (glucose), 89–90, 224; blood tests to measure, 92; glycemic index, 96–100, 104; low levels of (*see* hypoglycemia)

blood-thinning medications, 16, 162, 222, 317, 323, 344, 384, 421

blueberries, 442

BMI (body mass index), 45, 145

body mass index (BMI), 45, 145; heart disease risk and, 190

bone density, 16, 165; anti-thyroid drugs and, 384–85; GnRH drugs and bone loss, 353–54, 360, 417, 421–22, 424; osteoporosis (*see* osteoporosis); testing, 168–70, 185

boron, 184, 187

bottle feeding, pros and cons of, 290

botulism, infant, 298–99

bowel problems, endometriosis and, 406–407, 418–20, 424

BRCA1 and BRAC2 genes, 131

breakfast, 51, 345

breast cancer, 130–50, 349; alcohol and, 144–45, 149; BRCA1 and BRAC2 genes, 131; causes of, 130–31; diagnosis of, 133–34; dietary strategies,

135–45, 149; prevention, 134–49; recommendations for prevention of, 149–50; risk factors, 132–33; statistics, 130; vitamins and minerals and, 145–48, 150; weight control and, 145, 150

breastfeeding, 286–300, 304, 435; bottlefeeding, pro and cons of, 290; components of breast milk, 287; drawbacks of, 289–90; Graves' disease treatment while, 373; herbal remedies during, cautions about, 116, 222, 321–22, 323, 325, 342, 344, 435, 444; indications of successful, 291–92; infant benefits of, 288; iron deficiency risk for breastfed infants, 66; maternal benefits of, 289; nutrition while, 292–97; tips, 290–91; vitamin supplements while, 297; weaning to solids, 297–99

breasts, 286; cancer (*see* breast cancer); fibrocystic (*see* fibrocystic breast conditions); PMS and tender, 304, 322; self-examination, 134, 153

Brigham and Women's Hospital, 441

bulimia nervosa, 231–34

butter, 195

B vitamins, 3–6, 221–22, 316; Chronic Fatigue Syndrome and, 82–83, 88; heart disease and, 203–204, 209, 377–79. *See also individual B vitamins*

C

caffeine, 3, 38–40, 81, 442; while breastfeeding, 296; endometriosis and, 417–18, 424; fertility and, 249–50, 254–55, 255; fibrocystic breast conditions and, 159, 162; hypoglycemia and, 102, 105; insomnia and, 107, 110, 112, 116; migraines and, 120; osteoporosis and, 175, 186; perimenopause symptoms and, 334–35, 344; PMS and, 304, 314–15, 326; during pregnancy, 284–85

calcitonin, 166

calcium, 16–20, 288; absorption, 177, 179, 186; food sources, 17–18; hormones regulating, 165–66; iron absorption and, 70, 75; magnesium and, 20, 22, 179, 319, 321, 326; osteoporosis and, 16, 176–79, 186; PMS and, 304, 317–20, 326; RDA, 16, 422; supplements, 19–20, 177–79, 186, 318–20, 326, 355–56, 360, 385–86, 423, 424; vitamin D and, 20, 177, 179, 180, 186, 319, 326, 354–56, 360, 384–86, 387, 421–23, 424

calcium channel-blockers, 122

cAMP, 159

Canadian National Breast Screening Study, 134

Canadian Pediatric Society, 286

cancer, 11, 14, 131. *See also specific types of cancer*

Cancer Research Center of Hawaii, 400

Candida albicans (candidiasis), 272–73, 407, 415

canola oil, 197, 208, 219

carbohydrates, 90, 345; bedtime snack to enhance sleep, 113, 116, 337–38, 344; daily servings for weight loss, 55, 353; depression and, 218–19, 224; glycemic index, 96–100, 104, 309–10, 326, 353–54, 360; for perimenopause symptoms,

337–38, 344; PMS and, 308, 309–10, 326; reducing portion size, 48–49, 353, 360

Carnitine, 87, 88

carotenodermia, 382

carotenoids and breast cancer, 145–46

cataracts, 11, 14

catechins, 144, 149, 202, 209

cervical conization, 393

cervical dysplasia, 390–403; antioxidants and, 394–401, 402–403; causes of, 391; conventional treatment for, 393–94; diagnosis of, 390, 392–93; folate and, 6, 401–402; recommendations, 402–403; risk factors for, 392; symptoms of, 391

cervical mucous tests, 247

chasteberry *(Vitex angus-castus)*, 251, 255, 321–22, 327

chiropractic treatment, 123

chocolate, migraines and, 120

cholesterol, blood, 155, 355; garlic and, 207–208; HDL, 190, 191–92, 195, 198, 203, 349, 355; heart disease and, 190, 191–92, 376–77; LDL, 190, 191–92, 194, 195, 197, 198, 199, 203, 204, 206, 208, 209, 376–77, 383; total/HDL cholesterol ratio, 192

cholesterol, dietary, 197–98, 209

choline, 339, 345

chromium: food sources, 103, 105, 355; hypoglycemia and, 103, 105; for polycystic ovary syndrome, 355–56, 361; RDA, 103, 355; supplements, 103, 105, 355–56, 361

Chronic Fatigue Syndrome (CFS), 76–88; causes of, 76–78; conventional treatment of, 80; diagnosis of, 79–80;

dietary strategies for, 81–82, 88; essential fatty acids and, 81, 86–87, 88; herbal remedies for, 84–86, 88; L-carnitine and, 87, 88; managing, 81–88, 89; recommendations, 88; risk factors, 78–79; symptoms of, 78; vitamins and minerals and, 82–84, 88

cigarette smoking. *See* smoking

Clomid® (clomiphene citrate), 248, 351

coffee, 70, 102, 284–85; decaf, 102. *See also* caffeine

cold, common, 78, 88

collard greens, 31, 139, 140

conception, 241–42

congenital heart disease, 188

congestive heart failure, 188

conjugated linoleic acid (CLA), 136

copper, 184, 187

coronary heart disease. *See* heart disease

corpus luteum, 303, 329

cortisol, 228

cortisone, 368

Coumadin® (warfarin), 16, 162, 222, 317, 323, 344, 384, 421

cranberry extract, 443

cranberry juice, 441, 447

Crixivan® (indinavir), 222

Cyclomen® (danazol), 154

cyclosporin, 374

cystitis, 438

cystoscopy, 428

D

daidzein, 34, 136, 171, 335

dairy products, 177; daily servings for weight loss, 55; migraines and, 120; recommended daily servings, 37

Danazol, 409

Danocrine®, 307

dehydration: alcohol and, 112–13
depression, 107, 109, 212–25, 304; causes of, 212–13; conventional treatment of, 217–18; diagnosis of, 217; dietary strategies, 218–20, 224–25; eating disorders and, 228, 234, 235; ginkgo biloba for, 223; managing, 218–25; risk factors, 215–16; St. John's Wort for, 222, 225, 323; statistics, 212; symptoms of, 213–15; types of, 213; vitamins and minerals and, 220–22, 225; women and, 215, 216–17
DHA (docosahexaenoic acid), 86, 87, 219, 220, 225, 283
diabetes, 358; gestational, 276; heart disease and, 190; hypoglycemia and, 89, 90, 92, 94; type 2, 10, 349–50
diet. See nutrition
dietary approaches: to breast cancer, 135–45, 149; for breast-feeding mothers, 292–97; to Chronic Fatigue Syndrome, 81–82, 88; to depression, 218–20, 224–25; to endometriosis, 410–20, 424; to fibrocystic breast conditions, 155–59, 162; for healthy pregnancy, 280–85; to heart disease, 194–203, 377; to hypoglycemia, 95–103, 104; to insomnia, 107, 110, 112–13, 116; to interstitial cystitis, 430–35, 436; to migraines, 120, 123–25, 128; to osteoporosis, 171–76, 186; to perimenopause, 334–38, 344–45; to polycystic ovary syndrome, 352–54, 360; to premenstrual syndrome (PMS), 307–15, 326; to thyroid disease, 374–75, 376–77, 386; to urinary tract infections, 441–42, 447

dietitians, registered, 124, 227, 255, 352–53, 360
diffuse toxic goiter. See Graves' disease (Graves' hyperthyroidism)
dimethyl sulfoxide (DMSO), 429
dinner, 53–54; optimal time for, 47–48
diuretics, 307
DNA, 131; synthesis, folate and, 71, 401
Dr. Atkins' diet, 48, 353
dopamine, 303, 316, 321–22
dual-energy-x-ray absorptiometry (DEXA), 168–70, 185
Duke University, 159

E
eating disorders, 226–37; anorexia (see anorexia nervosa); binge eating disorder, 234–35; bulimia nervosa, 226, 231–34; treatment centers, listing of, 236–37
Echinacea, 84, 88
E. coli bacteria, 438, 445, 447
ectopic (tubal) pregnancy, 271–72
edema, 276–77
eggs, 197, 209
elderly, 215; anemia and, 64; insomnia and, 109; sleep patterns of, 107; urinary tract infections, 440
electroconvulsive therapy (ECT), 218
Elmiron ® (pentosan polysulfate sodium), 429
endocervical curettage, 393
endometrial cancer, 349, 351
endometriosis, 404–24; causes of, 404–405; conventional treatment of, 409–10; diagnosis of, 408; dietary strategies, 410–20,

424; managing, 410–24; recommendations, 424; risk factors, 408; symptoms of, 405–407; vitamins and minerals for, 420–23, 424
Endometriosis Society, 406
EPA (fatty acid), 86, 87, 219, 220, 225
epinephrine (adrenaline), 91
Epstein-Barr disease. See Chronic Fatigue Syndrome (CFS)
ergot drugs, 122
essential fatty acids, 3, 202, 304; Chronic Fatigue Syndrome and, 81, 86–87, 88; endometriosis and, 410–13; PMS and, 312–13
estrogen: bone health and, 166; depression and fluctuating levels of, 216; fibrocystic breast conditions and, 152, 155–58, 162; menstrual cycle and, 131, 303, 329, 332; metabolism, 155–56; perimenopause symptoms and, 330, 331, 332; PMS and, 303–304; polycystic ovary syndrome and, 346, 347, 349, 350
estrogen therapy. See hormone replacement therapy
evening primrose oil (Oenothera biennis), 86, 160–61, 163, 313, 326
Evista® (raloxifene), 171
exercise, 3, 274, 344, 355, 429; anemia risk and regular endurance, 66; Chronic Fatigue Syndrome and, 80; heart disease and, 190; hypoglycemia and, 103, 105; insomnia and, 110; osteoporosis and, 185; PMS and, 325; weight-bearing, 185; for weight control, 47
eyes, Graves' disease and the, 369, 370, 374

F

fallopian tubes, 243, 244, 248, 411; ectopic (tubal) pregnancy, 271–72

family history: breast cancer risk and, 132; of depression, 215; endometriosis risk and, 408; Graves' disease and, 371; heart disease risk and, 190

fatigue, 258; anemia-related (*see* anemia); Chronic Fatigue Syndrome (*see* Chronic Fatigue Syndrome [CFS])

fats, dietary, 2; breast cancer and, 135–36, 149; daily servings for weight loss, 49–50, 55; fibrocystic breast conditions and, 155–57, 162; heart disease and, 194–97; infants' needs, 298; lower-fat choices, chart of, 311; monounsaturated, 196–97; omega-3 (*see* omega-3 fats); omega-6, (*see* omega-6 fats); PMS and, 311–12, 326; polyunsaturated, 161, 196; recommended daily servings, 37–38; saturated, 135–36, 149, 194–95, 208; trans, 195–96, 208, 412

fermented milk, 143, 149, 273, 416, 424, 446

fertility, *see* infertility

fertility drugs, 351

feverfew *(Tanacetum parthenium)*, 127–28, 323, 327

fiber, dietary, 3, 27, 28–30, 202, 274; breast cancer and, 141–42, 149; endometriosis and, 413–14, 424; fibrocystic breast conditions and, 157–58, 162; heart disease and, 199–200; high-fiber foods, 29–30, 142, 157; hypoglycemia and, 101, 104; insoluble, 28, 141, 157, 413–14; soluble, 28, 101, 104,

141, 142, 157, 199–200, 209, 413, 414

fibrocystic breast conditions, 151–63; causes of, 152; conventional treatment of, 154; diagnosis of, 153–54; dietary strategies, 155–59, 162; evening primrose oil and, 160–61, 163; ginkgo biloba and, 161–62, 163; managing, 154–63; recommendations, 162–63; risk factors, 153; statistics, 151, 153; symptoms of, 152–53; vitamin E and, 159–60, 162–63

fish, omega-3 fats in, 136, 149, 196, 208, 219, 283, 413

fish oils, 86, 87, 181, 220, 225

flavonoids, 202

flaxseed, breast cancer and, 138–39

flaxseed oil, 86, 208, 219, 412–13, 424

fluids. *See* water and fluids

fluoride supplements, 299

folate, 6–8, 30, 223–24, 387; alcohol and absorption of, 72, 148, 150; cervical dysplasia and, 401–402, 403; depression and, 221, 225; folic acid supplements, 8, 72–73, 401–402, 403; food sources, 4, 7–8, 71–72, 148, 221, 284, 378, 402, 403; heart disease and, 203–204; megaloblastic anemia and deficiency of, 6, 62, 64, 67, 71–73, 75; neural tube defects and, 6, 278–79, 283–84; RDA, 4, 6; supplements, 75, 148, 221, 283–84; vitamin B12 and, 8, 9, 72, 73, 75, 147, 148, 221, 403

folic acid. *See* folate, folic acid supplements

follicle-stimulating hormone (FSH), 242, 248, 303, 329, 351

food allergies, 56–57, 78, 82, 88, 288

migraines and, 124

Food and Drug Administration (FDA), 196, 198, 412, 422

food sensitivities, 56–59, 298; elimination/challenge diet, 58–59, 432–33, 436; interstitial cystitis and, 430–34, 436

Fosamax® (aldendronate), 171

free radicals, 30, 145, 191, 204, 376, 377, 381, 383, 420. *See also* antioxidants

fructo-oligosaccharides (FOSs), 416

fruits: breast cancer and, 139–40, 149; daily servings, 31; daily servings for weight loss, 55; orange, 30–31, 395; pesticides, washing to remove, 3; phytochemicals in, 27, 31; recommended daily servings, 37

Fry, Dr. Kathleen, 341

fungal infections, 78

fuzzy thinking, 337–38

G

gamma-aminobutyric acid (GABA), 304

gamma-linoleic acid (GLA), 86, 161, 312–13, 326

garlic, 85–86, 88, 207–208, 209, 273, 443, 447

genistein, 34, 136–37, 171, 335

gestational diabetes, 276

ginger, 260

ginkgo biloba: fibrocystic breast conditions and, 161–62, 163; for memory, 343–44, 345; for PMS, 322–23, 327; sexual dysfunction and, 223, 225

ginseng: American (Canadian), 358; Panax (*see* Panax ginseng); Siberian (*see* Siberian ginseng)

GLA (gamma-linoeic acid), 86, 161, 312–13, 326
glucagon, 90
glucocorticoids, 166
glucose. *See* blood sugar (glucose)
glucose intolerance, 340
glucose tolerance factor (GTF), 103, 355
glucose tolerance test, 93, 266–67
glycemic index, 96–100, 309–10, 326, 353–54, 360; ranking of foods, 97–100, 310, 354
gonadotropin-releasing hormone (GnRH), 242, 248, 303, 351, 353, 409
gonadotropin-releasing hormone (GnRH) drugs, 353–54, 360, 417, 421–22, 424
grains, whole, 27, 36, 209; food sources, 201; heart disease and, 200–201; recommended daily servings, 36
Graves' disease (Graves' hyperthyroidism), 366–74; causes of, 368–69; conventional treatment of, 372–74; described, 367–68; diagnosis of, 371–72; dietary strategies for, 374–75, 386; recommendations, 386–87; risk factors, 371; symptoms of, 369–70; vitamins and minerals for, 375–76, 381–86, 387
green tea, 144, 149, 202

H
Harvard University, 139, 148, 197, 250, 417, 418, 441; Nurses' Health Study (*see* Nurses' Health Study)
Hashimoto's thyroiditis (chronic thyroiditis), 363, 365, 366
headaches, migraine. *See* migraine headaches

heart attacks, 188, 189, 205
heart disease, 188–209; antioxidants and, 11, 14; blood cholesterol levels and, 190, 191–92, 376–77; causes of, 188–89; dietary strategies, 194–203, 377; folate and, 6; high blood pressure and, 190, 192–93; homocysteine and, 193, 377–78; preventing, 193–209; recommendations, 224–25; risk factors, 189–90; statistics, 188; vitamins and minerals and, 203–207, 317, 377–79
hemoglobin, 63, 67, 68, 339
hemorrhoids, 273–74
heparin, 323
herbal remedies: during pregnancy or while breastfeeding, caution about, 116, 222, 279, 285, 321–22, 323, 325, 342, 344, 444. *See also specific remedies and medical conditions*
herbal teas, 144, 285
high blood pressure, 349; heart disease and, 190, 192–93
hirsutism, 346, 349, 351
histamine toxicity, 57
homocysteine, 193, 203, 209, 377–78
honey, botulism in infants and, 298–99
hormone replacement therapy, 216, 332–33; breast cancer risk and, 133; migraines and, 120; for osteoporosis, 170
hormones. *See specific hormones*
hot flashes, 109, 330; managing, 334–37, 340–41, 344
human papillomavirus (HPV), 391, 392, 401
hydrochloric acid, 147
hydrogenated fats, 195–96, 208, 220, 412, 424
hyperforin, 222, 324, 327

hypericin, 222, 324
hypertension. *See* high blood pressure
hyperthyroidism, 183, 368. *See also* Graves' disease (Graves' hyperthyroidism)
hypnosis, 123
hypnotic drugs, 111
hypoglycemia, 89–105, 304, 309; causes of, 89; chromium and, 103, 105; conventional treatment of, 89, 94; diagnosing, 92–94; dietary approaches to managing, 95–103, 104; exercise and, 103, 105; glycemic index, 96–100, 104; managing, 95–105; meal timing, 95–96, 104; prevention, 89; questionnaire, 93–94; reactive, 90–91; recommendations, 104–105; risk factors, 92; symptoms of, 91–92
hypothalamus, 287, 302, 303, 364
hypothyroidism, 243, 304, 362–67; causes of, 363–64; congenital, 366; conventional treatment of, 366; diagnosis of, 366; dietary strategies, 374–75, 376–77, 386; recommendations, 386–87; risk factors, 365–66; secondary, 364; symptoms of, 364–65; vitamins and minerals for, 375–76, 377–80, 387
hysterectomy, 410

I
Imitrex®, 122
immune system, 32, 443; Chronic Fatigue System and, 77, 78; food allergies and, 56; vitamins and minerals and, 12, 14, 145
infertility: causes of, 241–45, 363, 369; combined infertility

factors, 245; conventional treatment for, 247–48; diagnosis of, 246–47; dietary strategies, 249–50; endometriosis and, 406, 417, 418, 424; female, 240, 242–44, 249–52, 255; Graves' disease and, 373; herbal remedies for, 251, 255; lifestyle factors, 251–52, 254–55; male, 240, 244, 252–55; polycystic ovary disease and, 346, 347, 351; recommendations, 255; risk factors, 246; statistics, 240;symptoms of, 245–46; vitamins and minerals and, 252–54

inositol, 359–60, 361

insomnia, 106–16; causes of, 107–109, 116, 330; chronic, 107; convention treatment of, 110–11; diagnosis of, 110; dietary strategies, 107, 110, 112–13, 116; managing, 112–16; perimenopause and management of, 330, 334–35, 337–38, 341–42, 344; rebound, 111; recommendations, 116; risk factors, 109; transient, 107; valerian for, 115–16, 341–42; vitamin B12 and, 114–15, 116, 338

Institute of Medicine, 196, 412

insulin, 48, 90, 276, 353, 355, 358

insulin resistance, 103, 349, 352

interferon, 86

interstitial cystitis (IC), 425–36; causes of, 425–26; conventional treatment of, 429–30; diagnosis of, 428; dietary strategies, 430–35, 436; managing, 430–36; recommendations, 436; risk factors, 427; symptoms of, 427; uva ursi for, 435–36

in vitro fertilization, 248

iodine, 375–76; thyroid disease and, 366, 386

Iowa State University, 172

Iowa Women's Health Study, 200

ipriflavone, 173–74, 186, 358–59, 360

iron, 23–24, 68–71; absorption, 64, 70–71, 74; anemia, iron-deficiency, 62–71, 74–75, 288, 298, 332, 339, 345; calcium absorption and, 177; deficiency, 23, 62; enhancing absorption of nonheme, 70–71, 74, 339; food sources, 23–24, 68, 74, 339–40; -fortified infant formula, 290, 298; RDA, 23; supplements, 24, 69, 75, 274, 340, 345, 380, 387

irritable bowel syndrome (IBS), 407

isoflavones. *See* soy foods and isoflavones

J

Johns Hopkins University, 250

K

kale, 31, 139, 140

kava kava *(Piper methysticum),* 324–25, 327, 342–43

kefir, 143, 273, 415, 416, 446, 447

Kyolic® Estro-Logic™, 341, 344

L

lactase deficiency, 57

lactic acid bacteria, 142–43, 149, 415–16, 424

Lactobacillus acidophilus, 445–46, 447

lactose intolerance, 178, 415

Lanoxin® (digoxin), 222

laparoscopic surgery, 247, 248

laparoscopy, 408

L-arginine, 434–35, 436

L-carnitine, 87, 88, 255

lecithin supplements, 339

lignans, 138, 149

linoleic acid, 86, 202, 312, 410–11

lunch, 52–53

Lupron® (leuprolide), 351, 353, 358, 360, 409, 417, 421

lutein, food sources of, 146

luteinizing hormone (LH), 242, 248, 251, 303, 329; polycystic ovary syndrome and, 346, 350

lycopene, 206–207, 209; cervical dysplasia and, 397–99; food sources of, 146, 206, 398, 403; supplements, 207, 398–99, 403

M

magnesium, 20–22; calcium and, 20, 22, 179, 319, 321, 326; Chronic Fatigue Syndrome and, 83–84, 88; food sources, 21–22, 126, 183–84; for migraines, 126–27, 128, 320; osteoporosis and, 183–84, 187; PMS and, 304, 320–21, 327; RDA, 21, 183; supplements, 22, 83–84, 126, 128, 320–21, 327

mammography, 133–34, 154

manganese, 184, 187

manic depression. *See* bipolar disorder

margarine, 195, 196

meals: frequency of, 47, 95–96, 104, 309, 326; insomnia and content and timing of, 110–11; schedule for hypoglycemics, 95–96, 104

meats, 304; recommended daily servings, 37; saturated fats, and breast cancer, 135–36, 149

melatonin, 216, 338

memory problems, 331, 339, 343–44, 345

menopause: defined, 328; heart disease risk and, 190; insomnia and, 109; late, breast cancer risk and, 133; osteoporosis and (*see* osteoporosis); perimenopause (*see* perimenopause)

menstruation, 213, 302–303, 329, 405; age for first period, 132; eating disorders and cessation of, 228; fibrocystic breast conditions and, 152; Graves' disease and, 369; heavy bleeding, 331–32, 339–40, 345; insomnia and, 108; iron needs and, 23, 64; migraines during, 120; during perimenopause, 328, 331–32, 339–40, 345; polycystic ovary syndrome and, 346, 347, 351; premenstrual syndrome (*see* premenstrual syndrome [PMS])

Metformin®, 10, 72, 74, 352

MFP factor, 70

migraine headaches, 117–28; alternative treatments for, 123; causes of, 117, 118; conventional treatment of, 121–23; diagnosis of, 119–20; dietary approaches, 120, 123–25, 128; feverfew *(tanacetum parthenium)* for, 127–28, 323, 327; magnesium for, 126–27, 128, 320; managing, 123–28; medications for, 122–23; recommendations, 128; risk factors, 119; symptoms of, 118–19; triggers, 120–21; vitamin B2 (riboflavin) for, 125–26, 128

milk: breast cancer and, 136; formula, 290; sweet acidophilus, 143, 273, 416, 446, 447

minerals, 3. multivitamin and mineral supplements (*see* multivitamin and mineral supplements). *See also specific minerals*

miscarriage, 243, 271, 284–85, 348, 363, 369

monoamine oxidase inhibitors (MAOIs), 218

monounsaturated fats, 196

mood swings during perimenopause, 331 managing, 334–45

morning sickness, 259–60

Movana™, 324

multivitamin and mineral supplements, 3, 69, 74–75, 181, 221, 316, 340, 345; for breast-feeding mothers, 297; Chronic Fatigue Syndrome and, 82, 88; heart disease and, 203–204, 209, 377–79

mutations, 131

myoglobin, 68

N

National Institutes of Health, 170, 332

National Sleep Foundation, 109

needle aspiration of breast lump, 154

neural tube defects, 278–79

neurotransmitters, 112, 213, 221, 224, 228, 303, 331. *See also specific neurotransmitters, e.g.* serotonin

New England Journal of Medicine, 198, 205

niacin (vitamin B3), 4, 5, 204, 378–79

night sweats, 109, 330

nitrates and nitrites, 120

nonsteroidal anti-inflammatory drugs (NSAIDs), 80, 122, 307

North American Menopause Society, 332

Nurses' Health Study, 143–44, 145, 182, 195, 200, 201–202, 203, 205

nutrition, 2–43: basic principles, 2–3; dietary approaches to medical conditions (*see* dietary approaches); eating disorders (*see* eating disorders); fiber (*see* fiber, dietary); healthy diet plan, 35–38; phytochemicals and, 27; protein (*see* protein); soy foods (*see* soy); foods and isoflavones; substances to limit, 38–40; vitamins and minerals, 3–27; weight control (*see* weight control). *See also individual nutrients*

nuts, 201–202, 208

O

obesity: polycystic ovary syndrome and, 349, 352–53; weight control (*see* weight control)

olive oil, 196–97, 209

omega-3 fats, 86, 196, 208, 225, 283, 411–12, 413, 424; breast cancer and, 136, 149; depression and, 219–20, 225

omega-6 fats, 86, 196, 411–12

oral contraceptives, 72, 216, 222, 307, 351, 392, 409; breast cancer risk and, 133; heart disease and, 190; migraines and, 120

organic produce, 81

osteocalcin, 182

osteoclasts and osteoblasts, 165, 166, 181, 182

osteoporosis, 165–87, 318; boron and, 184, 187; calcium and, 16, 176–79; causes of, 165–66; conventional treatment for, 170–71; diagnosis of, 168–70, 185; dietary approaches, 171–76, 186; exercise and, 185, 187; hormones and bone health, 165–66; magnesium and, 183–84, 187; managing and preventing, 171–87; manganese, zinc and copper and, 184, 187; phosphorus and, 182–83, 187; recommendations, 185–87; risk factors, 167–68; statistics, 165; symptoms of, 166–67; vitamin A and, 181, 187; vitamin C and, 181–82, 187; vitamin D and, 179–81, 186; vitamin K and, 182, 187

ovarian cancer, 248, 349, 351

ovarian cysts, 248; polycystic ovary syndrome (*see* polycystic ovary syndrome [PCOS])

ovaries, 243, 252

ovulation and anovulation, 242, 243, 248, 347, 410

oxalic acid, 177

oxytocin, 287

P

Panax ginseng, 357–58, 361; for Chronic Fatigue Syndrome, 84–85, 88

pantothenic acid, 4

Pap smear, 390, 391, 392–93, 394, 402

parathyroid hormone (PTH), 165–66, 176, 182–83, 304

parthenolide, 127, 128

peanut oil, 197

Penn State University, 208

perimenopause, 328–45; cause of, 329; conventional treatment of, 332–33; defined, 328; dietary strategies, 334–38, 344–45; herbal remedies for symptoms of, 340–45; managing symptoms of, 334–45; the menstrual cycle, 329; recommendations, 344–45; risk factors for symptoms of, 331–32; symptoms of, 330–32; vitamins and minerals, 338–40, 344–45

personal trainers, 185

pesticides, 3

phosphorus, 176, 177, 182–83, 187, 288

phytate-rich foods, iron absorption and, 71

phytochemicals, 27, 140

pica, 65

pill, the. *See* oral contraceptives

pituitary gland, 242, 251, 287, 302, 321, 329, 364

plant foods: changing dietary habits, 69; Chronic Fatigue Syndrome and, 81; phytochemicals in, 27, 140; role in daily diet of, 2. *See also* vegetables; *specific types of plant foods, e.g.* fruits

PMS. *See* premenstrual syndrome (PMS)

PMS Escape™, 308

polycystic ovary syndrome (PCOS), 10, 249, 346–61; causes of, 347–48; conventional treatment of, 351–52; diagnosis of, 350–51; dietary strategies, 352–54, 360; herbal remedies for, 357–58; managing, 352–61; other natural health products for, 358–60, 361; recommendations, 360–61; risk factors, 350; symptoms and associated medical conditions, 348–50; vitamins and minerals for, 354–57, 360–61

polyunsaturated fats, 161, 196

postpartum depression, 216

prebiotics, 417

preeclampsia, 276–77

pregnancy, 256–85, 410, 435; age at first, 132; anemia risk during, 66, 267, 274–75; concerns and complications of, 270–80, 365–66, 439; confirming your, 257; depression and, 213, 216;

first trimester, 258–63; foods and beverages to avoid, 284–85; Graves' disease treatment during, 373; herbal remedies during, cautions about, 116, 222, 279, 285, 321–22, 323, 325, 342, 344, 435, 444; hypoglycemia and, 92; infertility (*see* infertility); insomnia during, 109, 267–68; iron needs during, 23, 64, 274–75; migraines during, 121; nutritional guidelines, 280–85; polycystic ovary syndrome and complications of, 348; second trimester, 263–67; third trimester, 267–70; weight gain during, 261–62, 265, 269; zinc needs during, 25

Prelief®, 434, 436

premenstrual dysphoric disorder (PMDD), 305

premenstrual syndrome (PMS), 216; causes of, 303–304; conventional treatment of, 306–307; diagnosis of, 306; dietary strategies, 307–15, 326; fibrocystic breast conditions and, 152; herbal remedies for, 321–25, 327; insomnia and, 108; lifestyle factors, 325, 326; monthly cycle, 302–303; recommendations, 326–27; risk factors, 305–306; symptoms of, 304–305; vitamins and minerals for, 221, 315–21

pretibial myxedema, 370

Princess Margaret Hospital, 138

proanthocyanins, 442

probiotics, 414–16; supplements, 143, 149, 416, 424, 445–46, 447

processed foods, sodium in, 176, 186, 314, 355

progesterone, 108, 251; menstrual cycle and, 108, 131, 303, 329, 332; PMS and, 303–304; polycystic ovary syndrome and, 347

progestins, 409

prolactin, 161, 242–43, 251, 287, 304, 316, 322

Propyl-Thyracil® (propylthiouracil), 385

prostaglandins, 86, 127, 312, 407, 411, 424

PGE, 161, 312, 411

protein, 32–33, 219, 345; complementary proteins, 32–33; daily servings for weight control, 48, 55; food sources, 33; hypoglycemia and, 101–102, 105; osteoporosis and, 174, 186; RDA, 33

Protein Power diet, 48, 353

psychotherapy, 111, 123, 218 for eating disorders, 231, 234, 235

psyllium, 199, 200, 209

punch biopsy, 393

R

radiation, 133

radioactive iodine, 372–73

rapini, 139

RDAs. *See individual nutrients*

rebound insomnia, 111

red blood cells: anemia and (*See* anemia); nutrients required for production of, 63, 64

relaxation, 111, 123, 325

Remifemin®, 341

retrograde menstruation theory of endometriosis, 405

RH factor, 267, 275–76

riboflavin (vitamin B2): for migraines, 125–26, 128;RDA, 4; supplements, 125–26, 128

risk factors. *See specific medical conditions*

romaine lettuce, 139

rubella (German measles), 279, 288

S

St. John's Wort *(hypericum perforatum)*, 222, 225, 323–24, 327

St. Michael's Hospital, 358

S-allyl cysteine (SAC), 207–208

salt. *See* sodium

SAMe (S-adenosylmethionine), 221, 223–24, 225

Sandimmune® (cyclosporine), 222

saturated fats, 135–36, 149, 194–95, 208

Seasonal Affective Disorder (SAD), 216, 222, 323

seeds, 202

selective estrogen receptor modulators (SERMS), 171, 217–18, 223, 225, 307

selenium: as antioxidant, 11; food sources of, 379–80, 387; male fertility and, 252, 253, 255; RDA, 379; supplements, 380, 387; thyroid hormone T3 and, 379–80

serotonin, 122, 216, 218–19, 221, 222, 228, 303, 304, 316, 326, 337

serotonin reuptake inhibitors (SSRIs), 80, 221

Setchell, Dr. Ken, 172

sexual dysfunction, ginkgo biloba and, 223, 225

sexually transmitted diseases, 243, 391, 392, 438; infertility and, 240

Siberian ginseng for Chronic Fatigue Syndrome, 85

sleep: bedtime routine, 111; environment, 111; problems (*see* insomnia)

smoking, 371; beta-carotene supplementation and, 382, 397, 403; blood levels of vitamin C and, 399; cervical dysplasia and, 392, 396, 402; depression and, 216; heart disease and, 190; infertility and, 251–52, 253, 255; insomnia and, 107; migraines and, 120

snacks, 48, 52, 53; for hypoglycemics, exercise and, 103; insomnia and carbohydrate-rich, 113, 116

sodium, 3, 40–43; osteoporosis and, 175–76, 186; PMS and, 304, 313–14, 326

soy foods and isoflavones, 34–35; breast cancer and, 136–38, 149; fibrocystic breast conditions and, 158–59; heart disease and, 198–99, 209, 377; for osteoporosis, 171–73, 186; for perimenopause symptoms, 335–37, 344; recommended daily servings, 37; thyroid gland and, 377

spicy foods, 111, 296, 442

spina bifida, 278

spinach, 31, 71, 139, 140

spinal cord defects, folate and, 6, 278–79, 283–84

spironolactone, 351, 355

staphylococcal infections, 288

Stein-Leventhal syndrome. *See* polycystic ovary syndrome (PCOS)

steroid drugs, 166, 374

stress management, 123, 325, 429

stroke, 188

Sudden Infant Death Syndrome (SIDS), 288

sugar: blood sugar (*see* blood sugar [glucose]); refined, 3, 49, 81, 353; sunscreen, 180

sweet acidophilus milk, 143, 273, 416, 446, 447
sweets, 49
Swiss chard, 31, 139, 140–41
Synarel® (nafarelin), 351, 353, 360, 409, 417, 421
Synthroid® (levothyroxin), 166, 380
syphilis, 279

T

tamoxifen, 154
tannins, 70
Tapazole® (methimazole), 372, 385
tea, 102; breast cancer and, 143–44, 149; calcium absorption and, 177; heart disease and, 202, 209; herbal, 144, 285; iron absorption and, 70–71, 74
teenage girls: anemia risk of, 66; eating disorders and, 226, 229–30, 233
tempeh, 138
tetany, 385
Theo-Dur® (theophylline), 222
thiamin (vitamin B1): food sources, 4; RDA, 4
thyroid disease, 362–87; Graves' disease (see Graves' disease [Graves' hyperthyroidism]); hypothyroidism (see hypothyroidism)
thyroidectomy, 373
thyroid gland, 363, 364, 366, 377
thyroid hormones, 243; bone loss and, 166; thyroxine (T4), 363, 364, 366, 368, 375; triiodothyronine (T3), 363, 364, 366, 368, 375, 379
thyroid-stimulating hormone (TSH), 364, 371
thyrotoxicosis. See Graves' disease (Graves' hyperthyroidism)

thyroxine (T4), 363, 364, 366, 368, 375
tofu, 138
Toronto General Hospital, 138
toxemia (preeclampsia), 276–77
transcutaneous Electrical Nerve Stimulation (TENS), 429
trans fats, 195–96, 208, 412
Trental®, 323
tricyclic antidepressants, 80, 218
triglycerides, 190, 191, 208, 349, 353, 355
triiodothyronine (T3), 363, 364, 366, 368, 375, 379
triterpene glycosides, 341
tryptophan, 218, 308, 337
Tufts University, 180
tyramine, 120

U

ultrasound, 154, 261–62, 265–66, 372
University of Cincinnati College of Medicine, 172
University of Massachusetts, 177
University of Minnesota, 136
University of Pennsylvania School of Medicine, 397
University of Reading, 315
University of Texas Southwestern Medical Center, 177
University of Toronto, 138
University of Wales, 313
urinary tract infections (UTIs), 437–47; causes of, 437–38; conventional treatment of, 440; diagnosis of, 440; dietary strategies, 441–42, 447; herbal remedies for, 443–44, 447; lifestyle factors and, 446; probiotics for, 445–46, 447; risk factors, 439–40; symptoms of, 439
urination: frequency, 258–59, 427; urgency or pain, 427, 439

uterus, 243, 244, 411; endometriosis and (see endometriosis)
uva ursi, 435–36, 444, 447

V

vaginal yeast infections, 272–73, 415
valerian (Valeriana officinalis), 115–16, 341–42, 344
vegans, vitamin B12 and, 10, 74, 75, 114, 148, 221–22, 297, 338
vegetables, 37; breast cancer and, 139–41, 149; daily servings, 31; daily servings for weight loss, 55; dark green, 30–31, 139–41, 219, 395; pesticides, washing to remove, 3; phytochemicals in, 27, 31; recommended daily servings, 37
vinegar in hypoglycemic's diet, 102, 105
vitamin A, 145, 279, 395; food sources of, 181; osteoporosis and, 181, 187
vitamin B1. See thiamin (vitamin B1)
vitamin B2. See riboflavin (vitamin B2)
vitamin B3. See niacin (vitamin B3)
vitamin B6, 4, 387; depression and, 220–21, 225; food sources of, 4, 5–6, 378; heart disease and, 203–204; PMS and, 304, 315–16, 326; supplements, 6, 225, 316, 326
vitamin B12, 9–10, 223–24, 387; breast cancer and, 147–48, 150; depression and, 221–22, 225; fertility and, 250, 253, 255; folate and, 8, 9, 72, 73, 75, 147, 148, 221, 403; food sources, 4, 9–10, 221, 253, 378; heart disease and, 203–204; for

vitamin B12 *(Continued):*
insomnia, 114–15, 116, 338, 344; male fertility and, 253; pernicious anemia and, 62, 64, 67, 73–74, 75, 250; RDA, 4, 9, 148, 253; supplements, 10, 74, 75, 115, 148, 204, 221–22, 297, 338, 344; vitamin C and, 115

vitamin B complex. *See* B vitamins

vitamin C, 30; absorption of nonheme iron and, 70, 74; as antioxidant, 11, 204, 383, 387, 399–400; breast cancer and, 146–47; cervical dysplasia and, 394, 399–400, 403; food sources of, 12, 182, 252–53, 399; heart disease and, 204–205, 209; male fertility and, 252–53, 255; osteoporosis and, 181–82, 187; RDA, 11, 182, 252; supplements, 12–13, 146–47, 205, 209, 383, 399–400, 403; vitamin B12 and, 115

vitamin D, 13–14, 166, 297; for breastfed infants, 299; calcium and, 20, 177, 179, 180, 186, 319, 326, 354–56, 360, 384–86, 387, 421–23, 424; food sources, 14; osteoporosis and, 179–81; RDA, 13, 422; supplements, 14, 180–81, 299, 355–56, 385–86, 423, 424

vitamin E, 14–16, 225, 288; as antioxidant, 11, 14, 205, 317, 383–84, 387, 400–401, 421, 424; cervical dysplasia and, 400–401, 403; fibrocystic breast conditions and, 159–60, 162–63; food sources, 15, 160, 202, 384, 400, 403, 421, 424; heart disease and, 205–206, 209, 317, 377; male fertility and, 252, 253, 255; PMS and, 316–17, 326; RDA, 15; supplements, 15–16, 160, 206, 209, 317, 326, 384, 400–401, 403, 421, 424

vitamin K, osteoporosis and, 182, 187

vitamins, 3; multivitamin and mineral supplements (*see* multivitamin and mineral supplements). *See also specific vitamins*

W

waist/hip ratio, 46

walnut oil, 208, 219

water and fluids, 38, 81, 274, 340, 436; daily requirements, 3, 38; fiber and, 158, 424; insomnia and intake of, 111; PMS and retention of, 303, 304–305, 313–14, 322, 327; urinary tract infections and, 442, 447

weight control, 44–56, 352–53, 360; body mass index (BMI),

45; breast cancer and, 145, 150; eating disorders (*see* eating disorders); exercise and, 47; fertility and, 249, 255; meal plan for healthy weight loss, 51–56; mind set for, 47; momentary lapses, dealing with, 50; realistic goal, setting a, 46–47; social support for, 47; strategies for losing weight, 46–50; thyroid disease and, 374–75, 386; waist/hip ratio, 46

wheat bran, 141, 142, 149, 157

Wingo, Claudia, 341

Women's Health Initiative (WHI), 133, 170, 332

Women's Hospital of Texas in Houston, 414

Wurtman, Dr. Judith, 308

Y

Yale University School of Medicine, 434

yeast infections, 272–73, 407, 415

yogurt, 142–43, 149, 273, 415, 416, 424, 446, 447

Z

zinc, 25–27, 184, 187; deficiency, 25; food sources, 26–27, 184, 254; male fertility and, 253–54, 255; PMS and, 304; RDA, 25, 254; supplements, 27, 254